AF515475

TRANSESOPHAGEAL ECHOCARDIOGRAPHY OF THE TRICUSPID AND PULMONARY VALVES

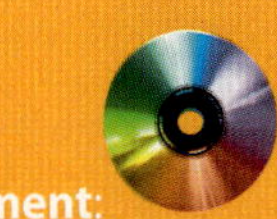

System requirement:

- Operating system—Windows XP or above
- Web browser—Internet Explorer 8 or above, Google Chrome, Mozilla Firefox
- Essential plugins—Java and Flash Player
  - Facing problems in viewing content—It may be your system does not have Java enabled.
  - If videos do not show up—It may be the system requires Flash Player or need to manage Flash setting. To learn more about Flash setting click on the link in the help section.
  - You can test Java and Flash by using the links from the help section of the CD/DVD.

Accompanying CD/DVD ROM is playable only in Computer and not in DVD player:

CD/DVD has autorun function—It may take few seconds to load on your computer. If it does not work for you, then follow the steps below to access the contents manually:

- Click on my computer
- Select the **CD/DVD drive** and click open/explore—This will show list of files in the CD/DVD
- Find and double click file—"launch.html"

For more information about troubleshoot of Autorun click on:
http://support.microsoft.com/kb/330135

TRANSESOPHAGEAL ECHOCARDIOGRAPHY OF THE TRICUSPID AND PULMONARY VALVES

EDITOR

POONAM MALHOTRA KAPOOR

MD DNB MNAMS FIACTA FTEE FISCU

Professor
Department of Cardiac Anesthesia
Cardiothoracic and Neurosciences Center
All India Institute of Medical Sciences, New Delhi, India
Secretary, Society of Cardiac Anesthesia
New Delhi and NCR Branch
Coordinator, Indian Association of Cardiovascular Thoracic Anesthesiologists (IACTA) Education and Research Cell
Co-editor, *Annals of Cardiac Anesthesia*

Forewords

Navin C Nanda
Balram Airan

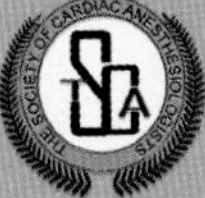

Under the Aegis of SCA—Delhi and NCR

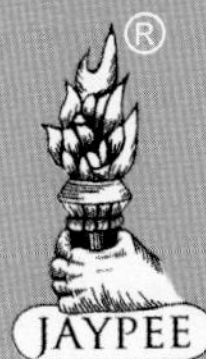

JAYPEE BROTHERS MEDICAL PUBLISHERS (P) LTD

New Delhi • London • Philadelphia • Panama

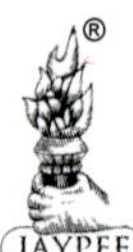

Jaypee Brothers Medical Publishers (P) Ltd.

Headquarters
Jaypee Brothers Medical Publishers (P) Ltd.
4838/24, Ansari Road, Daryaganj
New Delhi 110 002, India
Phone: +91-11-43574357
Fax: +91-11-43574314
Email: jaypee@jaypeebrothers.com

Overseas Offices

J.P. Medical Ltd.
83, Victoria Street, London
SW1H 0HW (UK)
Phone: +44-2031708910
Fax: +02-03-0086180
Email: info@jpmedpub.com

Jaypee-Highlights Medical Publishers Inc.
City of Knowledge, Bld. 237, Clayton
Panama City, Panama
Phone: +1 507-301-0496
Fax: +1 507-301-0499
Email: cservice@jphmedical.com

Jaypee Medical Inc.
The Bourse
111, South Independence Mall East
Suite 835, Philadelphia, PA 19106, USA
Phone: +1 267-519-9789
Email: jpmed.us@gmail.com

Jaypee Brothers Medical Publishers (P) Ltd.
17/1-B, Babar Road, Block-B, Shaymali
Mohammadpur, Dhaka-1207
Bangladesh
Mobile: +08801912003485
Email: jaypeedhaka@gmail.com

Jaypee Brothers Medical Publishers (P) Ltd.
Bhotahity, Kathmandu, Nepal
Phone: +977-9741283608
Email: kathmandu@jaypeebrothers.com

Website: www.jaypeebrothers.com
Website: www.jaypeedigital.com

Inquiries for bulk sales may be solicited at: jaypee@jaypeebrothers.com

Transesophageal Echocardiography of the Tricuspid and Pulmonary Valves

First Edition: **2014**

ISBN: 978-93-5152-129-7

Printed at Replika Press Pvt. Ltd.

Dedicated to

My father and family

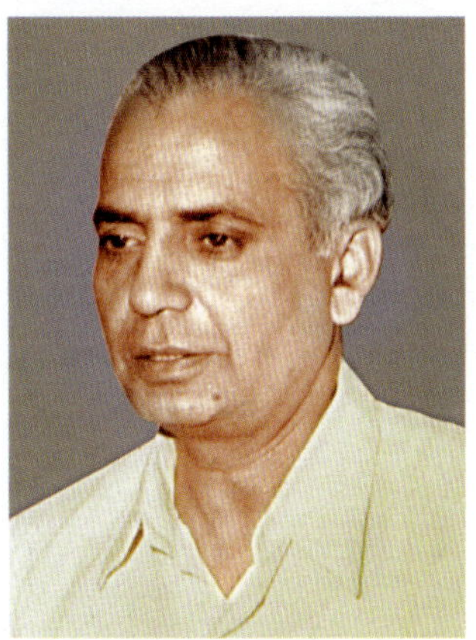

Dr KK Malhotra
(4.7.1929–4.1.2011)

My mentor, guide and inspiration in life

An extraordinary physician and human being with boundless affection, witty, hardworking and godly qualities who three years after he's gone, still inspires me to read and write

Contributors

Ajay Jha
Senior Resident
Department of
Cardiac Anesthesia
Cardio-Neuro Center (CNC)
All India Institute of
Medical Sciences
New Delhi, India

Arindam Choudhury
Assistant Professor
Department of
Cardiac Anesthesia
Cardio-Neuro Center (CNC)
All India Institute of
Medical Sciences
New Delhi, India

Arun Subramaniam
Senior Resident
Department of
Cardiac Anesthesia
Cardio-Neuro Center (CNC)
All India Institute of
Medical Sciences
New Delhi, India

BS Sethi
Senior Resident
Department of
Cardiac Anesthesia
Cardio-Neuro Center (CNC)
All India Institute of
Medical Sciences
New Delhi, India

Dharmesh Aggarwal
Consultant
Department of Anesthesiology
Fortis Hospitals
Bangaluru, Karnataka, India

Kalpana Irpachi
Senior Resident
Department of Cardiac Anesthesia
Cardio-Neuro Center (CNC)
All India Institute of
Medical Sciences
New Delhi, India

Mahesh Vakamudi
CEO and Chief
Department of
Anesthesia
Sri Ramachandra Medical
College (SRMC) and
Research Institute
Porur, Chennai, Tamil Nadu, India

Manju Mani
Senior Consultant and Head
Department of
Cardiac Anesthesia
Apollo Hospital
New Delhi, India

Muralidhar Kanchi
Director (Academic)
Head and Professor
Department of
Anesthesia and Intensive Care
International Health, University
of Minnesota, USA
Narayana Hrudayalaya Hospitals
Bommasandra Industrial Area
Bangaluru, Karnataka, India

Murali Chakarvarthy
Chief Consultant and Head
Department of Anesthesia
Critical Care and Pain Relief
Fortis Hospitals
Bangaluru, Karnataka, India

Navin C Nanda
Distinguished Professor of
Medicine and Cardiovascular
Disease
Director
Heart Station/Echocardiography
Laboratories University of
Alabama at Birmingham
Birmingham, Alabama, USA

Poonam Malhotra Kapoor
Professor
Department of Cardiac Anesthesia
Cardiothoracic and
Neurosciences Center
All India Institute of Medical
Sciences, New Delhi, India
Secretary
Society of Cardiac Anesthesia
New Delhi and NCR Branch
Coordinator
Indian Association of
Cardiovascular Thoracic
Anesthesiologists (IACTA)
Education and Research Cell
Co-editor
Annals of Cardiac Anesthesia

Rajiv Juneja
Director
Medanta Institute of
Anesthesioloy and Critical Care
Medanta—The Medicity
Gurgaon, Haryana, India

Ramchandran Gopinath
Head
Department of Anesthesia and
Research
Nizam's Medical College
Hyderabad, Andhra Pradesh, India

Sameer Taneja
Senior Resident
Department of
Cardiac Anesthesia
Cardio-Neuro Center (CNC)
All India Institute of
Medical Sciences
New Delhi, India

Sarvesh Pal Singh
Senior Resident
Department of
Cardiac Anesthesia
Cardio-Neuro Center (CNC)
All India Institute of
Medical Sciences
New Delhi, India

SN Das
Additional Professor
Department of
Cardiac Anesthesia
Cardio-Neuro Center (CNC)
All India Institute of
Medical Sciences
New Delhi, India

Suruchi Hasija
Assistant Professor
Department of
Cardiac Anesthesia
Cardio-Neuro Center (CNC)
All India Institute of
Medical Sciences
New Delhi, India

Suruchi Ladha
Senior Resident
Department of
Cardiac Anesthesia
Cardio-Neuro Center (CNC)
All India Institute of
Medical Sciences
New Delhi, India

Usha Kiran
Professor and Head
Department of
Cardiac Anesthesia
Cardio-Neuro Center (CNC)
All India Institute of
Medical Sciences
New Delhi, India

Vishwas Malik
Additional Professor
Department of
Cardiac Anesthesia
Cardio-Neuro Center (CNC)
All India Institute of
Medical Sciences
New Delhi, India

Yatin Mehta
Chairman
Medanta Institute of
Anesthesioloy and Critical Care
Medanta—The Medicity
Gurgaon, Haryana, India

Foreword

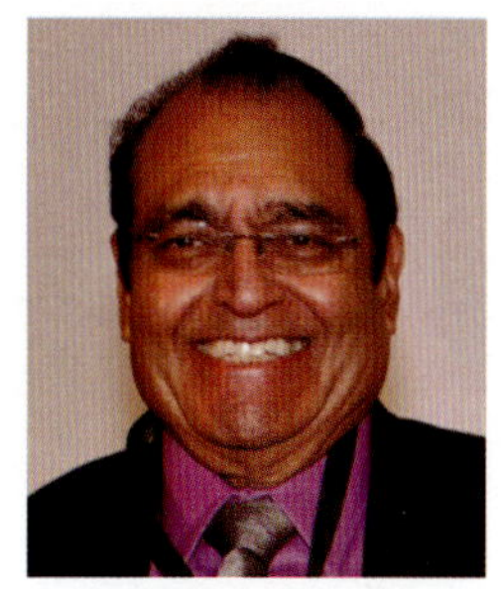

Echocardiography is an integral part of clinical cardiological range of cardiovascular diseases. In addition to examination in clinical settings, it is essential for better outcomes in the ICU and Operating Room.

Transesophageal Echocardiography of the Tricuspid and Pulmonary Valves is aimed primarily for cardiology, cardiac anesthesia and cardiac surgery fellows as it also has a 3D TEE aspect to most disease of the right ventricle. We are well aware, that 3D TEE is a now a potent visual medium which can be used by the novice or experienced echocardiographer and also beautifully complements the traditional 2D imaging and it also permits visualization of any cardiac structure of interest from multiple perspectives. The chapters in the book encompass information on all aspects of the two valves of the right side with for the first time, a chapter each on their respective pathologies. The details of each lesion on TEE for the right ventricle are very beautifully illustrated with tables, figures and adequate videos which are self-explanatory.

The wealth of information provided in the book is truly awesome. For the first time, there is a book only for a particular part of the cardiac anatomy which is what makes reading this book a must for every echocardiographer. Every clinician who sees patients with right sided lesions of the heart would want a copy of the book, close at hand. I wish the editor all success in her endeavor, in bringing about detailed advances on *Transesophageal Echocardiography of the Tricuspid and Pulmonary Valves*.

Navin C Nanda
Distinguished Professor of
Medicine and Cardiovascular Disease
Director
Heart Station/Echocardiography Laboratories University of
Alabama at Birmingham
Birmingham, Alabama, USA

Foreword

Transesophageal Echocardiography of the Tricuspid and Pulmonary Valves is an important and admirable book. It is thorough, lucid and extremely practical and is a manual of all, the echocardiographer needs to know about their proper role in the operative room and the ICU postoperatively as regards the adequacy of the cardiac surgery for the right sided valves.

It is not only a very practical guide to best practice in *Transesophageal Echocardiography of the Tricuspid and Pulmonary Valves*, but also sets out the procedure to be used to reach the diagnosis of disease and also manage the clinically negligent cases. The text is expressed in clear and accessible terms and offers useful practical guidance on many of the difficult issues that arise in obtaining good views of these two valves, which are mostly neglected by many cardiac surgeons. Repair of the tricuspid valve with a good outcome requires good TEE all throughout the procedure and this is precisely, what this book aims to provide to the novice and advanced echocardiographer, in honing his skills.

There are myriad ways in which echocardiography can be used to solve clinical problems in the perioperative OR and the ICU. Those of us who have spent our careers in the field of cardiac surgery, have long marveled at the capacity of echo for reinvention, most obviously in its technical capabilities but even more impressive in its expended clinical applications. By publishing the book *Transesophageal Echocardiography of the Tricuspid and Pulmonary Valves*, Dr Poonam Malhotra Kapoor has filled a lacuna in this field. I recommend this resource to you with great enthusiasm.

Balram Airan
Professor and Head
Department of Cardiothoracic and Vascular Surgery (CTVS)
Chief
Cardiac Center
All India Institute of Medical Sciences (AIIMS)
New Delhi, India

Preface

Worldwide, valvular heart disease remains a major cause of morbidity and mortality. In India, 20 percent of all cardiac surgical cases are valvular in nature and Rheumatic Heart Disease is like an epidemic as far greater number of patients have disease that is managed medically. Transesophageal echocardiography (TEE) is an invaluable tool to diagnose valve lesions today preoperatively, perioperatively, and postoperatively and TEE for the right sided valves is an important armamentarium cardiac surgery field.

Transesophageal echocardiography (TEE) has brought together many medical disciplines and no other technology in recent times has evoked such an impact on clinicians and a change in their practice as much as TEE, particularly in the operating room and intensive care unit.

At AIIMS, lesions of right side of the heart with rheumatic etiology presents with large numbers and what struck me was that literature on these valves—the tricuspid and pulmonic valves was sketchy unlike that for the mitral and aortic valves. Hence, the concept, I wrote this book to give you a complete introduction to the subject, from the views for TEE of TV and PV to the images you need to recognize and the hemodynamic calculations you can make with TEE, for the right side of heart—the whole nine yards. It is to deepen your understanding of TEE of these neglected valves.

The book has three sections one each on the detailed TEE of the TV and PV and a quick revision with MCQs as a short 3rd section of the book is a treatise to the reader in the form of multiple choice questions—without explanation. It will also help in preparing for the examination. Transesophageal echocardiography (TEE) is the perfect launch pad for better understanding especially now the 3D TEE for TV repair.

The book is for the medical students, anesthesiologists, the surgeons, intensivists, and anyone else who needs to enhance his knowledge on this subject.

A new companion DVD with videos which is hyperlinked to the text aid in better understanding of the subject.

There is so much yet to be discovered and invented by the younger generation of doctors who choose to use this technology judiciously with their minds and aim to chisel TEE for TV and PV to its finest glory.

The ball has been set rolling.

I am deeply indebted to the section editors for their prompt replies and all the support from the institution (Professor Usha Kiran) and from the Delhi Branch Society, Founder President, Dr Yatin Mehta and Associate Vice President, Dr Rajiv Juneja for their everlasting faith in me. This is an ode to AIIMS and Society of Cardiac Anesthesiology (SCA)—Delhi and NCR.

I hope the reader will enjoy reading the book as much as I have loved writing it.

Happy reading.

Poonam Malhotra Kapoor

Acknowledgments

It is with God's blessing that this book is being released and seeing the light of the day.

It would be difficult to list individually the people who have given encouragement and support during the writing of the book, so I offer my thanks to the whole team connected to cardiac services at the AIIMS-CN Center not only are they loyal, but also indeed they must be the best team in the country for cardiac services. Special mention must go to Professor Usha Kiran, Professor Balram Airan, Dr Sandeep Chauhan, Dr Suruchi Hasija and Dr Sarvesh Pal Singh the last two along with Dr Dharmesh Aggarwal, and Dr Kanchi Murlidhar have given great inputs in the form of videos. Special thanks to them all.

My heartfelt gratitude to Dr Yatin Mehta and Dr Rajiv Juneja for their untiring effort and support for SCA—Delhi and NCR and this book. They are most encouraging and inspirational seniors; one has a rare privilege like me to work with a stalwart like Dr Yatin Mehta, who is a true maestro.

I am deeply indebted and obliged to Dr Navin C Nanda, and Dr Balram Airan, for writing foreword(s) for the book and encouraging me with expert suggestions. They are God's blessings as seniors and encouraging supporters.

My office team Mr Sandeep, Mr Manoj Mishra, Mr Pradeep, Mr Sachin Balyan, and Miss Poonam are to be especially thanked for their data and reference input and typing and preparation of this manuscript in such a short time. I owe a big thank you to Pranav Kapoor for the wonderful illustrations in the book. God bless them all.

I am heartily thankful to Shri Jitendar P Vij (Group Chairman), Mr Ankit Vij (Managing Director), Mr Tarun Duneja (Director-Publishing), Mr KK Raman (Production Manager), Mr Sunil Kumar Dogra (Production Executive). Mr Neelambar Pant (Production Coordinator) Mr Chandra Dutt (Typesetter), Mr Manoj Pahuja, Mr Sumit Kumar, Mr Satender Singh (Graphic Designers), Mr Gyanendra Kumar, Mr Akhilesh Kumar Dubey (Proofreaders), M/s Jaypee Brothers Medical Publishers (P) Ltd, New Delhi, India, and their highly professional publishing team to whom I am most grateful for their third time within a year speedy work in such a professional manner. Thanks to their editorial efforts to improve the book overall.

My special thanks go to my wonderful family—my husband, son and my sisters, and my mother who are all my moral and emotional supporters at all adverse moments. I thank almighty for his utmost blessings on me for a family like mine, AIIMS and SCA—Delhi and NCR. Thank you *God* for everything.

Contents

DVD Contents

Chapter 1

S. No.	Video Name
1.	*Video 1:* Direct planimetry of the TV can be done on 3D echo
2.	*Video 2:* Moderator band in RV and the anterior and posterior leaflets on enface view on 3D echo
3.	*Video 3:* Annular contraction of the TV annulus in systole, due to its fibrous and muscular nature
4.	*Video 4:* The TV with its 3 leaflets in case of a 18 years old in deep TQ view, showing its position to the mitral valve
5.	*Video 5:* ME 4 chamber views the TV but not the PV
6.	*Video 6:* IVC diameter measurement in lower esophageal TEE view
7.	*Video 7:* The TG midpapillary can be used to measure the distensibility index

Chapter 2

S. No.	Video Name
1.	*Video 1:* ME four chamber view
2.	*Video 2:* ME four chamber view
3.	*Video 3:* ME bicommissural view
4.	*Video 4:* ME ascending aortic SAX
5.	*Video 5:* ME ASC aortic LAX
6.	*Video 6:* ME right pulmonary vein view
7.	*Video 7:* ME AV SAX view
8.	*Video 8:* ME RV inflow-outflow view
9.	*Video 9:* ME RV inflow-outflow view
10.	*Video 10:* ME RV inflow-outflow view
11.	*Video 11:* ME modified bicaval view
12.	*Video 12:* UE right and left PV view
13.	*Video 13:* TG basal SAX
14.	*Video 14:* TG basal SAX
15.	*Video 15:* TG basal SAX
16.	*Video 16:* TG basal SAX
17.	*Video 17:* TG midpapillary SAX view
18.	*Video 18:* TG midpapillary SAX view
19.	*Video 19:* TG midpapillary SAX view
20.	*Video 20:* TG apical SAX view
21.	*Video 21:* TG RV basal view
22.	*Video 22:* TG RV inflow view
23.	*Video 23:* Deep TG 5–chamber view
24.	*Video 24:* TG RV inflow
25.	*Video 25:* UE aortic arch SAX
26.	*Video 26:* Pulmonic valve and RVOT 70–110
27.	*Video 27:* Tricuspid inflow and pulmonic regurgitation in diastole
28.	*Video 28:* Pulmonary valve in RT sided inflow-outflow view

Chapter 3

S. No.	Video Name
1.	*Video 1:* Bicaval view
2.	*Video 2:* Midesophageal (ME) four-chamber view
3.	*Video 3:* Midesophageal right ventricle (ME RV) inflow outflow view
4.	*Video 4:* TV septal leaflet which straddles the VSD and this point measures the gradient across the VSD

Chapter 4

S. No.	Video Name
1.	*Video 1:* Functional tricuspid regurgitation with severe mitral restenosis following a CMV done on this patient in dysphonic with mitral area of 0.6 and moderate tricuspid regurgitation. TV annulus measures 32 mm and anterior papillary muscle is tethered
2.	*Video 2:* Functional tricuspid regurgitation with severe mitral restenosis following a CMV done on this patient in dysphonic with mitral area of 0.6 and moderate tricuspid regurgitation. TV annulus measures 32 mm and anterior papillary muscle is tethered
3.	*Video 3:* Functional tricuspid regurgitation with severe mitral restenosis following a CMV done on this patient in dysphonic with mitral area of 0.6 and moderate tricuspid regurgitation. TV annulus measures 32 mm and anterior papillary muscle is tethered
4.	*Video 4:* Functional tricuspid regurgitation with severe mitral restenosis following a CMV done on this patient in dysphonic with mitral area of 0.6 and moderate tricuspid regurgitation. TV annulus measures 32 mm and anterior papillary muscle is tethered
5.	*Video 5:* Functional tricuspid regurgitation with severe mitral restenosis following a CMV done on this patient in dysphonic with mitral area of 0.6 and moderate tricuspid regurgitation. TV annulus measures 32 mm and anterior papillary muscle is tethered
6.	*Video 6:* Functional tricuspid regurgitation with severe mitral restenosis following a CMV done on this patient in dysphonic with mitral area of 0.6 and moderate tricuspid regurgitation. TV annulus measures 32 mm and anterior papillary muscle is tethered
7.	*Video 7:* Functional tricuspid regurgitation with severe mitral restenosis following a CMV done on this patient in dysphonic with mitral area of 0.6 and moderate tricuspid regurgitation. TV annulus measures 32 mm and anterior papillary muscle is tethered
8.	*Video 8:* Functional tricuspid regurgitation with severe mitral restenosis following a CMV done on this patient in dysphonic with mitral area of 0.6 and moderate

tricuspid regurgitation. TV annulus measures 32 mm and anterior papillary muscle is tethered

9. *Video 9:* Functional tricuspid regurgitation with mitral stenosis
10. *Video 10:* Tricuspid valve 4 chamber view
11. *Video 11:* ME RV inflow—outflow view
12. *Video 12:* Mid-esophageal bicaval modified view
13. *Video 13:* View of coronary sinus
14. *Video 14:* ME-AV SAX (Midesophageal aortic valve short axis view)
15. *Video 15:* TG-TV SAX (Transgastric tricuspid valve short axis view)
16. *Video 16:* Transgastric-RV inflow view
17. *Video 17:* The ruptured papillary muscle
18. *Video 18:* The carcinoid heart disease.
    The tricuspid valve seen "enface" with all 3 leaflet with thickened and shortened leaflets causing stenosis and/or regurgitation and ultimately right heart failure
19. *Video 19:* Laminar tricuspid regurgitation in transthoracic view
20. *Video 20:* The laminar flow in tricuspid regurgitation, wherein, the regurgitant volume is much greater for a given transvalvar pressure gradient. The velocity of the jet is around 2 m/s
21. *Video 21:* Severity of RVOT obstruction should be ruled out with Doppler. This may dilate the TV annulus and cause a TR as in this 22-year-old male
22. *Video 22:* TR coexisted with PS in this 24-year-old patient who underwent a DCRV repair with a diverge repair for the TV
23. *Video 23:* Tricuspid regurgitation in a patient with chronic constrictive pericarditis
24. *Video 24:* Double outlet right ventricle with ventricle septal defect with mitral stenosis
25. *Video 25:* Ebstein anomaly of the tricuspid valve
26. *Video 26:* Three dimension (3D) echo cardiogram of Ebsteins' anomaly of tricuspid valve regurgitation
27. *Video 27:* Tricuspid atresia with ASD and VSD
28. *Video 28:* 3D tricuspid atresia
29. *Video 29:* Mild tricuspid regurgitation with mitral valve repair
30. *Video 30:* Huge tricuspid regurgitation
31. *Video 31:* Tricuspid regurgitation with mitral stenosis
32. *Video 32:* Mitral stenosis with TR
33. *Video 33:* Three dimensional echocardiography of tricuspid regurgitation

Chapter 5

S. No. Video Name

1. *Video 1:* Tricuspid stenosis on 3D TEE with thickened TV cusps

Chapter 6

S. No. Video Name

1. *Video 1:* TEE of pulmonary valve stenosis
2. *Video 2:* Tetralogy of Fallot in pulmonary stenosis
3. *Video 3:* Double chamber right ventricular in pulmonary stenosis
4. *Video 4:* Pulmonary insufficiency
5. *Video 5:* Associated lesions in pulmonary stenosis
6. *Video 6:* Arterial septal defect in pulmonary stenosis
7. *Video 7:* Fetal echocrdiography in pulmonary stenosis
8. *Video 8:* Severe pulmonary stenosis with color Doppler
9. *Video 9:* Double outlet right ventricle (DORV) with pulmonary stenosis

Chapter 7

S. No. Video Name

1. *Video 1:* Pulmonic valve and RVOT at 70°–110°
2. *Video 2:* Pulmonary valve in right sided inflow-outflow view
3. *Video 3:* Tricuspid inflow and pulmonic regurgitation in diastole
4. *Video 4:* PPHN, pulmonary regurgitation

Chapter 9

S. No. Video Name

1. *Video 1:* The marked distortion of right ventricular and right atrial geometry. The approx position of the mitral annulus is noted by the broad arrow at the lower right.
2. *Video 2:* Ebstein anomaly in adult patient with continuous wave Doppler
3. *Video 3:* Ebstein anomaly in adult patient with continuous wave Doppler
4. *Video 4:* Ebstein anomaly in adult patient with continuous wave Doppler
5. *Video 5:* A long snake-like posterior leaflet
6. *Video 6:* A long snake-like posterior leaflet

Chapter 10

S. No. Video Name

1. *Video 1:* Real time 2D and 3D transthoracic echocardiography in right ventricular thrombus

Above videos do not have voice over

I

TRANSESOPHAGEAL ECHOCARDIOGRAPHY OF TRICUSPID VALVE

yatin mehta
section editor

1 Anatomy of Tricuspid and Pulmonary Valves

Poonam Malhotra Kapoor, Ajay Jha

- Anatomy of the Tricuspid Valve
- Chordae
- Pulmonic Valve Anatomy
- Anatomy of the Right Heart
- Physiology of the Right Heart
- Application of Tricuspid Valve and Pulmonary Anatomy
- Right Ventricular Diastolic Function

INTRODUCTION

The tricuspid and pulmonic valves serve to separate the right heart structures and regulate the flow of blood from the periphery to the pulmonary vascular bed. Both valves are well assessed with transesophageal echocardiography (TEE) through multiple views and the full range of ultrasound **(Fig. 1)**. Detailed TEE assessment can elucidate the pathologic conditions and mechanisms that affect these cardiac structures.

ANATOMY OF THE TRICUSPID VALVE

The tricuspid valve (TV) is a multicomponent complex structure.[1,2] It represents an important site of confluence between a vast venous system and the right heart and is an important structure for its own pathology as well as the insight. It can offer to the pulmonary circulation.[3] Unlike the aortic and mitral valve it is not possible to visualize all TV cusps simultaneously in one cross-sectional view by standard transesophageal two-dimensional echocardiography (2DE).[4]

Tricuspid valve disease can result from malformation or malfunction of any of a number of interrelated structures referred to as the tricuspid valve "complex". The tricuspid valve complex is composed of several structures whose integrated function is essential for tricuspid valve competence. For the tricuspid valve to remain

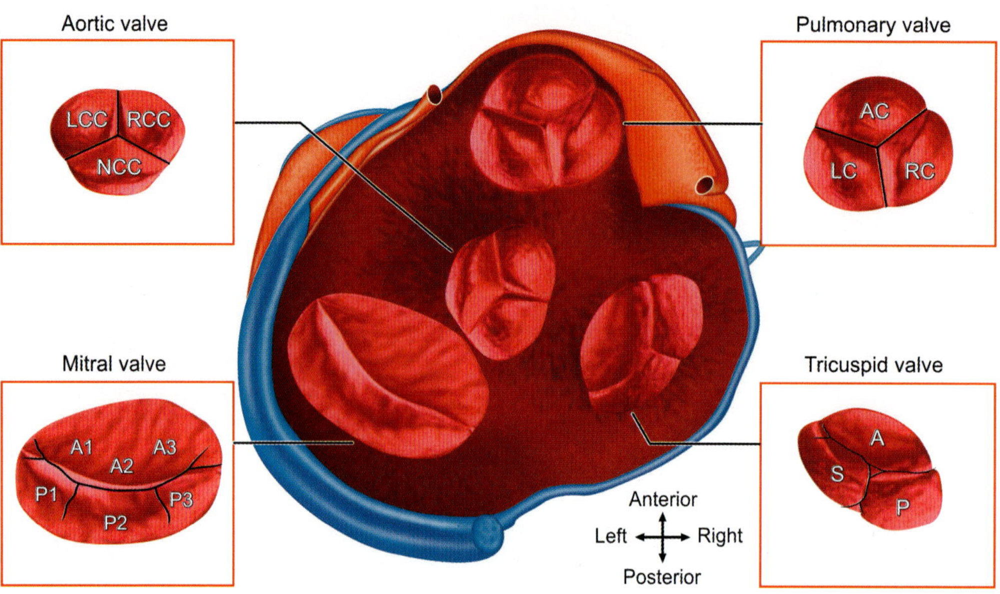

Figure 1

Nomenclature of the major cardiac valves

competent, not only the leaflets, but also the chordae, papillary muscles, annulus and the right atrial and right ventricular myocardium must all be anatomically and physiologically sound. The tricuspid annulus is "D" shaped, with the straighter portion falling along the septal leaflet **(Fig. 2)**.

Tricuspid Leaflets

The 3D TEE data set could be cropped to view all the three leaflets of the tricuspid valve from both the ventricular and atrial aspects in all patients, including the posterior tricuspid leaflet that is sometime difficult to characterize with 2D TTE. It is possible to perform direct planimetry of the tricuspid valve orifice area in patients with TS. By cropping from the ventricular aspect in a plane that was exactly parallel to the tricuspid valve orifice, a short axis or en face view of the flow limiting orifice was confidently imaged. Direct planimetry of the orifice area in the maximal systolic frame in two patients yielded measures consistent with mild TS[5] **(Fig. 3)**.

The normal tricuspid leaflets are delicate translucent structures that have a scalloped appearance when closed. The name of the valve is derived from the presence of three leaflets: anterior, septal and posterior **(Fig. 4)**.

The anterior leaflet is the largest and the septal leaflet the smallest. The posterior leaflet is intermediate in size and is characterized by the presence of from one to three clefts. The clefts in the posterior leaflet can be quite prominent, creating the illusion of multiple tricuspid valve leaflets. The free edges of the three leaflets are

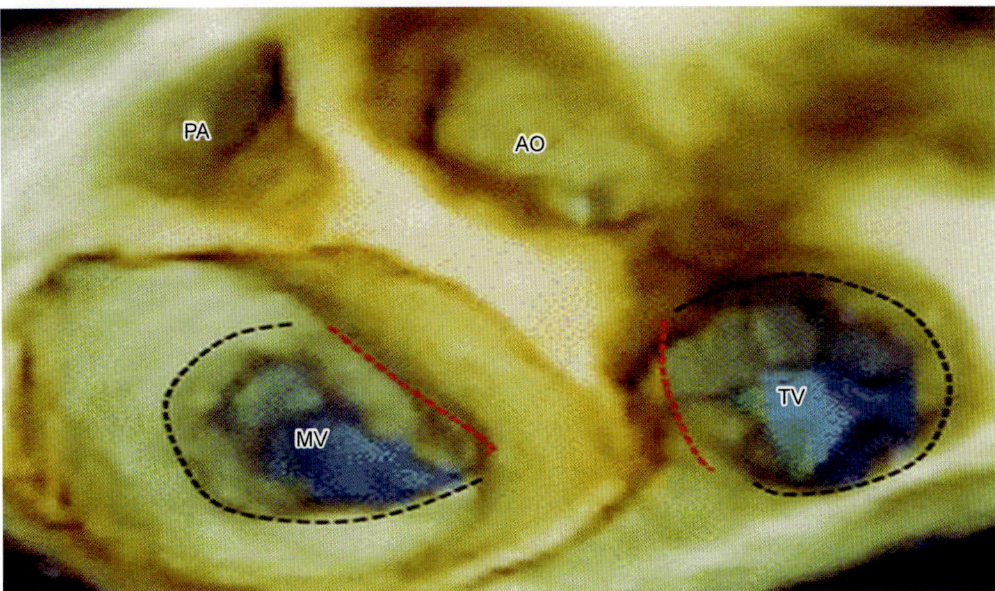

Figure 2

Three-dimensional transesophageal echocardiography (3D TEE) images of the base of the heart in full volume modality. The shape of the tricuspid annulus roughly mirrors that of the mitral annulus with a straight septal component (red dotted line) and a curved mural component (Black dotted line)

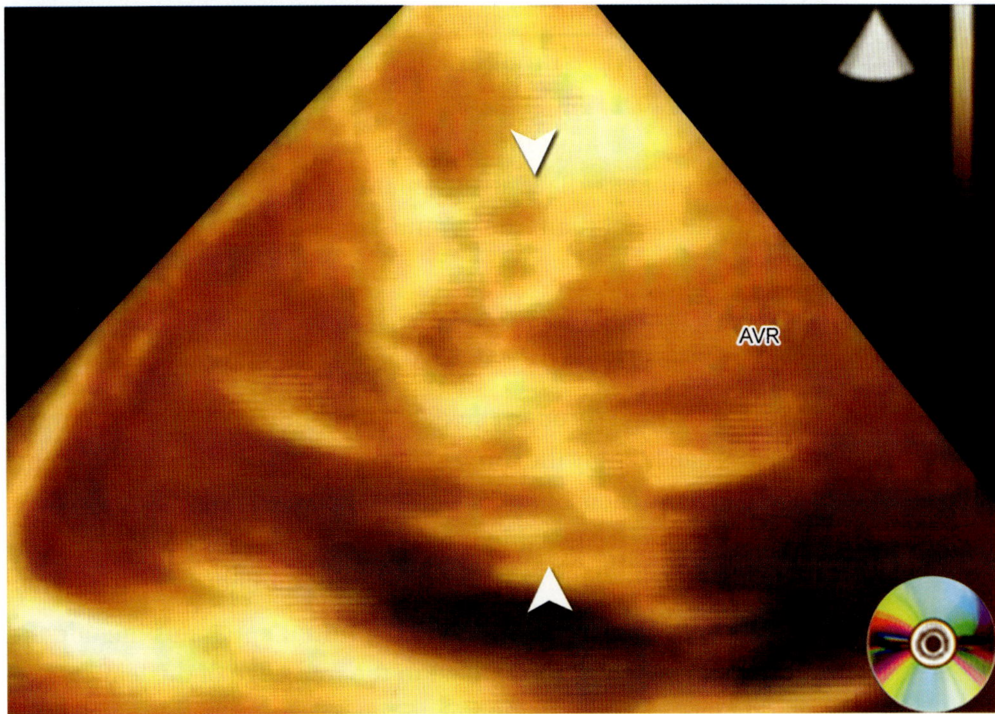

Figure 3 (VIDEO 1)

Direct planimetry of the TV can be done on 3D echo

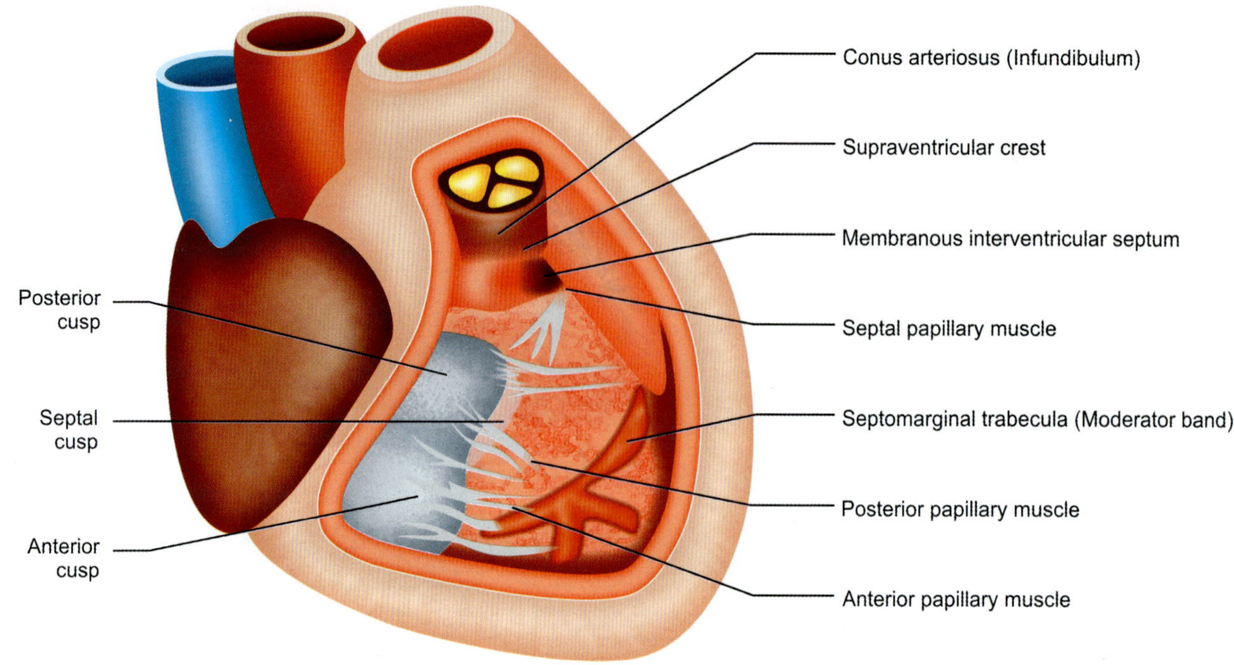

Figure 4

The detailed anatomy of the right ventricular inlet showing the 3 cusps of the tricuspid valve and the 3 papillary muscles

longer than the circumference of the annulus, thereby providing a complete and unobstructed opening as the leaflets drop curtain like into the right ventricle during diastole **(Fig. 5)**. In contrast to the other cardiac valves, the three thin membranous leaflets are not supported by a substantial fibrous annulus. The leaflets are less distinct than those of the other cardiac valves, separated more by indentations in a continuous sheet of tissue rather than true commissures. This makes up the entire tricuspid apparatus.

CHORDAE

When the right heart is opened through the acute margin **(See Fig. 1)**, the three largest fan-shaped chordae identify the three commissures. An average of 25 chordae tendineae attaches to the tricuspid valve leaflets. In contrast to mitral chordae, the chordae tendineae to the tricuspid leaflets are quite variable. The scalloped appearance of the tricuspid valve is due to the variability of the chordal attachments.

Two interesting types of chordae not seen in the mitral apparatus include the "free-edge chordae", which are long and attach to the free edge of the leaflets and the "deep chordae", which are short and attach to the basal portion of each leaflet. Of greatest interest are the short chordae that arise directly from the muscle of the septum and posterior wall and attach to the septal leaflet. This configuration limits the mobility of the septal leaflet and may predispose the tricuspid valve to

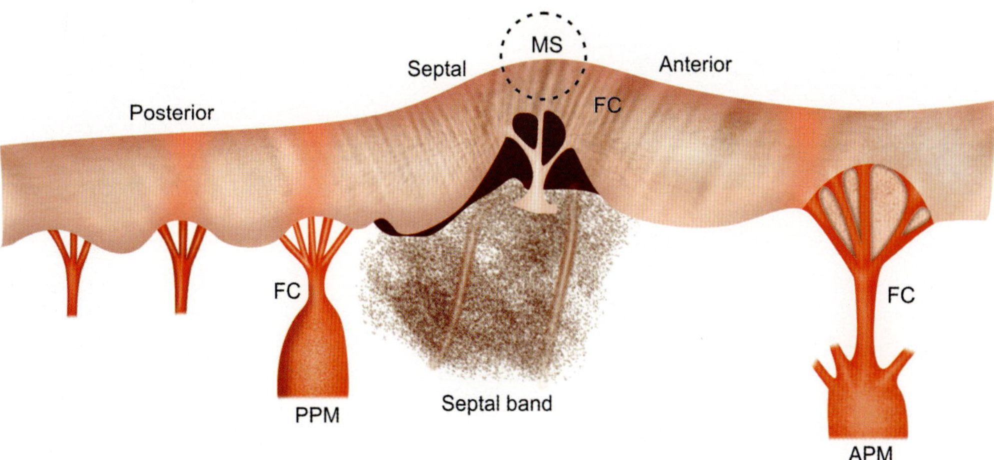

Figure 5

The tricuspid valve as viewed after incision through the acute margin of the right heart. The posterior, septal and anterior leaflets are identified the anteroposterior commissure. FC, Fan-shaped chordae; MS, membranous septum; APM, anterior papillary muscle; PPM, posterior papillary muscle; Small fan-shaped chordae indentify clefts in the posterior leaflet

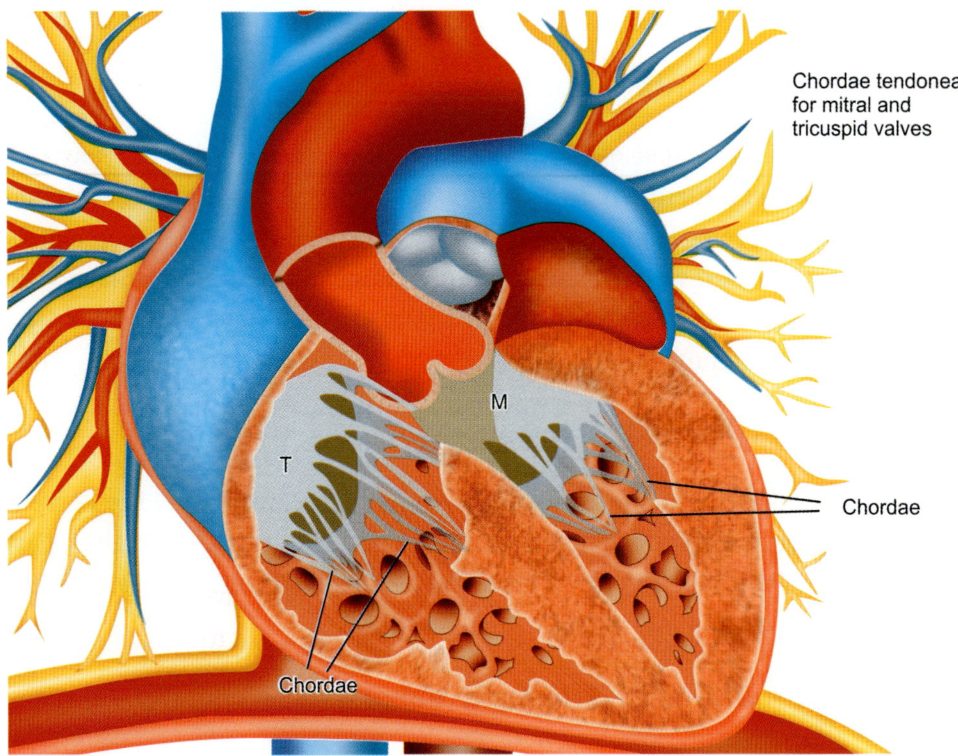

Figure 6

The chordae in the RV and LV have a big role to play in case of ventricular dilatation

incompetence. The fixed small septal leaflet allows for little compensation should the free wall of the right ventricle dilate **(Fig. 6)**.

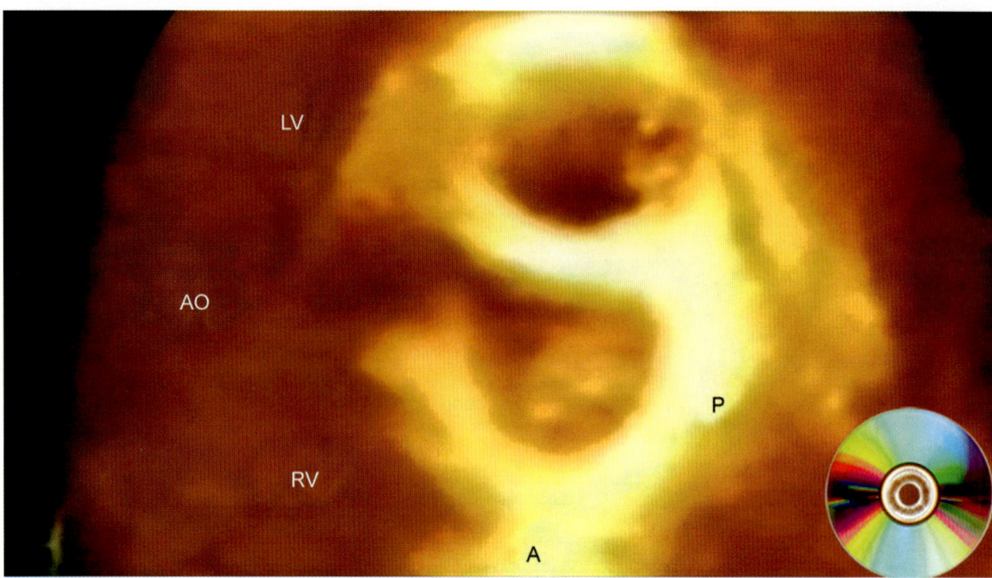

Figure 7 (VIDEO 2)

Moderator band in RV and the anterior and posterior leaflets on enface view on 3D echo

Papillary Muscles: Anterior and Medial

The anterior papillary muscle supplies fan-shaped chordae to the anterior and posterior leaflets, identifying the anteroposterior commissure. The medial papillary muscle supplies fan-shaped chordae to the posterior and septal leaflets and identifies the posteroseptal commissure. The large fan-shaped chordae to the anterior and the septal leaflets arise from the septal wall. A moderator band is seen and is a hallmark to identify the RV **(Fig. 7)**.

Dimensions of Tricuspid Valve

The normal circumference of the tricuspid valve annulus in an adult is 11 to 12 cm^2.[6] The tricuspid valve leaflets attach to the annulus at different levels. The highest part of the tricuspid valve's attachment occurs at the anteroseptal commissure, which is located near the membranous interventricular septum.

Supporting Structures of Tricuspid Valve

The supporting structures of the TV tend to be more complex and variable than those of the mitral valve. The anterior papillary muscle is large and gives rise to

- **An average of 25 chordae tendineae attaches to the tricuspid valve leaflets**

the moderator band, a linear band of cardiac muscle that runs perpendicular to the papillary muscle, attaches to the septum near the apex of the RV, and may be mistaken for an intracardiac mass. The posterior papillary muscle is frequently small and at times even absent.

The tricuspid annulus lies in a more apical position than that of the mitral valve, with its inferior margin adjacent to the junction of the inferior vena cava and coronary sinus. Beyond assessment of the anatomic structure and position of the tricuspid annulus, its systolic motion may be analyzed to provide important information about RV systolic function. Downward or apical movement of the annulus significantly augments RV stroke volume, even more than the corresponding effect of the mitral annulus on left ventricular ejection. With loss of annular motion, systolic shortening of the RV free wall decreases substantially, diminishing effective right heart function.[7]

Commissures and Leaflets of Tricuspid Valve

The commissures between each of the leaflets are less well-defined than those of the mitral valve. The annulus of the tricuspid valve is partially fibrous and partially muscular which allows annular contraction during systole **(Fig. 8)**.

The membranous septum and the bundle of His are near the commissure between the anterior and septal leaflets, which explains the shape of tricuspid ring prostheses. The plane of the TV annulus is slightly apical (6–10 mm) relative to the plane of the mitral valve—this is recognized echocardiographically by the TV septal leaflet's more apical attachment to the ventricular septum than the anterior mitral leaflet's **(Fig. 9)**. Greater apical displacement of the septal leaflet is seen in Ebstein's anomaly; absence of apical displacement indicates an AV canal defect **(Fig. 10)**.

As seen in **Figure 11**, the three TV leaflets are separated from each other by three commissures.

The commissures and the direction of closure lines are visualized. Visualization and measurement of commissures are relatively easy for the anteroseptal commissure and most difficult for the anteroposterior commissure **(Fig. 12)**.

Structure and Function of the Tricuspid Valve

The TV annulus also exhibits a horizontal, sphincter like motion during RV contraction. In healthy subjects, the TV annular area is maximal during atrial

- **The supporting structures of the TV tend to be more complex and variable than those of the mitral valve**

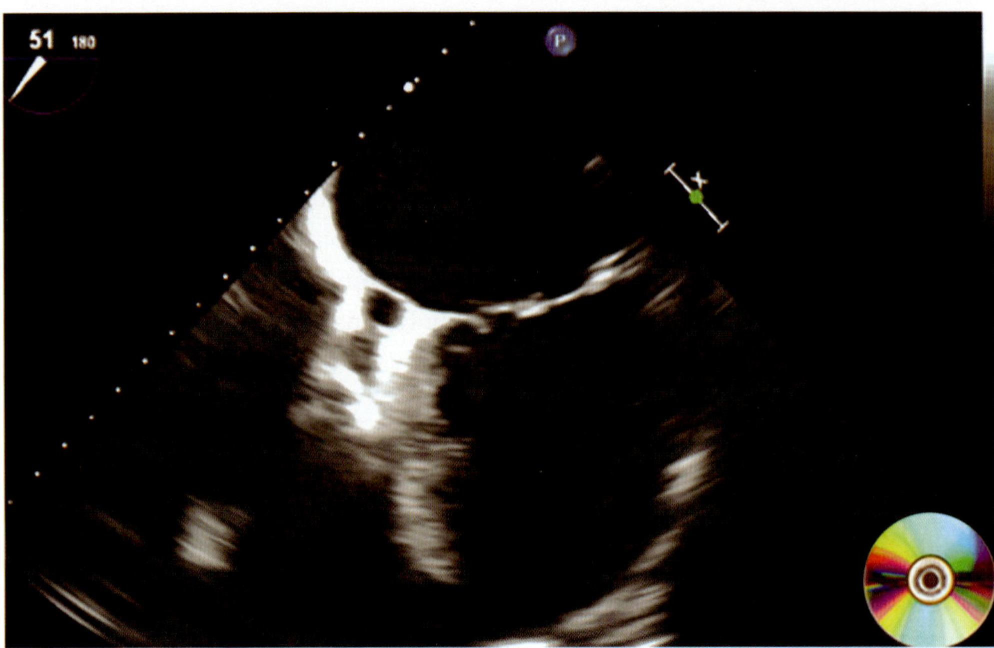

Figure 8 (VIDEO 3)

Annular contraction of the TV annulus in systole, due to its fibrous and muscular nature

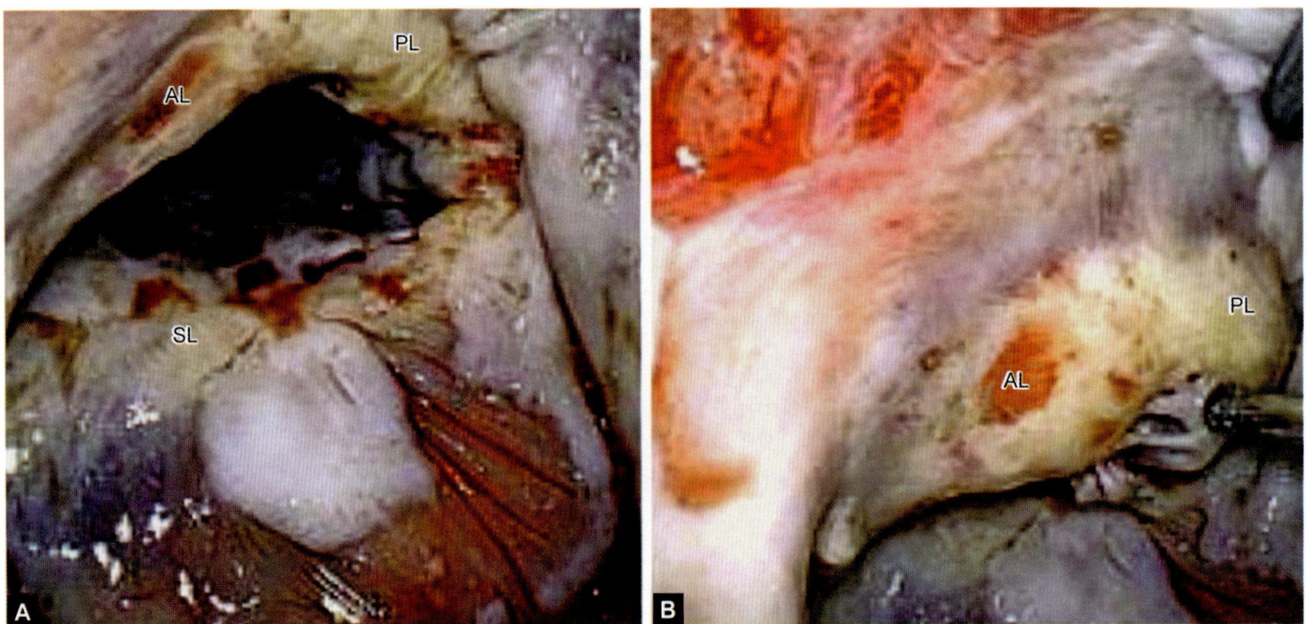

Figures 9A and B

The 3 leaflets of the tricuspid valve in surgical cross-section view

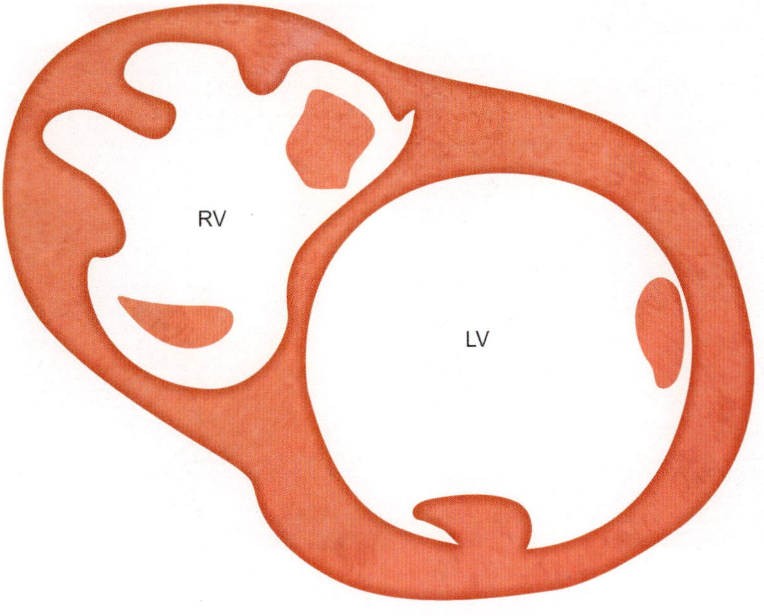

Figure 10

Apical view showing the more apical position of the TV than the MV

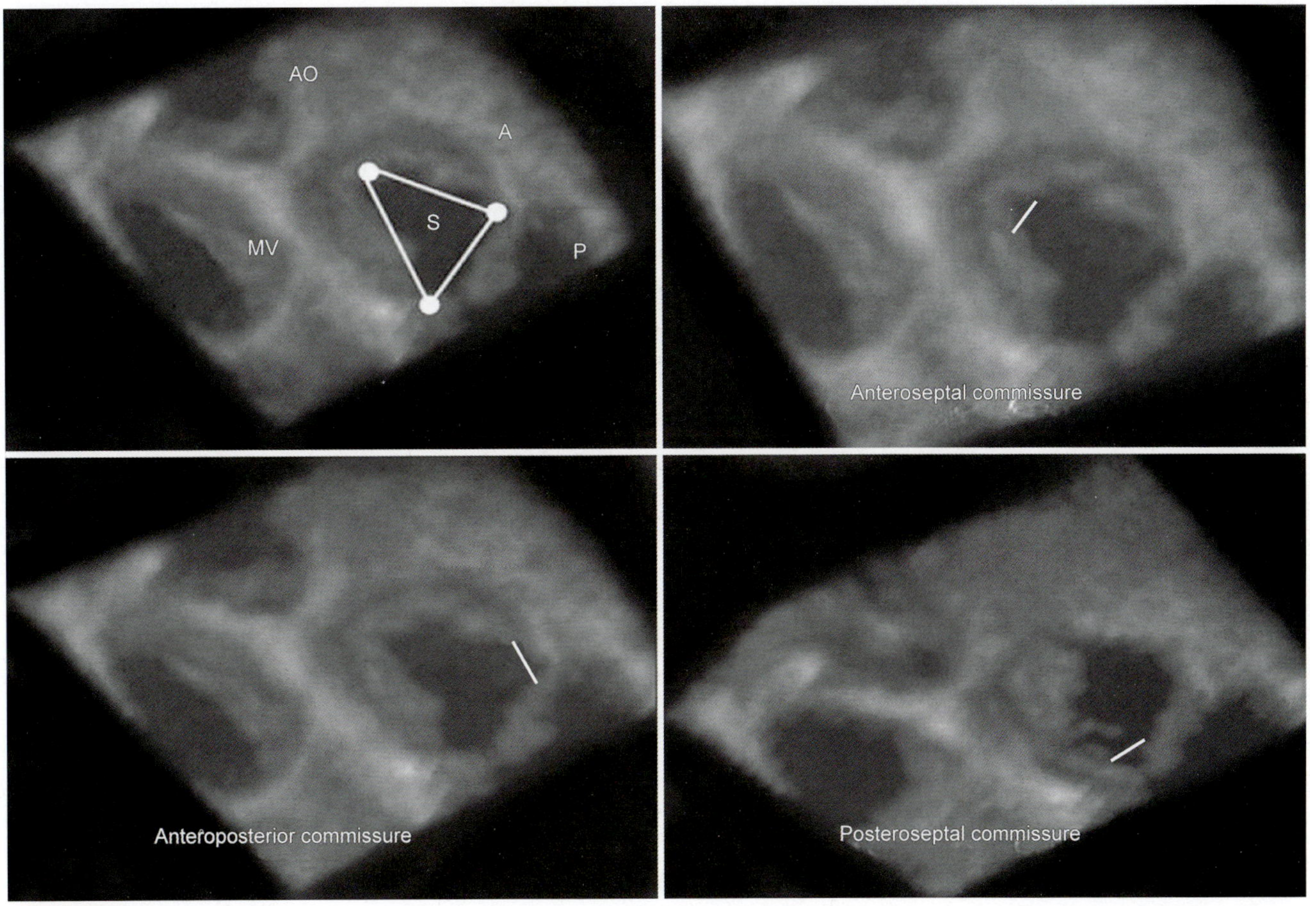

Figure 11

Triangular shaped area and the enface views of the leaflets and 2 commissures anteroseptal and posteroseptal commissures

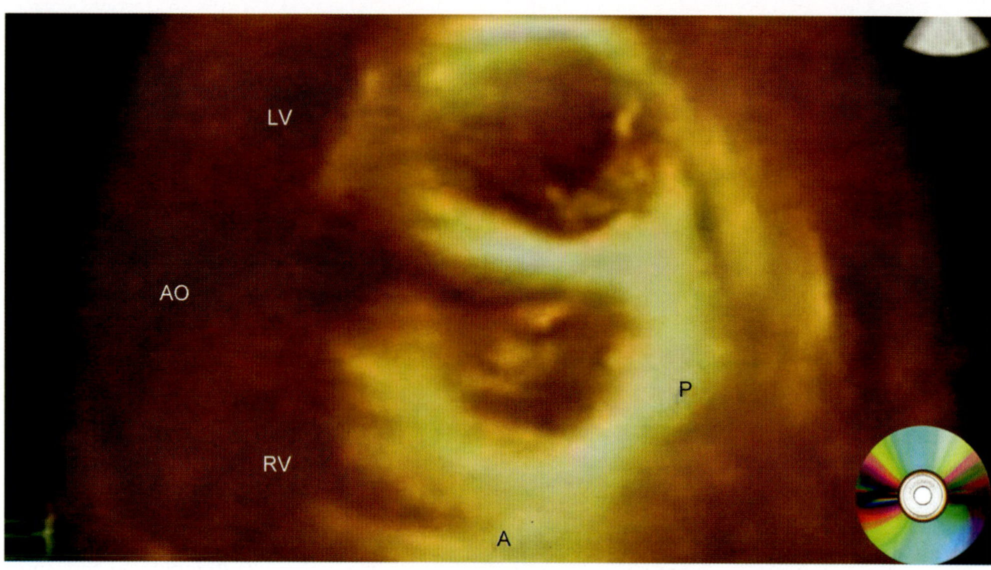

Figure 12 (VIDEO 4)

The TV with its 3 leaflets in case of a 18 years old in deep TQ view, showing its position to the mitral valve

contraction in late diastole, then decreases during early and midsystole and increases again during late systole and early dystole.[8] With more of its circumference in contact with the right ventricular myocardium, the tricuspid annulus exhibits and increased systolic area reduction when compared with the MV annulus (mean 33% reduction vs 26% reduction).[7] The difference between the systolic and diastolic annular diameters expressed as a fraction of the maximal (diastolic) diameter is known as tricuspid annulus fractional shortening (TAFS) and provides additional information regarding RV systolic function.[9]

The subvalvular apparatus of the TV, while similar to that of the MV, is more complex and variable in structure. The anterior papillary muscle is the largest muscle supporting the TV leaflets. It arises from the moderator bond, a linear band of cardiac muscle that runs perpendicular to the papillary muscle, attaches to the ventricular septum near the apex of the RV and may be mistaken for an intracardiac mass **(Figs 13 and 14)**. The posterior papillary muscle is frequently small and times even absent. A diminutive septal papillary muscle is also present **(Fig. 4)**.

- **The plane of the TV annulus is slightly apical (6–10 mm) relative to the plane of the mitral valve—this is recognized echocardiographically by the TV septal leaflet's more apical attachment to the ventricular septum than the anterior mitral leaflets**

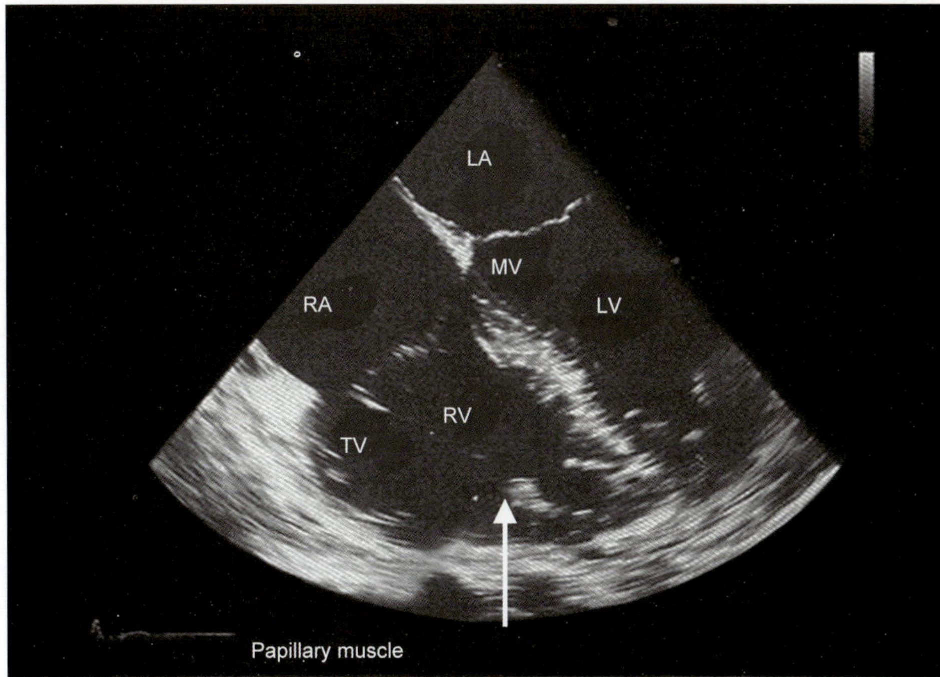

Figure 13

Transesophageal echocardiography image of a modified midesophageal 4-chamber (ME-4-C) view showing a prominent papillary muscle in the RV near the apex

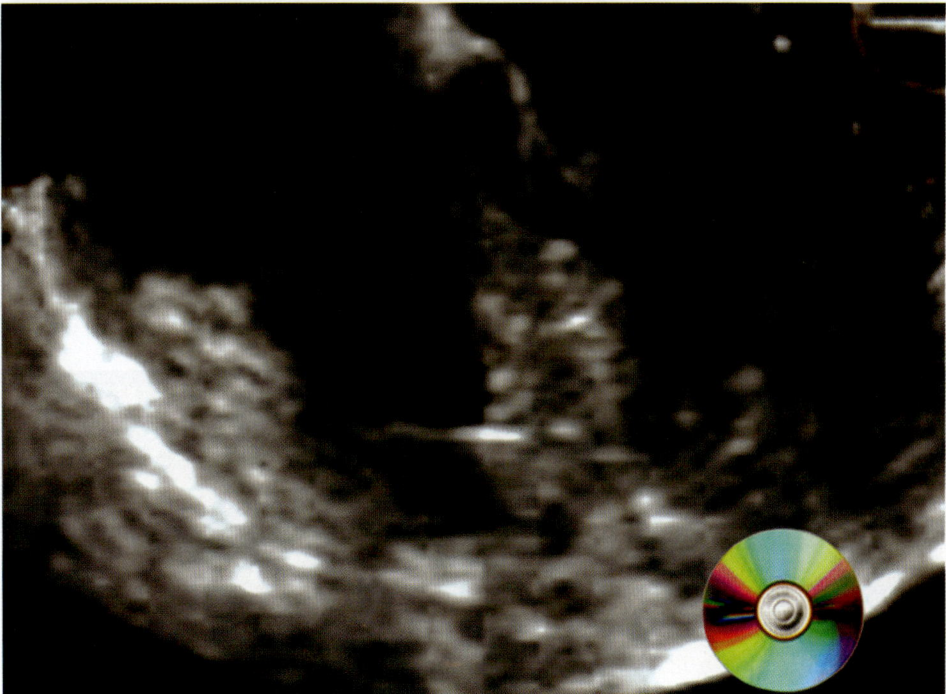

Figure 14 (VIDEO 5)

ME 4 chamber views the TV but not the PV

An alternative nomenclature describes two papillary muscles: a right anterior muscle and a posterior muscle that may have multiple heads.

PULMONIC VALVE ANATOMY

The pulmonic valve, being the most anterior valve, is well seen by transthoracic approaches but not TEE. This scalloped trileaflets semilunar valve is composed of smooth, thin cusps that form upon the smooth walled muscular infundibulum. The complex morphogenesis of the conotruncus creates a site for a number of congenital malformations associated with high morbidity and mortality. In this chapter, we will focus on assessment of normal structure affected by degenerative or acquired processes. The three leaflets of the pulmonic valve are pocket like cusps of approximately equal size that are supported by the sinotubular junction. The normal pulmonic valve is perpendicular and anterior to the aortic valve. While the other three cardiac valves are in fibrous continuity, the pulmonic valve stands alone, separated by the infundibulum.

3D TEE of Pulmonary Valve

In the aortic valve (AV) and aorta are located anterior and to the right of the pulmonary valve (PV) and pulmonary artery **(Fig. 15A)**. All four cardiac valves are visualized in this view. In **Figure 15B**, the AV and aorta are located directly anterior to the PV and pulmonary artery. The arrow points to the intra-arterial baffle. **Figure 15C** shows normal relationship of the semilunar valves and the great arteries in a patient without transposition of the great arteries. The PV and the pulmonary artery are located anterior and to the left of the aorta and the AV. All four cardiac valves are visualized **(Figs 15A to C)**.

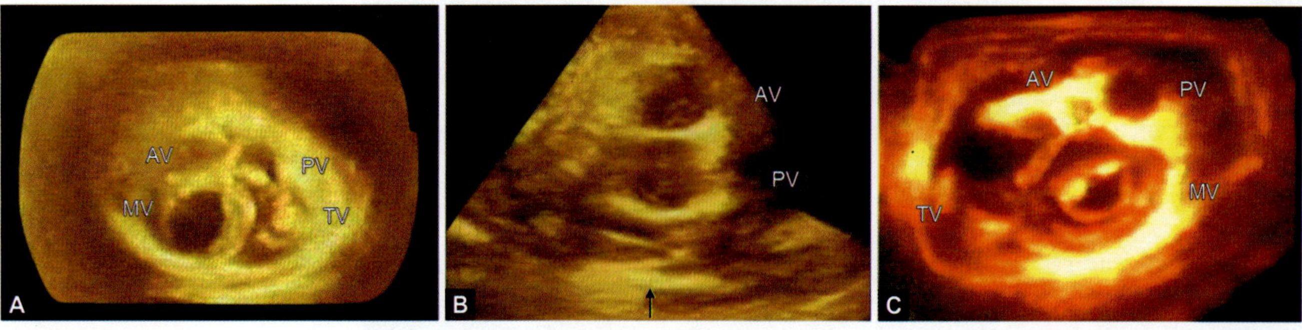

Figures 15A to C

3D TEE of pulmonary valve in different views

- **The posterior papillary muscle is frequently small and times even absent**

Structure and Function

The pulmonic valve (PV) is most similar in structure and the pulmonic valve (PV) is most similar in structure and function to the AY. Due to its position on the lower pressure right side of the heart, the pulmonic leaflets are somewhat thinner than those of the A Y. The three PV leaflets are termed anterior, left, and right. The latter two are situated posterior to the anterior leaflet and may be more correctly termed the right posterior and left posterior **(See Fig. 5)**. The valvular apparatus of the PV consists of the three leaflets or cusps, their associated sinuses of Valsalva, and structural similarity is a consequence of their common embryologic origin. Both semilunar valves develop from ridges of subendocardial tissue that form at the orifices of the aorta and the pulmonary trunk after partition of the bulbus cordis and the truncus arteriosus has occurred.[10] The annulus of the PV is much more ill defined and distensible than that of the AV because the pulmonary root attaches directly to RV muscle rather than to a fibrous annular ring. The geometric relationships between the valve annulus and sinotubular junction are similar on the right and left sides of the heart, resulting in a pulmonic sinotubular junction that is 10 to 15 percent smaller than the PV annulus diameter.[11] The PV area is similar to that of the AV, approximately 2 cm^2/m^2 body surface area. The anterior and right posterior PV leaflets and their associated sinuses of Valsalva are slightly larger than the left posterior.[12] Other features common to both the PV and the AV are the nodulus Arantii (small fibrous nodules in the free margin of the cusp) and the lunula (thin half-moon-shaped areas along the free edge of each cusp that can have perforations not considered clinically important.[13]

- **Pulmonary valvular apparatus consists of the 3 cusps, associated sinuses of Valsalva and a sinotubular junction similar to aortic valve.**
- **The 3 cusps are named the anterior, the left and right. Valve area is approximately 2 cm/m^2**
- **Anterior structure**
- **Difficult to image on TEE valve: 3 semi-lunar cusps:**
- **Right, left, anterior**
- **PA: Slightly dilated forming sinus**
- **Normally AV and PV lie at 90° planes to each other. Imaging:**
  - **RV inflow-outflow**
  - **ME AV Short axis view**
  - **ME ASV Long axis view**
  - **UE Ascending aorta short axis view**
- **The three leaflets of the pulmonic valve are pocket like cusps of approximately equal size that are supported by the sinotubular junction**

ANATOMY OF THE RIGHT HEART

The systemic venous return enters the right atrium via SVG and IVC, and the coronary venous blood via the coronary sinus. The hepatic veins insert into the IVC 2 to 3 cm distally from the insertion of the latter into the right atrium. A muscular ridge extending downward the IVC is called the crista terminalis and makes the border between the posterior, smooth walled part atrium. The right atrial (RA) appendage is located medially on right atrium adjacent to the ascending aorta. Anterior to the insertion of the IVC, a rudimentary but variable valve (Eustachian valve) can be seen. Occasionally, this valve is large and perforated, giving rise to a lace-like structure known as network of Chiari. Another small valvular structure is located at the orifice of the coronary, posterior, and septal leaflets that are connected to anterior, and medial papillary muscles, respectively.

The right ventricle can be depicted as a tetrahedron in which tricuspid ostium, interventricular septum, and anterior and inferior parts of the free wall represent the four walls, and margo acutus is the connection between the anterior and inferior walls. A strong muscle band divides the RV cavity into two parts: the RV inflow tract and the RV outflow tract. This U shaped band is called crista supraventricularis septum along the upper interventricular septum along the anterior tricuspid annulus into the RV free wall. A smaller (moderator) band also connects the distal interventricular septum with the free wall of the right ventricle. In contrast to the trabeculated inner wall of the inflow tract, the surface of the outflow tract (remnant of the bulbus cordis) is smooth.

The outflow tract is separated from the trunk of the PA by the pulmonary valve with right, left, and anterior cusps. The bifurcation of the PA is located to the left of the ascending aorta, with the right PA traversing toward the right hilus behind the aorta **(Fig. 16)**.

PHYSIOLOGY OF THE RIGHT HEART

Most of the venous return collected in the right atrium during RV systole enters the right ventricle in early diastole, immediately after opening of the tricuspid valve. The RA contraction completes the RV diastolic filling. The right ventricle operates as a low pressure, thin walled volume pump, moving the blood across the low resistance pulmonary bed into the left heart. After the onset of RV contraction, the RV pressure quickly exceeds the diastolic PA pressure, and consequently the time

- **Pulmonary valvular apparatus consists of the 3 cusps, associated sinuses of Valsalva and a sinotubular junction similar to aortic valve.**

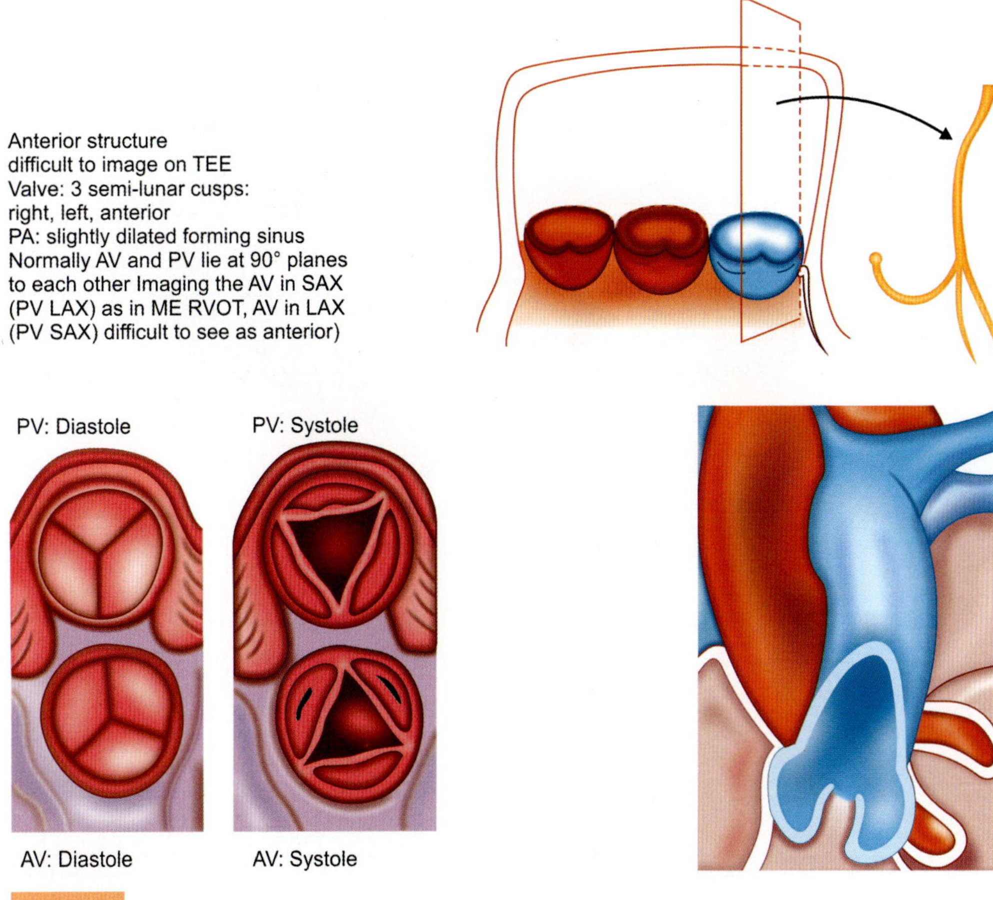

Figure 16

The 3 semilunar cusps of the pulmonary valve in systole and diastole

between the closure of the tricuspid valve and the opening of the pulmonary valve (isovolumic contraction period) is very short. The peak RV pressure is reached early during ejection, which—in contrast to left ventricular (LV) ejection—continues even during the late systolic decline in RV pressure. Therefore, the isovolumic relaxation period is also short and often absent. The global systolic function of the right ventricle is determined by RV preload (according to the Frank-Starling law), afterload, and contractility. The thin and compliant wall of the normal right ventricle allows a large increase in end-diastolic volume (preload) without a corresponding increase in RV end-diastolic and RA mean pressures. During acute increase in RV volume it is not only the RV wall but also the pericardium that increasingly opposes further filling and causes a steep increase in right filling pressures. The impedance of the pulmonary vascular bed represents the afterload of the right ventricle. The low pressure pump of the right ventricle is very sensitive to any increase in afterload, and thus there is a close correlation between pulmonary vascular resistance and

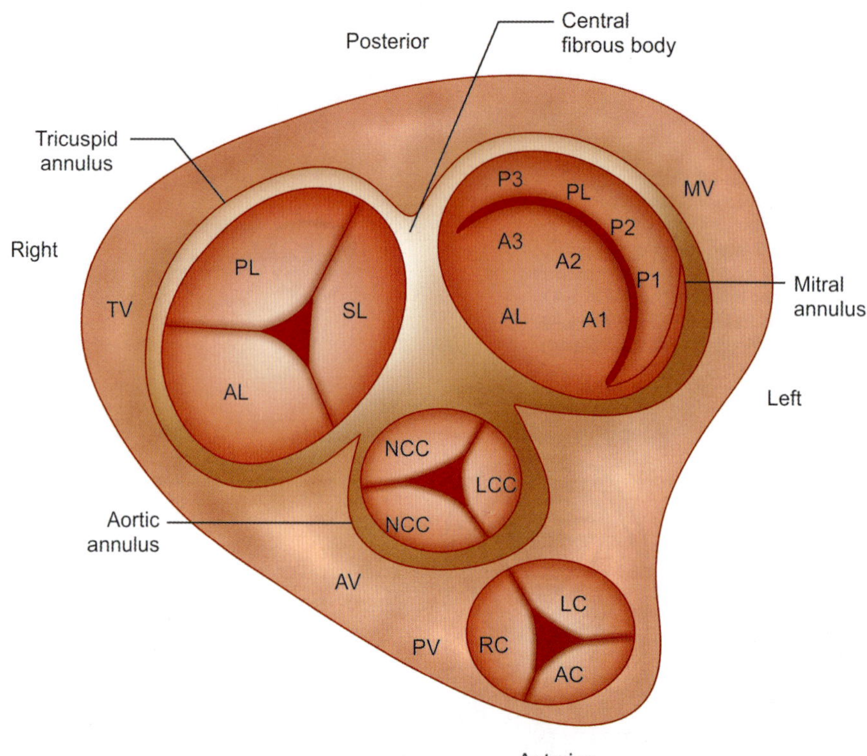

Figure 17

The pulmonary valve is the most anteriorly placed valve amongst the four valves as shown above

systolic function of the right ventricle **(Fig. 17)**. It is difficult to assess RV contractility directly at the bedside because it requires construction of RV pressure-volume or pressure-area loops, and calculation of RV end-systolic elastance. An improvement in wall motion associated with increase in stroke volume, decrease in RV size, and unchanged or decreasing filling pressures can be interpreted as indirect evidence of increased contractility.

The contraction of the right ventricle follows a specific, "peristaltic" pattern with the outflow tract contracting 25 to 50 ms after the inflow, giving rise to an intraventricular systolic pressure gradient between the proximal and distal parts of the right ventricle. The crista supraventricularis plays an important role during RV ejection by pulling in most of the RV free wall from margo acutus and anterior interventricular sulcus toward the apex. The effects of its contraction include systolic narrowing of the tricuspid orifice and displacement of the RV free wall toward the septum. The right and left ventricles operate in series, and the function of one

- **The right ventricle operates as a low pressure, thin walled volume pump, moving the blood across the low resistance pulmonary bed into the left heart.**

ventricle affects the function of the other. This phenomenon is called ventricular interdependence (cross-talk) and takes place in both systole and diastole. Because the ventricles share common myocardial fibers in the septal region, the contraction of one ventricle contributes to the force of contraction of the other. Naturally, the "help" of the left ventricle is much stronger. Both ventricles compete for space within the pericardium, and therefore the filling of one ventricle affects, by septal shift, the filling of the other. For instance, a marked dilatation of the right ventricle shifts the septum toward the left ventricle and impairs LV compliance and diastolic filling.

The upstream position of the right ventricle renders its pump function sensitive to changes in intrathoracic pressure and lung volume. During spontaneous inspiration, venous return, filling of the right heart, early and late diastolic filling velocities, RV end-diastolic volume, PA flow, and consequently RV stroke volume all increase. In maximal inspiration, even an increase in RV ejection fraction is observed. The respiratory variation in transtricuspid flow velocity (early (E) and late [A] waves) during quiet breathing is in the range 13 to 17 percent, whereas excessive variation (>50%) is an important sign of cardiac tamponade. "Opposite changes occur during mechanical ventilation. The intrathoracic pressure increase associated with the mechanical inspiration impairs venous return, reduces RV filling (E and A velocities), PA flow, and RV stroke volume. This inspiratory decrease in RV preload can combine with an increase in RV afterload (by compression of the pulmonary vascular bed due to high inspiratory pressures and/or additional positive end-expiratory pressure) to impair RV ejection."

Normal RV function implies transfer of venous return across pulmonary circulation into the left heart with physiological right heart volumes and pressures. RV dysfunction means that the right ventricle is still able to fulfill its physiological pumping function but only by activating its reserve or compensatory mechanisms, basically by the Frank-Starling mechanism as well as by development of myocardial hypertrophy in the long-term. RV dysfunction is suggested by symptoms and signs occurring under exercise or other forms of stress, and it is confirmed by hemodynamic and/or echocardiographic measurements. RV failure develops when the right ventricle is unable to function properly despite fully activated compensatory mechanisms and causes systemic venous congestion, under filling of the left ventricle, low cardiac output syndrome, or cardiogenic shock.

- **The intrathoracic pressure increase associated with the mechanical inspiration impairs venous return, reduces RV filling (E and A velocities), PA flow and RV stroke volume.**

APPLICATION OF TRICUSPID VALVE AND PULMONARY ANATOMY

Criteria for volume overload on the right side: transesophageal echocardiography of right side is important for measuring the following hemodynamic indices:

- Diastolic flattering of the septal wall giving a **D** shaped appearance to the LV is a subtle indicator of volume overload on the right side.
- **Eccentricity index:** Eccentricity index is the geometric index of septal shifting which may help in distinguishing between pressure and volume overload in the right ventricular. It is measured from left ventricular dimensions in the TG mid short-axis (SAX) view as the ratio of the inferoanterior internal diameter to the septolateral diameter measured at both end systole and end diastole. A ratio **>1 at end systole** indicates **RV** pressure overload, whereas a ratio **> 1 at end diastole** indicates volume overload. The index need not be calculated as it can be appreciated without making measurements.
  - A ratio >1 would give the LV a characteristic **D** shape. This is easy to appreciate in this patient in the picture **(Figs 18A and B)** who has history of breathlessness with chest pain and a SPO_2 of 88 percent requiring mechanical ventilation.

Measurements and indices are used for the purpose of measuring fluid responsiveness in a cardiac patient, perioperatively:

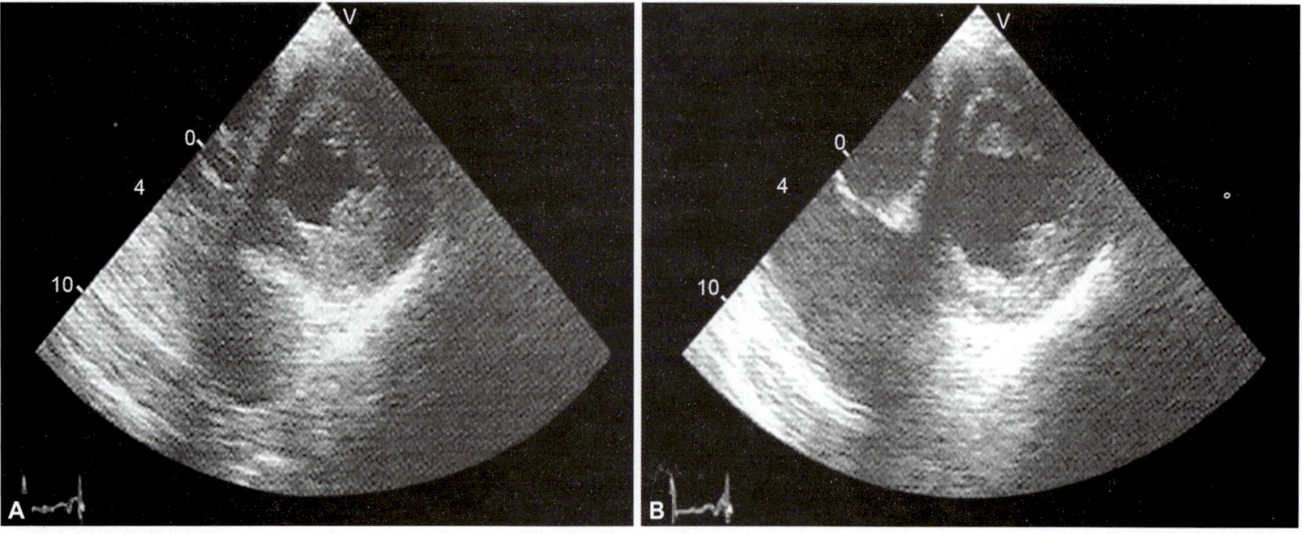

Figures 18A and B

TG midpapillary short axis view (TG mid SAX) in systole (A) and diastole (B) for many hemodynamic measurements as well

- IVC diameter
- IVC collapsibility index and distensibility index
- LV end diastolic area and volume
- LVOT VTI variation with respiration
- Peripheral artery V_{max} variation
- LVOT VTI variation with passive leg rise

IVC Diameter: This can be Measured in TEE in the LE Hepatic Vein View

- Low CVP likely as IVC diameter (IVCD) gets smaller than 1 cm and
- High CVP increasingly likely as IVCD increases above 2 cm.
- However, there is wide variation and the absolute measurements are not applicable with positive pressure ventilation.
- The examination of the IVC is particularly easy and can be done by someone with limited experience in echocardiography.

Respiratory Variations in IVC Diameter in a Patient on Controlled Ventilation (Fig. 19)

In a patient requiring ventilatory support, the inspiratory phase induces an increase in pleural pressure, which is transmitted to the right atrium, thus reducing venous return. The result is an inversion of the cyclic changes in IVC diameter, leading to increases in the inspiratory phase and decreases in the expiratory phase. These variations are also abolished by dilatation of the vena cava, indicating high right atrial pressure for the same reason as before. The respiratory variations in IVC diameter in a mechanically ventilated patient are therefore only observed when right atrial pressure is normal, that is low. In a patient presenting with signs of circulatory insufficiency, this finding may indicate hypovolemia. Measurement of IVC diameter in a patient receiving mechanical ventilation does not accurately predict right atrial pressure **(Figs 20 and 21)**.

Absence of respiratory variations in IVC diameter in a mechanically ventilated patient presenting with signs of circulatory insufficiency suggests that volume expansion will be ineffective in 90 percent of cases

Distensibility Index

This differs from ΔIVC (collapsibility index) in that the denominator is the minimum diameter. The cutoff for this index is 18 percent. In mechanically ventilated

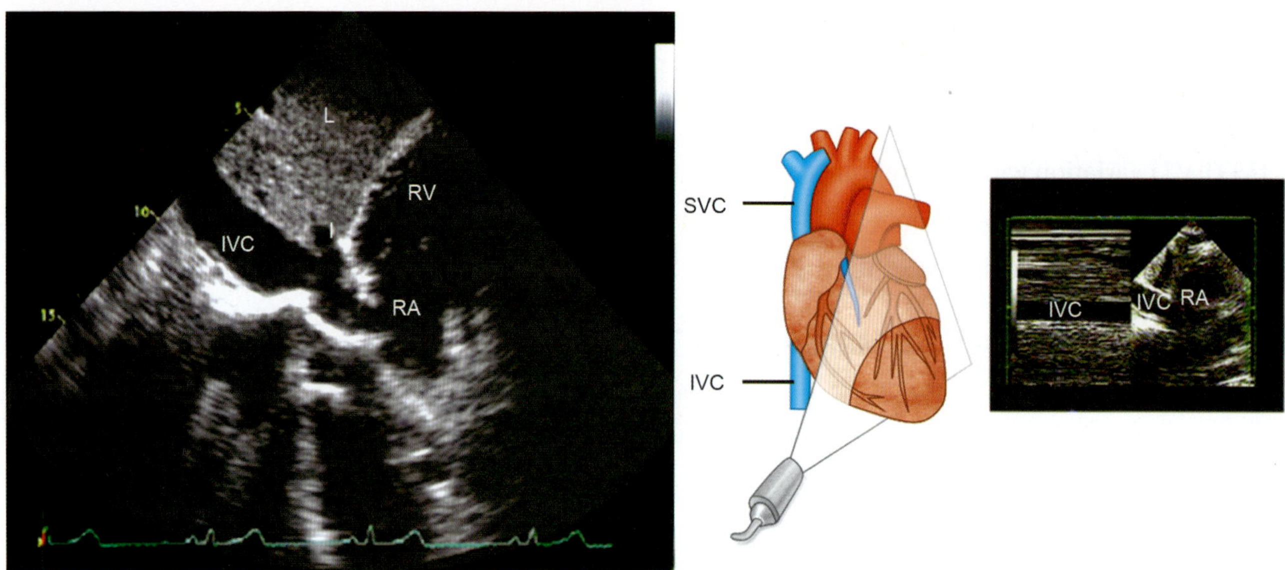

Figure 19

Measurement of IVC diameter in LE hepatic vein view

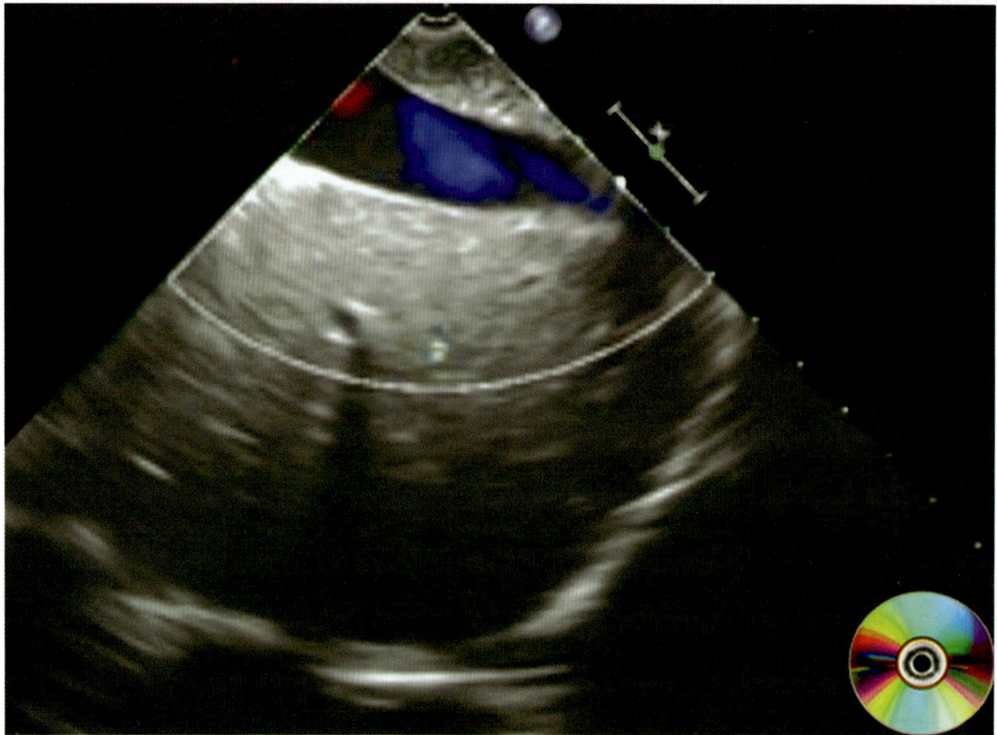

Figure 20 (VIDEO 6)

IVC diameter measurement in lower esophageal TEE view

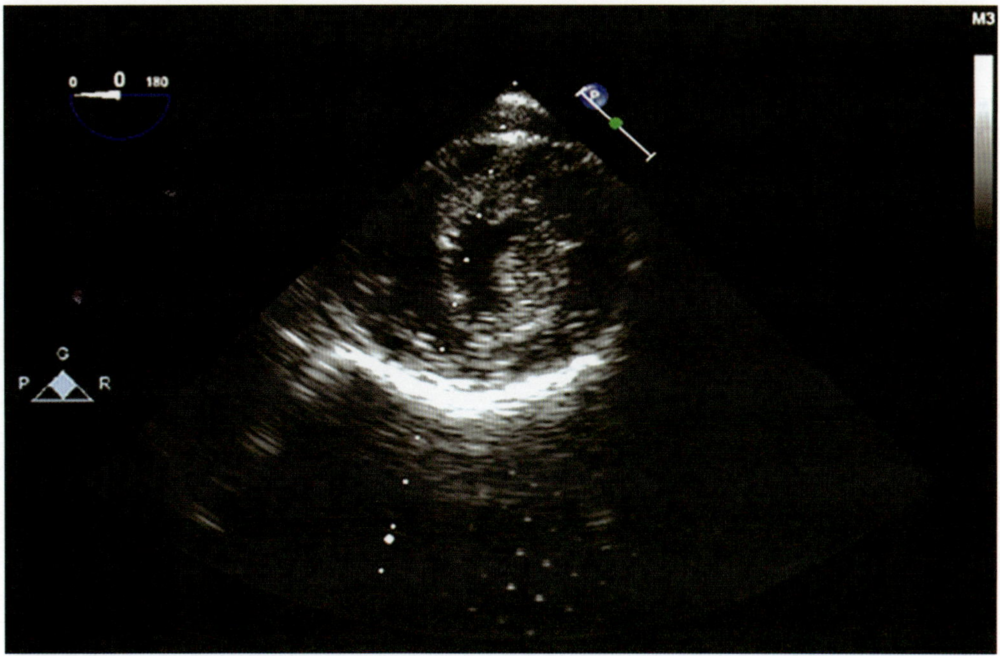

Figure 21

Left ventricular end-diastolic volume (LVEDV) can be measured and "kissing papillary" sign in transgastric midpapillary view for optimal fluid responsiveness in patients with near obliteration of the LV cavity

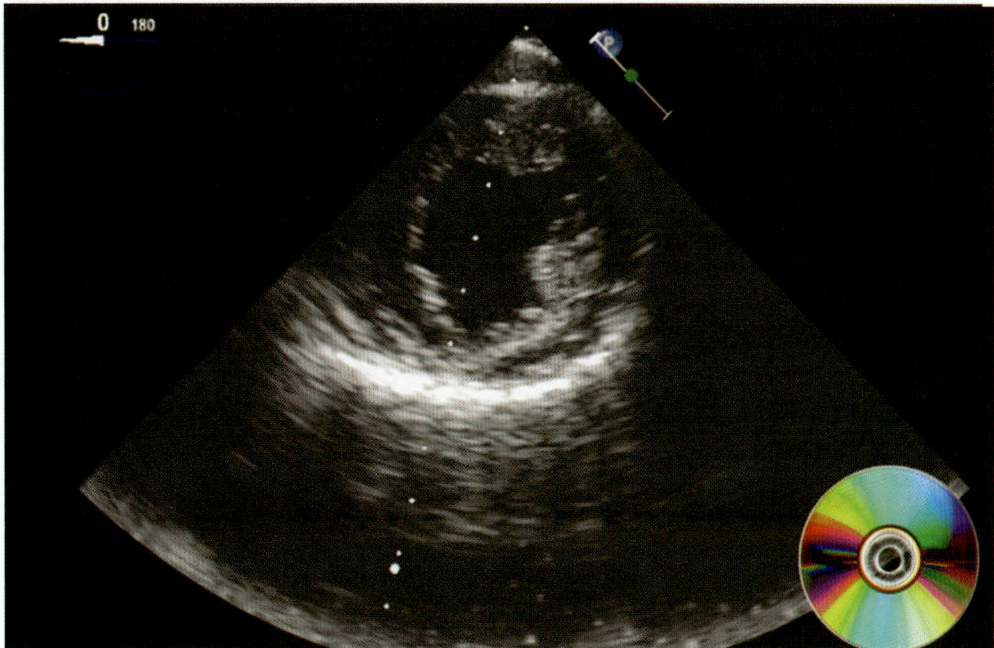

Figure 22 (VIDEO 7)

The TG midpapillary can be used to measure the distensibility index

patients, a 12 percent or more variation identified patients likely to respond to vascular filling, in terms of increased cardiac output, from those who would not respond, with a positive predictive value of 93 percent and a negative predictive value of 92 percent. It must be remembered that the measurements should be taken during mandatory ventilator breaths and the tidal volume should be at least 8 mL/kg. The great merit of this technique is that it is a dynamic, noninvasive parameter to evaluate the potential benefit of volume expansion **(Fig. 22)**.

Left Ventricular End-diastolic Volume and Kissing Papillary Muscle Sign

View shows hypovolemia.

- An LVEDA <10 cm^2 or a left ventricular end-diastolic area (LVEDA) index (LVEDA/BSA) of <5.5 cm^2/m^2 indicates Hypovolemia.
- Another sign that suggests severe hypovolemia is the "kissing papillary muscle sign" at end systole.

Collapsibility Index

Measurement of IVC diameter in different positions differentiates normal subjects from patients with elevated right atrial pressure. In a spontaneously breathing, healthy subject, cyclic variations in pleural pressure, which are transmitted to the right atrium, produce cyclic variations in venous return, which is increased by inspiration, leading to an inspiratory reduction of about 50 percent in IVC diameter. It should be noted that the denominator here is the mean diameter and not the maximum diameter.

Limitations of IVC Collapsibility Index

These variations are also abolished by dilatation of the vena cava, indicating high right atrial pressure for the same reason as before. The respiratory variations in IVC diameter in a mechanically ventilated patient are therefore only observed when right atrial pressure is normal, that is low.

In a patient presenting with signs of circulatory insufficiency, this finding may indicate hypovolemia. Measurement of IVC diameter in a patient receiving mechanical ventilation does not accurately predict right atrial pressure. However,

- **In terms of increased cardiac output, from those who would not respond, with a positive predictive value of 93 percent and a negative predictive value of 92 percent.**

there is wide variation and the absolute measurements are not applicable with positive pressure ventilation.

Fractional Area Change

To calculate RV fractional area change:

1. **In the modified apical 4-chamber view**, trace the RV endocardium to obtain an area measurement (in cm) at end-diastole and end-systole.
2. **RV fractional area change** can then be calculated (as a percentage) from:

RV fractional area change

$$= \frac{\text{End diastolic area–End systolic area}}{\text{End diastolic area}} \times 100 \text{ (to express as a percentage)}$$

Tricuspid Annular Plane Systolic Excursion

Tricuspid annular plane systolic excursion (TAPSE) is a simple and well-validated method of assessing RV function. The underlying principle is based on measuring how much the lateral tricuspid annulus moves vertically during systole—the more impaired the RV, the less annular displacement is seen. To measure TAPSE:

1. Obtain a modified apical 4-chamber view of the RV.
2. Using M-mode, place the cursor so that it passes through the lateral tricuspid annulus. Obtain an M-mode trace.
3. Measure the vertical displacement of the lateral tricuspid annulus from the M-mode trace **(Fig. 23)**.

- **TAPSE Ⓝ value is 16 to 20 mm and a TAPSE ≤ 5 mm is indicative of severe disease (BSE recommendations)**

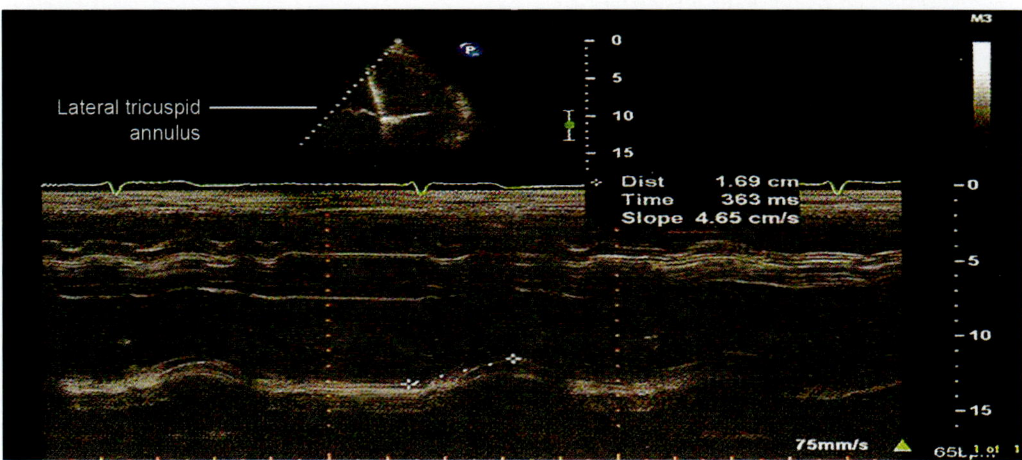

Figure 23

Measurement of tricuspid annular plane systolic excursion

Tei Index

The Tei index (myocardial performance index) is a measure of myocardial function that takes into account both systolic and diastolic function and is independent of heart rate (but cannot be used in an irregular rhythm such as AF). It is based upon the ratio between the sum of RV isovolumic contraction time (ICT) and isovolumic relaxation time (IRT), divided by ejection time (ET). To calculate the Tei index:

1. Use PW Doppler to obtain a trace of forward flow through the tricuspid valve, and measure the duration (in s) of RV systole. This is measured from the end of the forward flow trace in one cardiac cycle to the start of the forward flow trace in the next cycle. This is 'a' and represents ICT, ET and IRT.
2. Use PW Doppler to obtain a trace of forward flow through the pulmonary valve, and measure the duration (in s) of ejection. This is measured from the start to the end of a single forward flow trace in one cardiac cycle. This is 'b' and represents ET alone.

Volume and Pressure Overload

Assessing the IVS in the parasternal short axis view can provide useful information about RV hemodynamics. Normally septal motion is dominated by the LV, and the septum bulges towards the RV in the short axis views. If the RV is overloaded this septal bulge starts to flatten, and in the short axis views this gives the LVa 'D' shape rather than its usual circular appearance. In the presene of chronic RV volume overload (e.g. severe tricuspid regurgitation), the RV is dilated and the septum is pushed towards the LV in diastole. In RV pressure overload (e.g, severe pulmonary hypertension), the RV is hypertrophied and the septum is pushed towards the LV in systole. Coexistent volume and pressure overload will flatten the septum in both systole and diastole.

The LV eccentricity index can be used to quantify these changes in the RV. In the parasternal short axis view, at the papillary muscle level, the LV septolateral cavity diameter is measured across the LV cavity at right angles to the interventricular septum **(Fig. 24)**. The LV anteroposterior diameter is then measured at right angles to the first measurement, to give two perpendicular cavity diameters which are then expressed as a ratio (of the anteroposterior diameter to the septolateral diameter). The measurements are taken at end-systole and at end-diastole. Normal individuals have a circular LV cavity and therefore have a ratio of 1 in both systole and diastole.

In RV volume overload, the flattening of the septum in diastole means that the septolateral LV diameter becomes smaller than the anteroposterior diameter, and so the diastolic ratio is > 1. In RV pressure overload, the ratio is > 1 in both diastole and systole.

- **Tei index is < 0.40 with a higher value indicating worsening RV function**

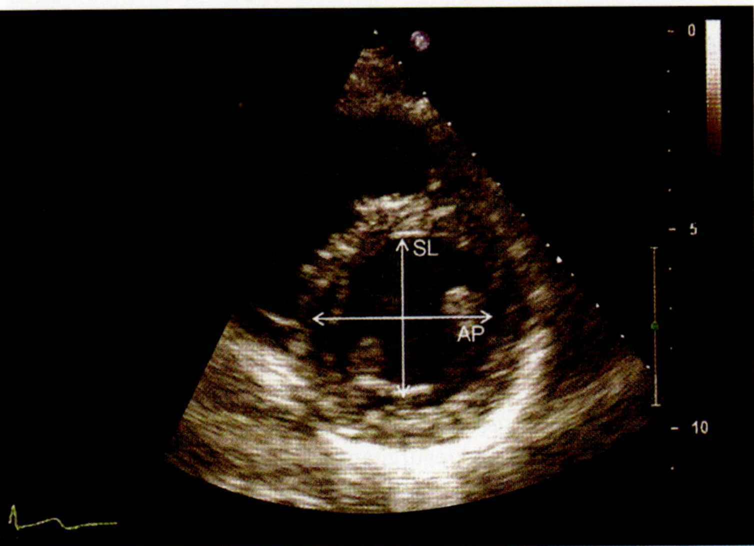

Figure 24

Measurement of LV septolateral (SL) and anteroposterior (AP) cavity-diameters in order to calculate the LV eccentricity index in the assessment of RV volume and pressure overload

RIGHT VENTRICULAR DIASTOLIC FUNCTION

Diastolic function of the RV is not commonly assessed in everyday clinical practice. Nonetheless, it is possible to gain valuable insights into RV diastolic function using simple echo parameters. PW Doppler of tricuspid inflow permits measurement of the tricuspid E and A waves and tricuspid E wave deceleration time (the time period between the peak of the E wave and the end of the E wave). The tricuspid E:A ratio (the ratio between peak E and A wave velocities) can be calculated:

$$\text{E: A ratio} = \frac{\text{Peak E wave velocity}}{\text{Peak A wave velocity}}$$

Tissue Doppler imaging can be performed at the lateral tricuspid annulus to yield a value for tricuspid early myocardial velocity (E').

A tricuspid E:A ratio <0.8 indicates impaired RV relaxation, while an E:A ratio of 0.8-2.1 plus an E:E' ratio of >6 indicates pseudonormal RV filling. Restrictive RV filling is indicated by an E:A ratio >2.1 with an E wave deceleration time of <120 ms.

REFERENCES

1. Lamers WH, Viragh S, Wessels A, Moorman A FM, Anderson RH. Formation of the tricuspid valve in the human heart. Circulation. 1995;91:111-21.
2. Silver MD, Lam JH, Ranganathan N, Wigle ED. Morphology of the human tricuspid valve. Circulation. 1971;43:333-48.

3. Wafae N, Hayashi H, Gerola LR, Vieira MC. Anatomical study of the human tricuspid valve. Surg Radiol Anat. 1990;12:37-41.
4. Maslow AD, Schwartz C, Singh AK. Assessment of the tricuspid valve: a comparison of four transesophageal echocardiographic windows. J Cardiothorac Vase Anesth. 2004; 18:719-24
5. Navin C Nanda, Ming Chon Hsiung, Andrew P Miller, Fadi J Hage. Tricuspid and pulmonary valves chapter 6 in "Live/Real Time 3D Echocardiography, 1st edn. Wiley Blackwell Publication. 2010. pp. 99-113.
6. Hauck A, Freeman D, Ackerman D, et al. Surgical pathology of the tricuspid valve: a study of 363 cases spanning 25 years. Mayo Clin Proc. 1988;63:851.
7. Isaaz K, Munoz L, Lee E, et al. Quantitation by Doppler echo of the motion of the cardiac base in normal man [Abstract]. Circulation. 1989;80(Suppl II):169.
8. Tei C, Pilgrim JP, Shah PM, et al. The tricuspid valve annulus: study of size and motion in normal subjects and in patients with tricuspid regurgitation. Circulation. 1982;66:665-71.
9. Colombo T, Russo C, Ciliberto GR, et al. Tricuspid regurgitation secondary to mitral valve disease: tricuspid annulus function as guide to tricuspid valve repair. Cardiavasc Surg. 2001;9:369-77.
10. Gersony W, Pruitt A, Riermenschneider T. The cardiovascular system. In: Behrman R, Kliegman R, Nelson W et al. (Eds). Nelson Textbook of Peadiatrics, 13th edn. Philadelphia: WB saunders. 1987. pp. 943-1032.
11. David TE, Omran A, Webbg, et al. Geometric mismatch of the aortic and pulmonary roots causes aortic insufficiency after the ross procedure. J Thorac Cardiovasc Surg. 1996;112:1231-7; discussion 1237-9.
12. Brickner ME, Hellis LD, Lange Ra. Congenital heart disease in adults. First of two parts. N Engl J Med. 2000;342:256-63.
13. Netter F. Atria and ventricles. In: Yonkman F (Ed). The Heart. New York: CIBA-GEIGY corporation. 1891:8.

2 Transesophageal Echocardiography Views of Tricuspid and Pulmonary Valves

Murali Chakarvarthy, Poonam Malhotra Kapoor, SN Das

- Mid-Esophageal Four-Chamber View
- Mid-Esophageal Mitral Commissural View
- Mid-Esophageal Ascending Aorta: Short Axis View
- Mid-Esophageal Ascending Aorta: Long Axis View
- Mid-Esophageal Right Pulmonary Vein View
- Mid-Esophageal Aortic Valve Short Axis View
- Mid-Esophageal Right Ventricular Inflow-Outflow View
- Mid-Esophageal Modified Bicaval View
- Upper-Esophageal Right and Left Pulmonary Veins View
- Transgastric Basal Short Axis View
- Transgastric Mid Papillary Short Axis View
- Transgastric Apical Short Axis View
- Transgastric Right Ventricular Basal View
- Transgastric Right Inflow-Outflow View
- Deep Transgastric 5–Chamber View
- Transgastric Right Ventricular Inflow View
- Upper-Esophageal Aortic Arch: Short Axis View
- Transesophageal Echocardiography Views to Assess Pulmonary Valve
- ASE/SCA 2013 Guidelines for Tricuspid Valve 3D TEE
- Pulmonary Valve 3D TEE

INTRODUCTION

Transesophageal echocardiography (TEE) has the unique advantage of portability and the ability to obtain high-resolution images of the abnormal cardiovascular anatomy, function and is relatively easy to perform with a low risk of complications.

Transesophageal echocardiography use has become an integral part in the care of cardiac surgical patients. This is evolving to be used in other subspecialties. The purpose of this article is to introduce the novice echocardiographer to a stepwise approach in image orientation and acquisition.

The American Society of Echocardiography (ASE) and the SCA have suggested a set of standard views and the nomenclature for those views **(Figs 1A to T)**. This nomenclature should be followed whenever possible to minimize confusion. Generally, a combination of these views allows for a complete diagnostic examination. However, deviation from these standard views may be necessary to obtain images appropriate to the individual patient **(Table 1)**. It is beneficial

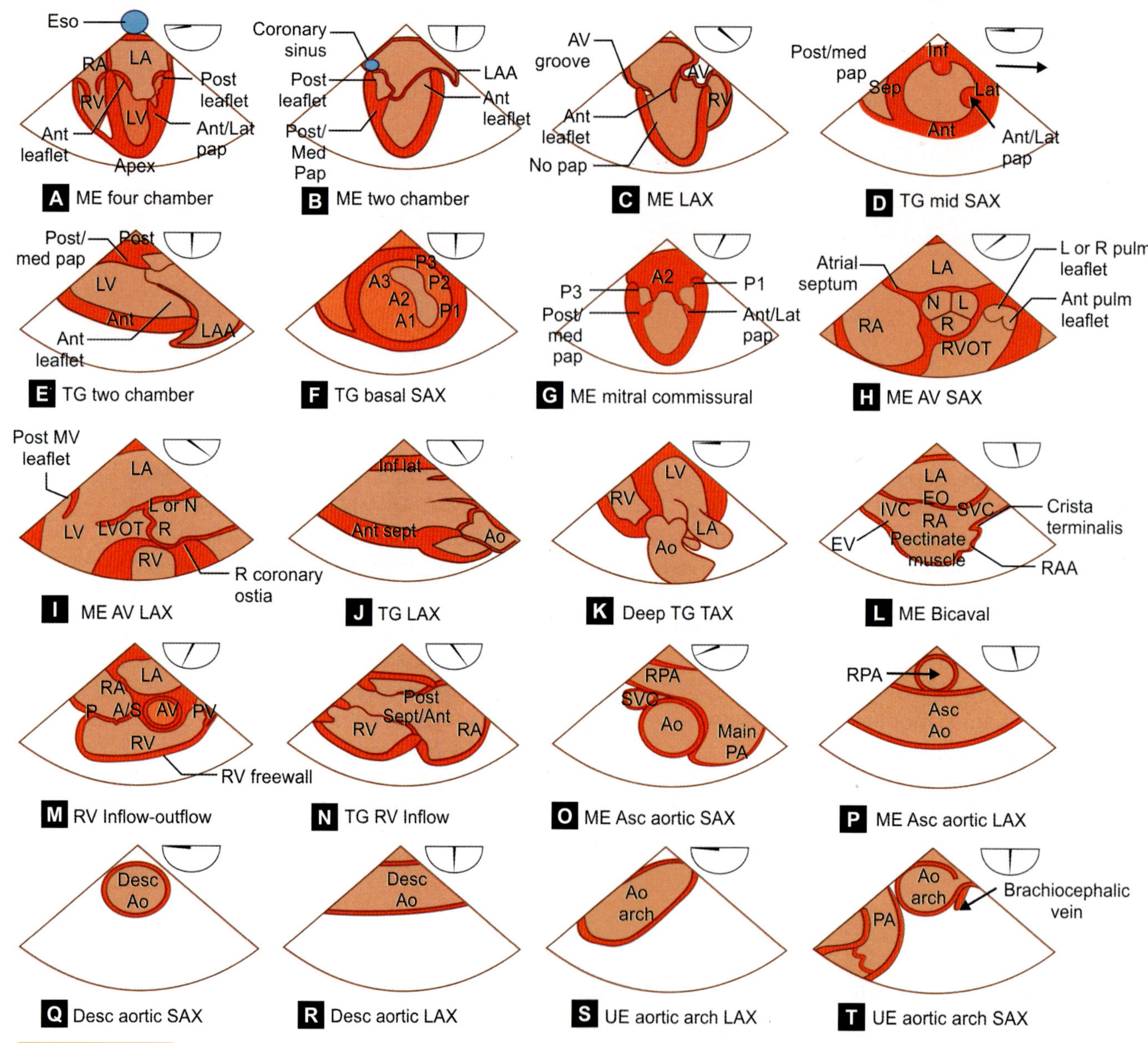

Figures 1A to T

The following is a suggestion for how to perform a focused 20-view TEE exam. There are many ways to do the exam, and ultimately the order of the exam depends on the preference of the examiner and the specific conditions of the patient. After you become familiar with the views, you can devise an order that works for you. Doing the exam in a similar fashion every time will ensure that you examine all 20 views and cover all the basics of the TEE exam for every patient. A basic 20 view exam can easily be expanded to the full ASE/SCA views with more experience (*Source*: ASE/SCA "Guidelines for performing a comprehensive intraoperative multiple TEE examination" Shanewise, et al. 1999)

to be flexible about the order in which the views are obtained to allow focusing on a specific clinical question in a timely manner. Each echocardiographer should develop a systematic order for routine diagnostic TEE. This not only allows for increased speed and efficiency but also ensures that an important finding will not be missed simply because a view was forgotten.

TEE Views for TV and PV (Figs 2A to I)

Table 1: List of focused views for tricuspid and pulmonary valve
• Mid-esophageal 4-chamber view
• Mid-esophageal mitral commissural view
• Mid-esophageal ascending aorta long axis view
• Mid-esophageal ascending aorta short axis view
• Mid-esophageal right pulmonary vein view
• Mid-esophageal aortic valve short axis view
• Mid-esophageal right ventricular inflow-outflow view
• Mid-esophageal modified bicaval TV view
• Upper esophageal right and left pulmonary veins view
• Transgastric basal short axis view
• Transgastric mid papillary short axis view
• Transgastric apical short axis view
• Transgastric right ventricular basal view
• Transgastric right inflow-outflow view
• Deep transgastric 5-chamber view
• Transgastric right ventricular inflow view
• Upper esophageal aortic arch short axis view

Probe Manipulation

Once in the esophagus, the transducer should be gently guided and the operator should never apply undue force.

There are 4 probe manipulations for optimal image acquisition. The probe manipulation described here is made with reference to the operator standing at the patient's head and looking towards the patient's feet.

1. *Advance, withdraw:* Pushing or pulling the tip of the TEE probe.
2. *Turn to right, turn to left (also referred to as clockwise and anticlockwise):* Rotating the anterior aspect of the TEE probe to the right or left of the patient.
3. *Anteflex, retroflex:* Anteflex is flexing the tip of the TEE probe anteriorly by turning the large control wheel clockwise. Retroflex is flexing the tip of the TEE probe posteriorly by turning the large wheel anticlockwise.
4. *Flex to right, flex to left:* Flexing the tip of the TEE probe with the small control wheel to the patient's right or left. The probe flexion to the right and left may not be necessary and should be avoided to minimize trauma to the esophagus **(Figs 4A to D)**.

- **The same has been revised in 2013. Eleven basic views should be followed by an echocardiographer and of these 9 ME and UE views (Figs 2A to I) and 8 TG views (Figs 3A to H) are important for detailed evaluation of tricuspid and pulmonary valve.**

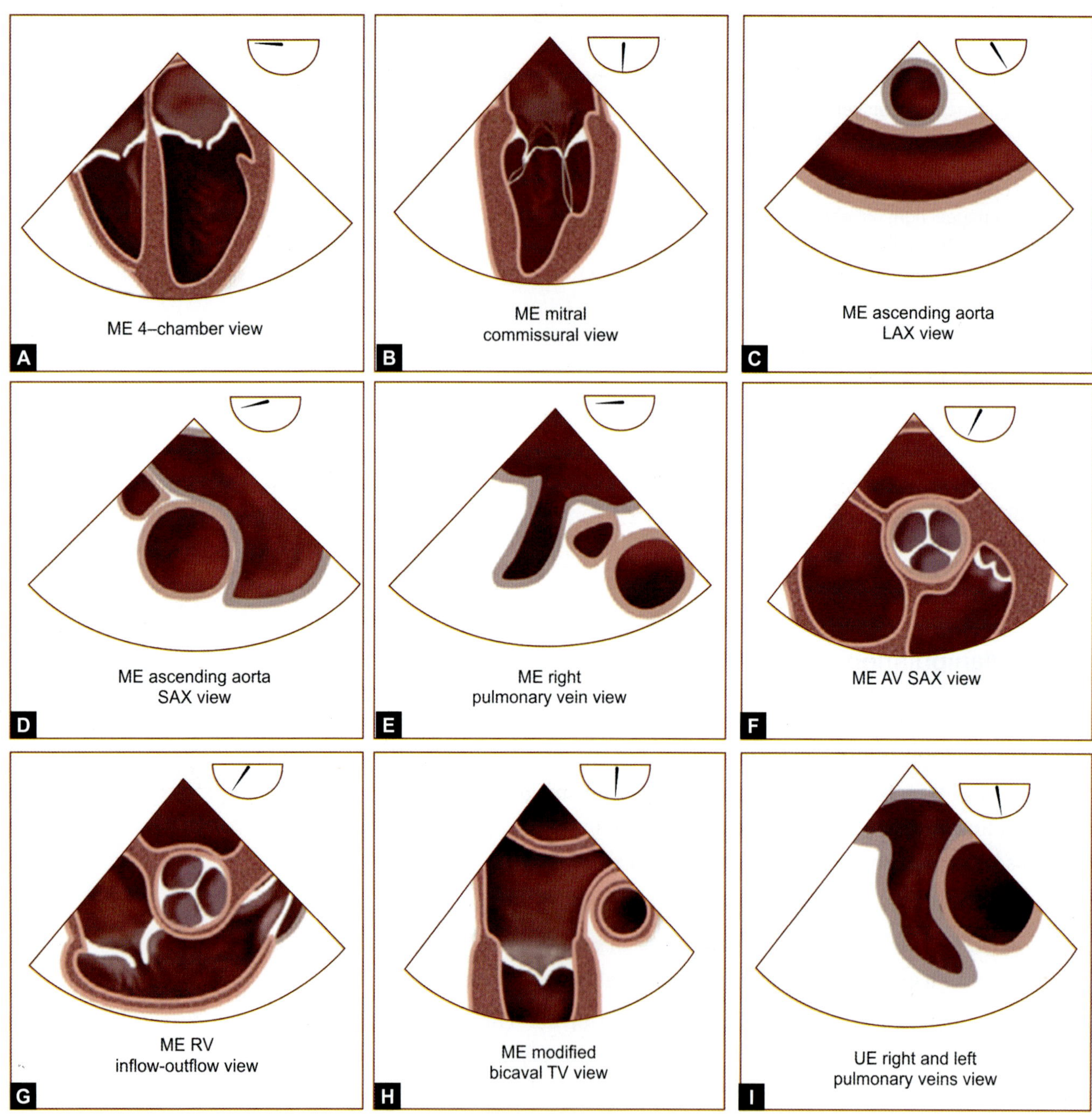

Figures 2A to I

Nine mid-esophageal views on TEE for quick assessment of tricuspid and pulmonary valve

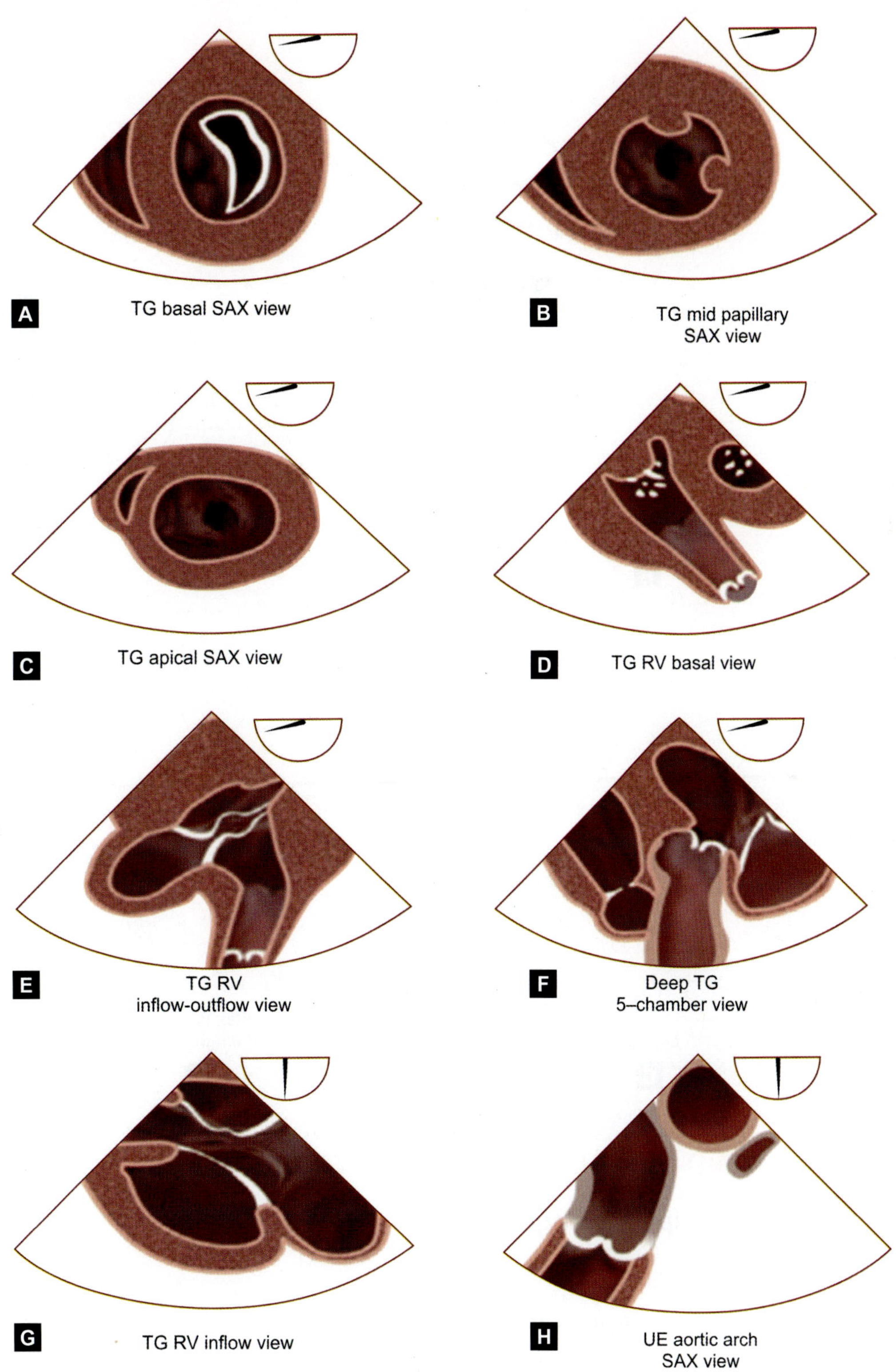

Figures 3A to H

Eight transgastric views on TEE for quick assessment of tricuspid and pulmonary valve

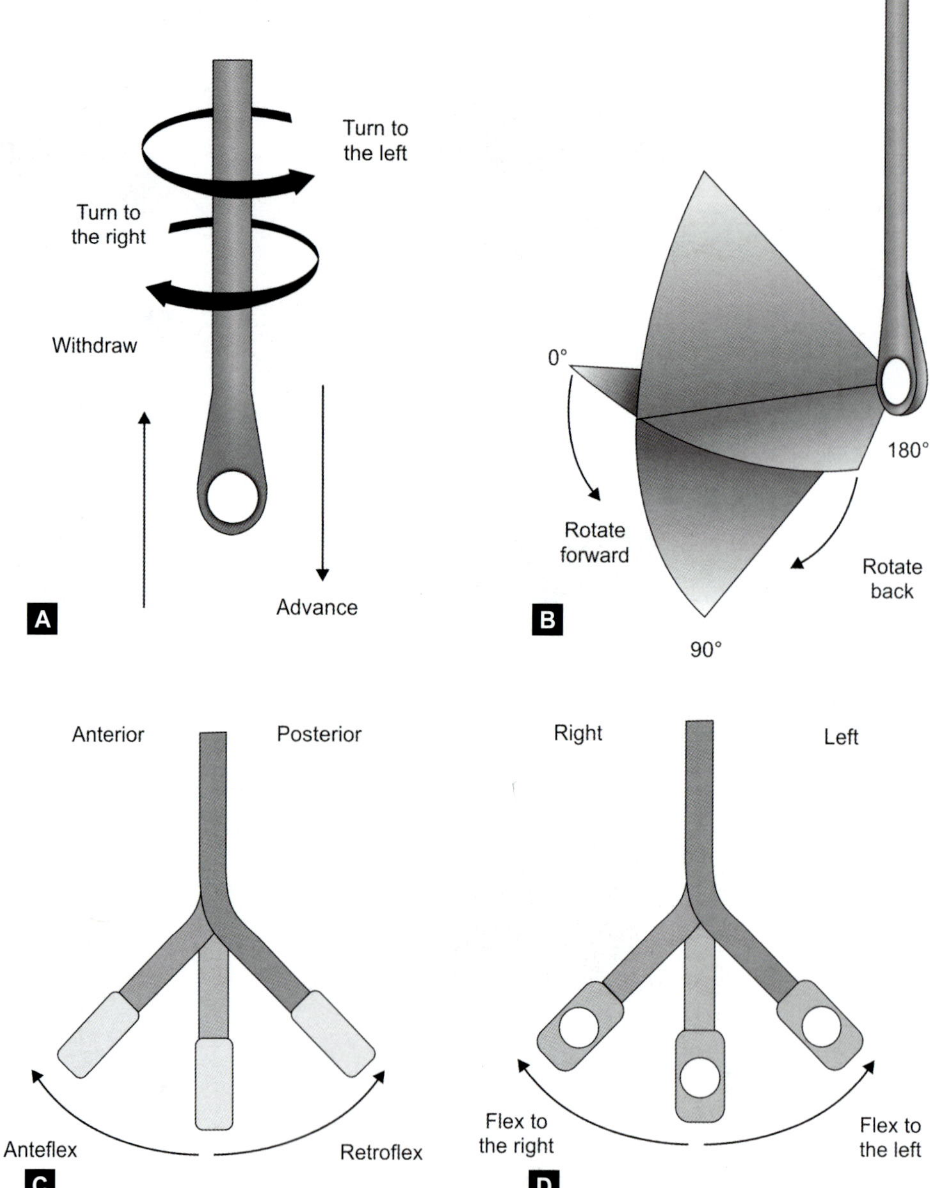

Figures 4A to D

Terminology of TEE probe manipulation

MID-ESOPHAGEAL FOUR-CHAMBER VIEW (FIGS 5A to E)

Multiplane Angle Range

- 0 to 20°
- *Sector depth:* ~ 12 to 14 cm

Anatomy Imaged

- Left ventricle and atrium
- Right ventricle and atrium

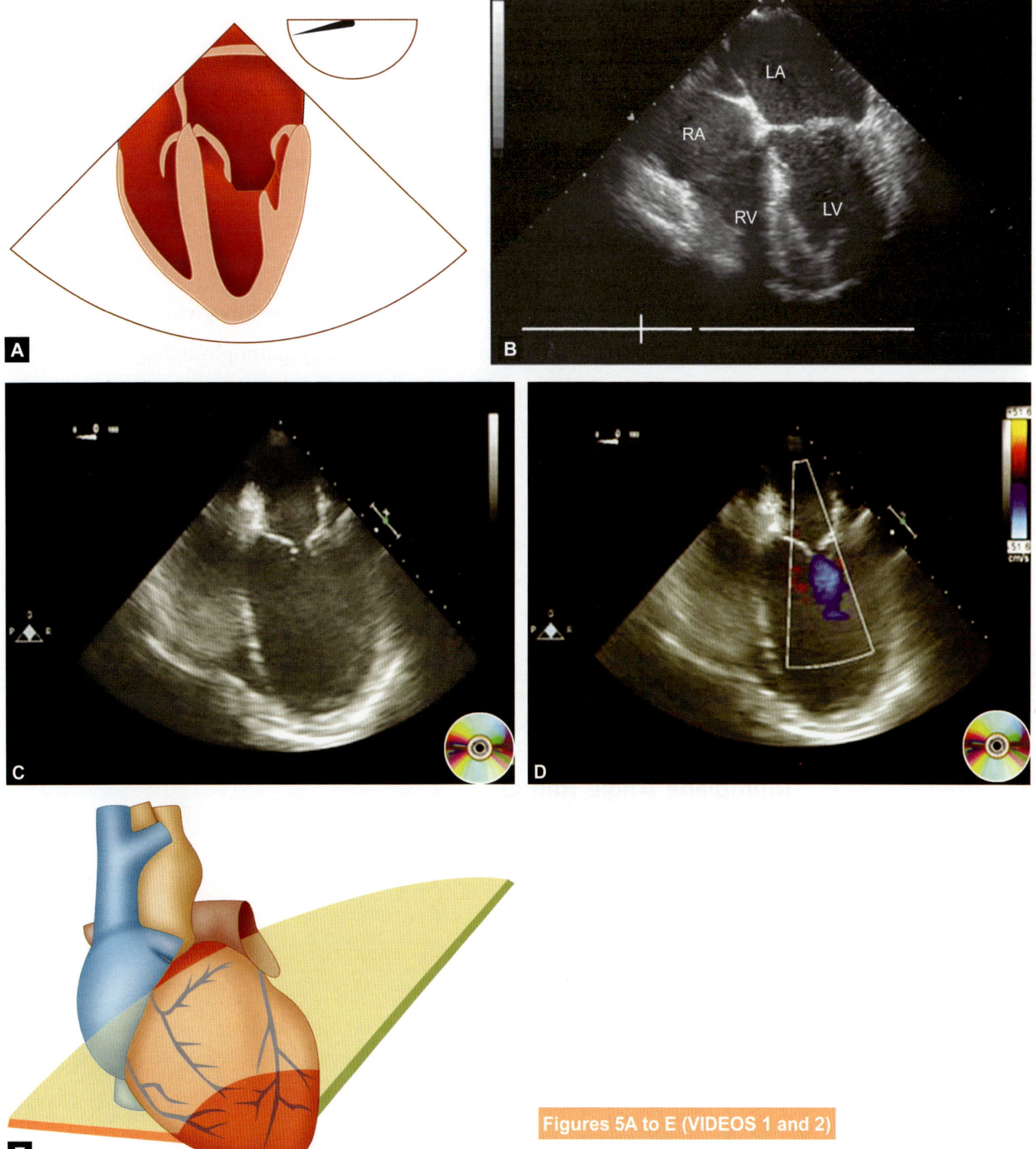

Figures 5A to E (VIDEOS 1 and 2)

ME four chamber view

- Mitral and tricuspid valves
- Interatrial and interventricle septa
- *Left pulmonary veins:* Slight probe withdrawal and turning to left
- *Right pulmonary veins:* Slight probe withdrawal and turning to right
- *Coronary sinus:* Slight probe advancement and turn to right.

Clinical Utility

- *Ventricle function:* Global and regional
- *Intracardiac chamber masses:* Thrombus, tumor, air; foreign bodies
- *Mitral and tricuspid valve evaluation:* Pathology, pathophysiology
- Congenital or acquired interatrial and ventral septal defects
- Hypertrophic obstructive cardiomyopathy evaluation
- Ventricular diastolic evaluation via transmitral and pulmonary vein Doppler flow profile analysis
- *Pericardial evaluation:* Pericarditis; pericardial effusion
- *Coronary sinus evaluation:* Coronary sinus catheter placement; dilation secondary to persistent left superior vena cava

MID-ESOPHAGEAL MITRAL COMMISSURAL VIEW (FIGS 6A TO D)

Multiplane Angle Range

- 60 to 70°
- *Sector depth*: ~ 12 cm

Anatomy Imaged

- Left ventricle and atrium
- Mitral valve

Clinical Utility

- *Left ventricle function:* Global and regional
- *Left ventricle and atrial masses:* Thrombus, tumor, air; foreign bodies
- *Mitral valve evaluation:* Pathology, pathophysiology
- Ventricular diastolic evaluation via transmitral Doppler flow profile analysis.

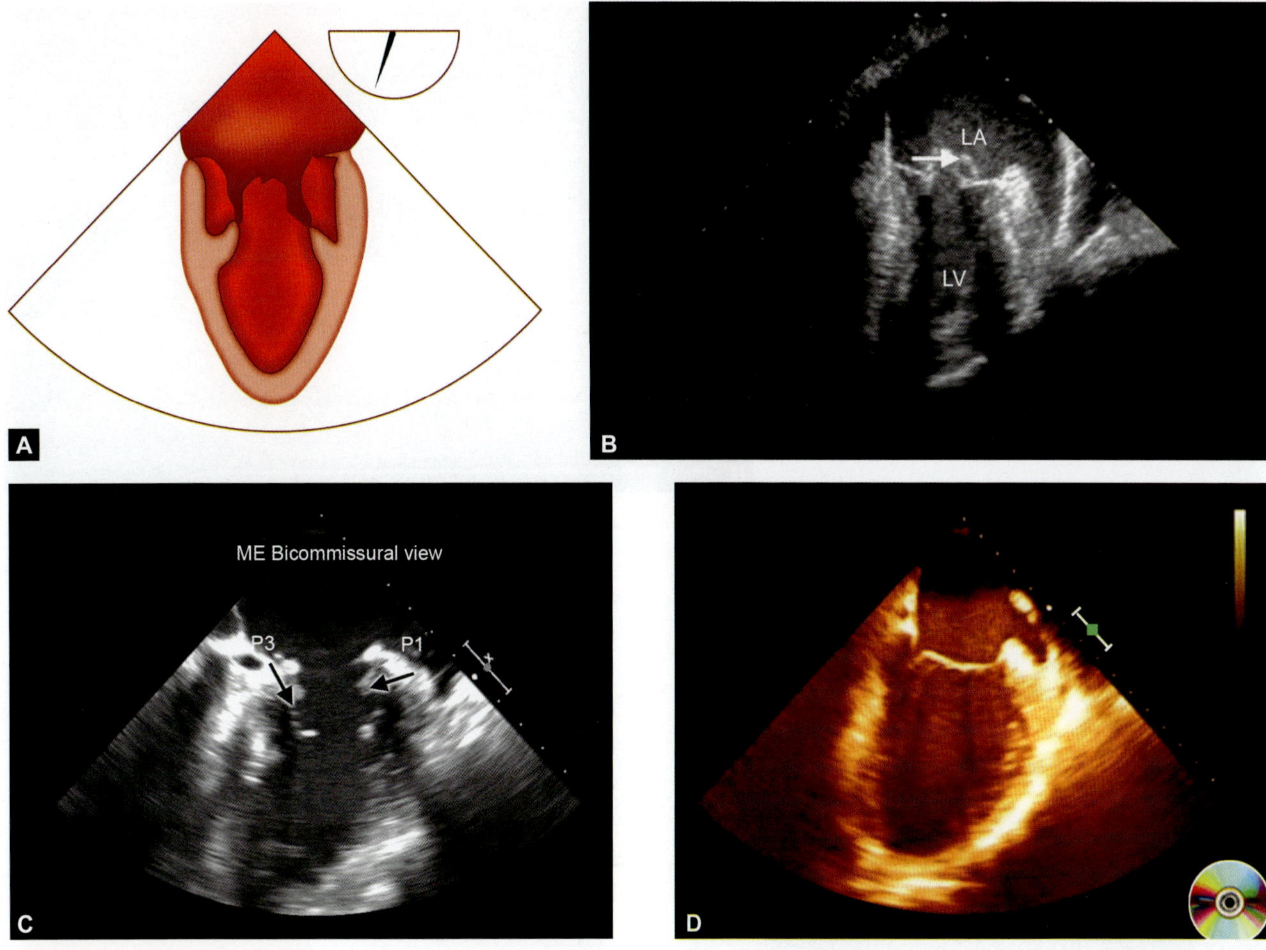

Figures 6A to D (VIDEO 3)

ME bicommissural view

MID-ESOPHAGEAL ASCENDING AORTA: SHORT AXIS VIEW (FIGS 7A TO C)

Multiplane Angle Range

- 0 to 60°
- *Sector depth:* ~ 12 cm.

Anatomy Imaged

- Ascending aorta
- Superior vena cava (short axis)

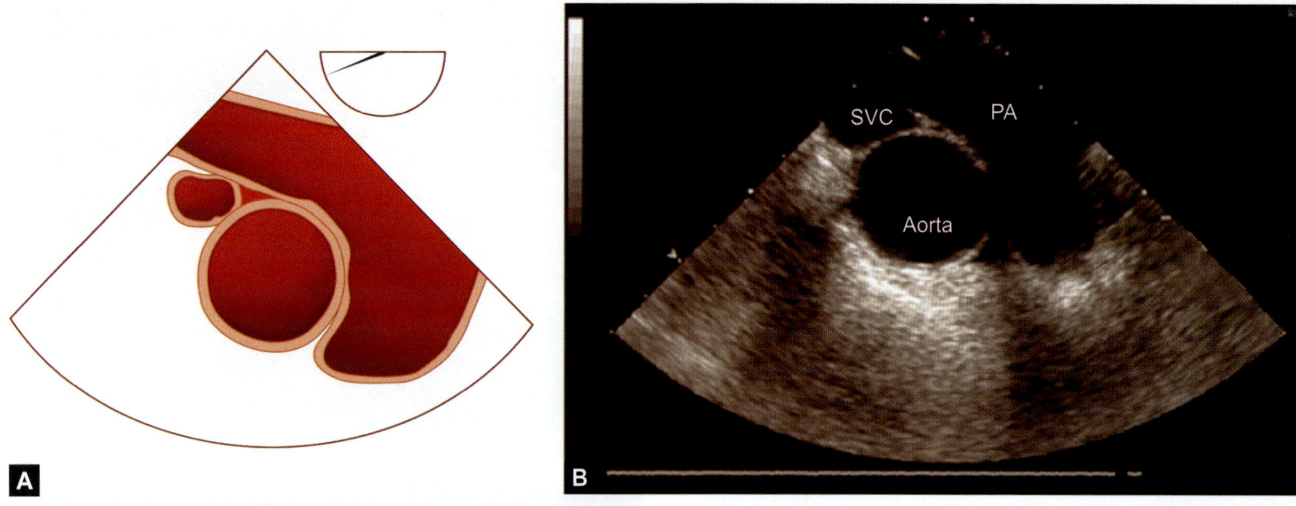

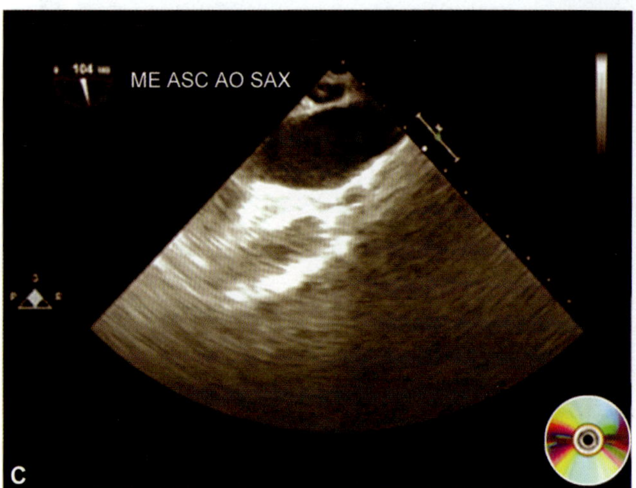

Figures 7A to C (VIDEO 4)
ME ascending aortic SAX

- Main pulmonary artery
- Right pulmonary artery
- Left pulmonary artery (turn probe tip to left)
- Pulmonic valve.

Clinical Utility

- *Ascending aorta pathology:* Atherosclerosis, aneurysms, and dissections
- *Pulmonic valve:* Pathology; pathophysiology
- Pulmonary embolus/thrombus evaluation
- *Superior vena cava pathology:* Thrombus, sinus venosus atrial septal defect
- Pulmonary artery catheter placement.

MID-ESOPHAGEAL ASCENDING AORTA: LONG AXIS VIEW (FIGS 8A TO C)

Multiplane Angle Range

- 100 to 150°
- *Sector depth*: ~ 12 cm

Anatomy Imaged

- Ascending aorta
- Right pulmonary artery

Clinical Utility

- *Ascending aorta pathology:* Atherosclerosis, aneurysms, and dissections
- Anterograde cardioplegia delivery evaluation

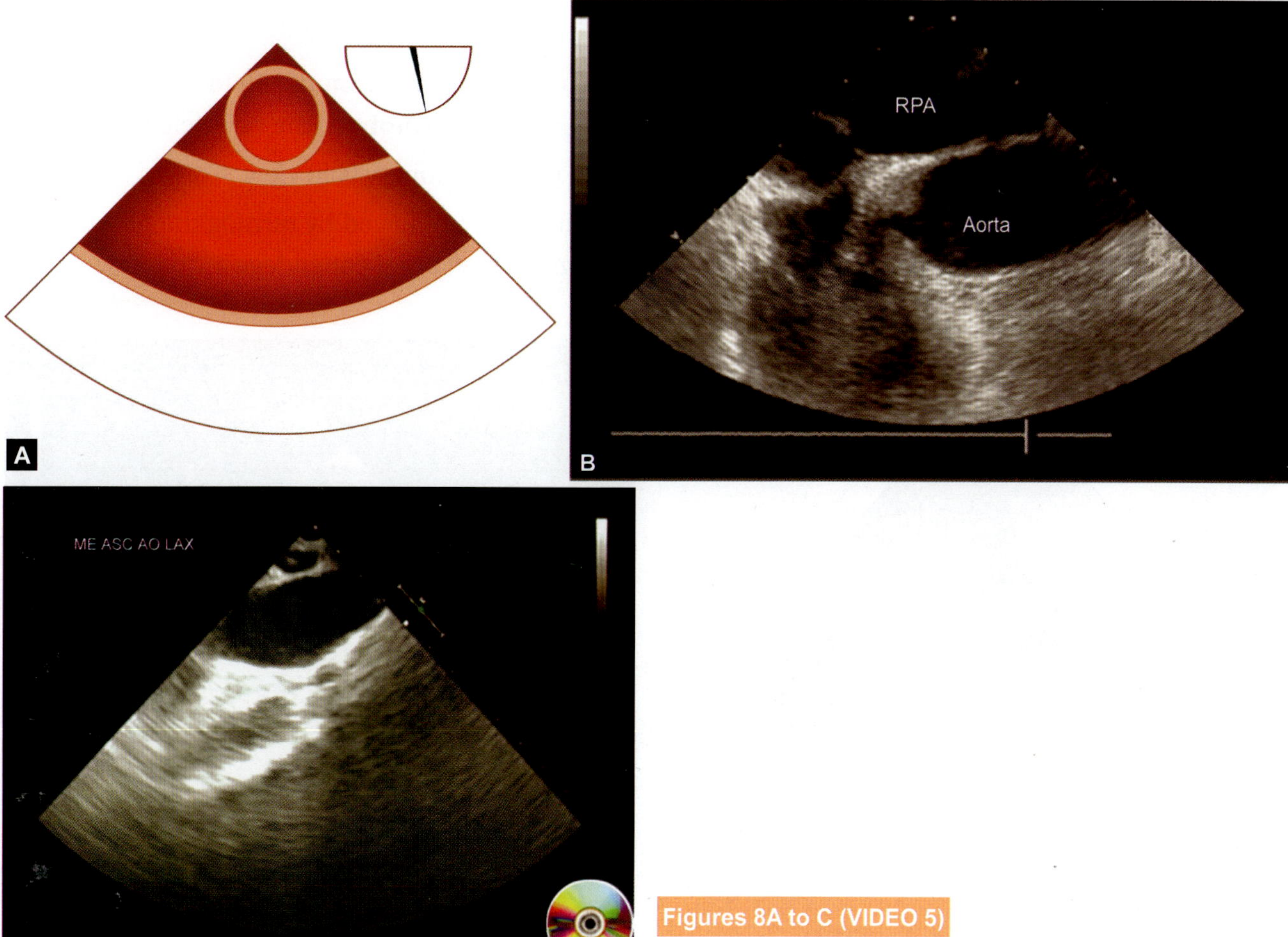

Figures 8A to C (VIDEO 5)
ME ASC aortic LAX

- Pulmonary embolus/thrombus
- Probe tip depth (from lips) upper esophageal (20–25 cm)

MID-ESOPHAGEAL RIGHT PULMONARY VEIN VIEW (FIGS 9A AND B)

Transducer Angle

- 0 to 30°
- Upper esophageal

Anatomy Imaged

- Mid-ascending aorta
- Superior vena cava
- Right pulmonary veins

In addition to the right pulmonary veins:

- The superior vena cava (SAX view) and ascending aorta (SAX view) are also imaged.
- The right pulmonary veins can also be imaged from the 90 to 110 view by first obtaining a ME bicaval view and turning the probe to the right (clockwise).
- This orthogonal image is the ME right pulmonary vein view.
- Note that the left pulmonary veins may be imaged by turning the probe to the left (counterclockwise) just beyond the left atrial appendage.

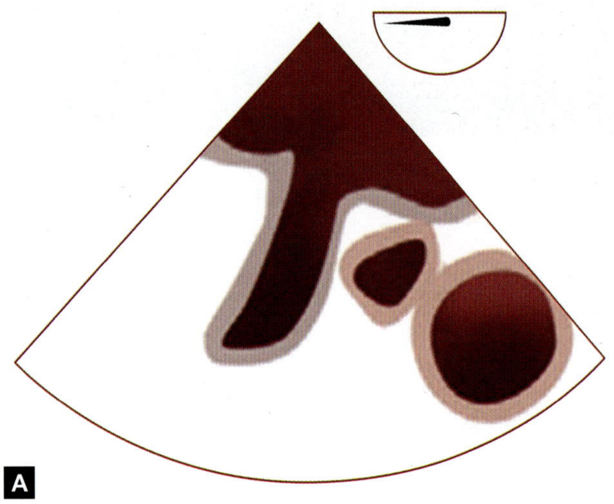

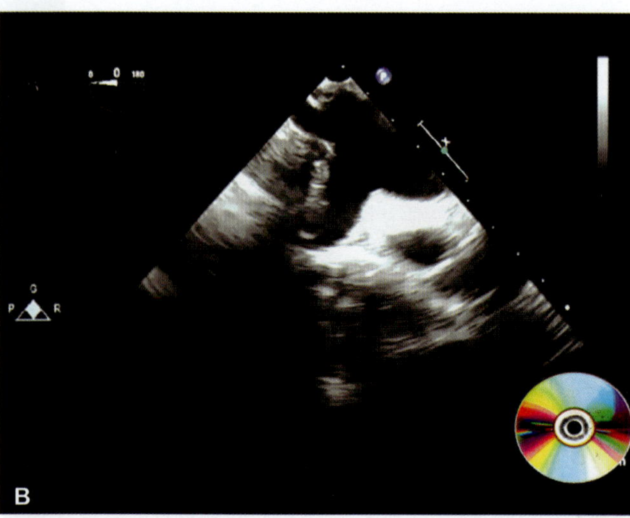

Figures 9A and B (VIDEO 6)

ME right pulmonary vein view

MID-ESOPHAGEAL AORTIC VALVE SHORT AXIS VIEW (FIGS 10A AND B)

Transducer Angle

- 25 to 45°
- Mid-esophageal

Anatomy Imaged

- Aortic valve
- Right Atrium
- Left Atrium
- Superior IAS
- RVOT
- Pulmonary valve

From the Mid-esophageal Right Pulmonary Vein View

- Reposition the probe (turning to the left, counterclockwise) to center the aorta in the display (as in the ME ascending aorta SAX view)
- Advance and rotate the transducer angle to between 25 and 45 to obtain the ME AV SAX view. Slight anteflexion may be required.

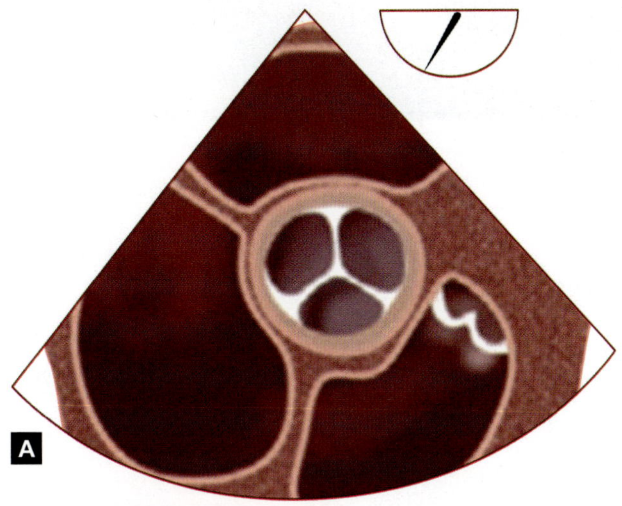

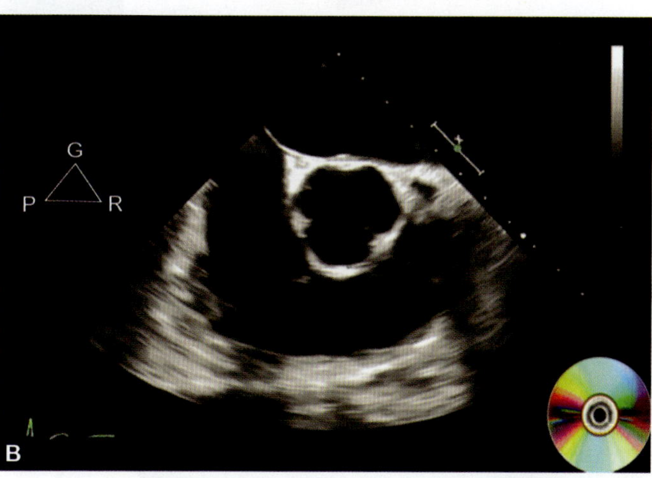

Figures 10A and B (VIDEO 7)

ME AV SAX view

MID-ESOPHAGEAL RIGHT VENTRICULAR INFLOW-OUTFLOW VIEW (FIGS 11A TO E)

Multiplane Angle Range

- 60–90°
- *Sector depth*: ~ 10 to 12 cm

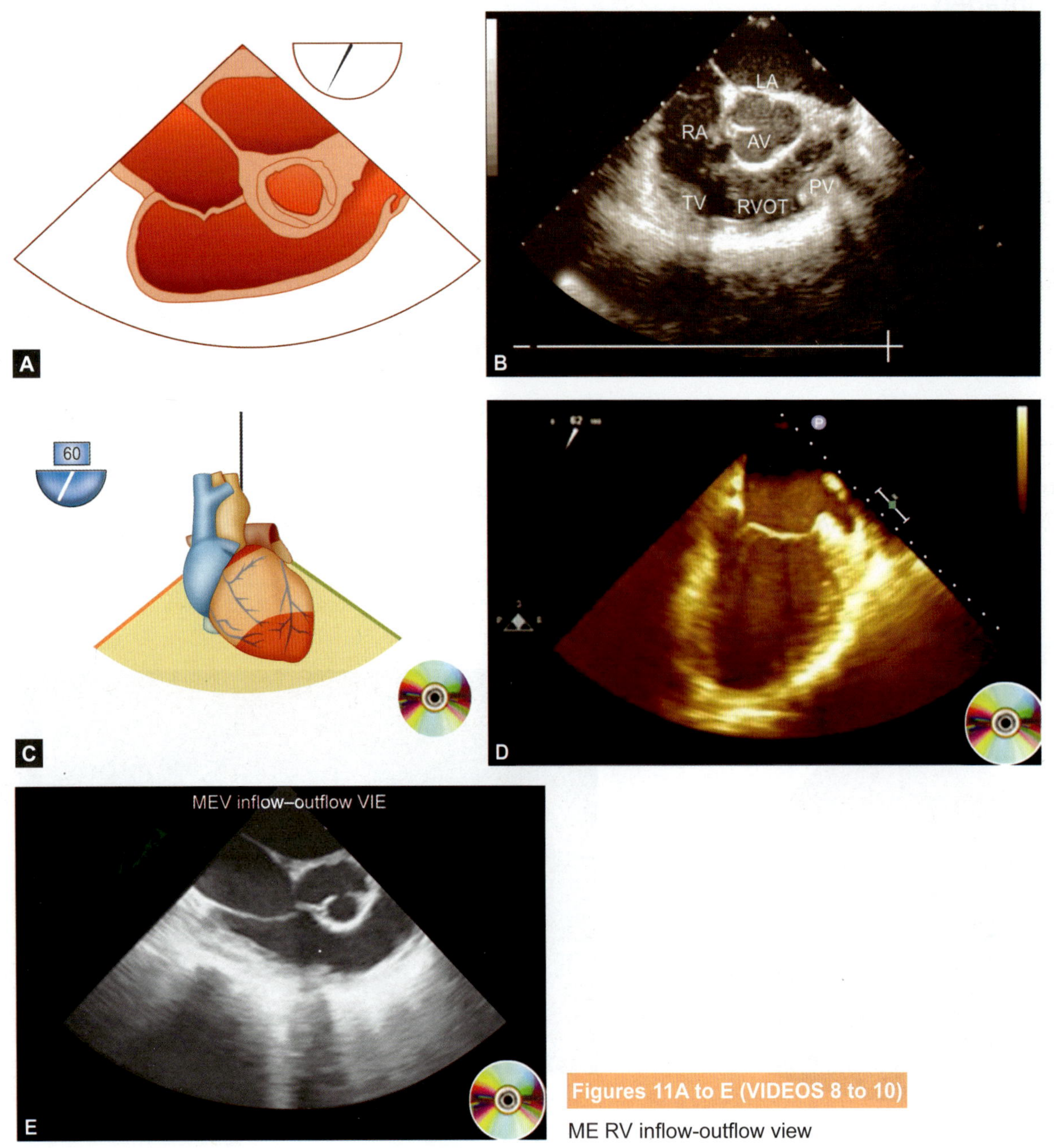

Figures 11A to E (VIDEOS 8 to 10)

ME RV inflow-outflow view

Anatomy Imaged

- Right ventricle and atrium
- Left atrium
- Tricuspid valve
- Aortic valve
- Right ventricular outflow tract
- Pulmonic valve and main pulmonary artery.

Clinical Utility

- *Right ventricle and atrial masses and left atrial:* Thrombus, embolus, tumor, foreign bodies
- *Pulmonic valve and subpulmonic valve:* Pathology; pathophysiology
- Pulmonary artery catheter placement
- *Tricuspid valve:* Pathology; pathophysiology

MID-ESOPHAGEAL MODIFIED BICAVAL VIEW (FIGS 12A TO C)

Structures Imaged

- Right atrium
- Left atrium
- Interatrial septum
- Inferior vena cava
- Tricuspid valve

Probe Adjustments

Probe rotated toward right as in bicaval view.

Clinical Utility

For cannula placement in the SVC/IVC in all minimally invasive procedures, e.g. Robotic Group

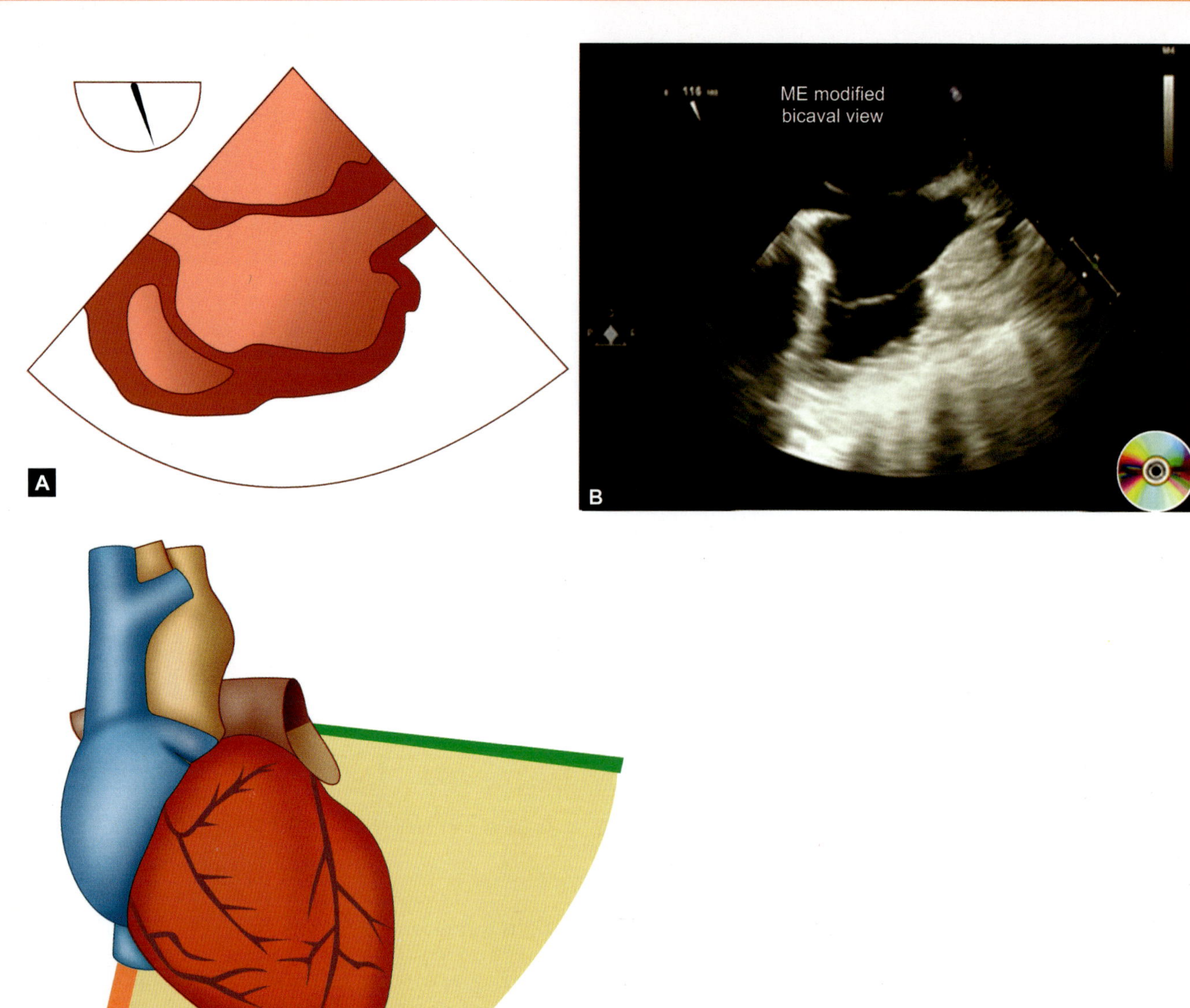

Figures 12A to C (VIDEO 11)

ME modified bicaval view

UPPER-ESOPHAGEAL RIGHT AND LEFT PULMONARY VEINS VIEW (FIGS 13A AND B)

Transducer Angle

- 90 to 110°
- Upper-esophageal

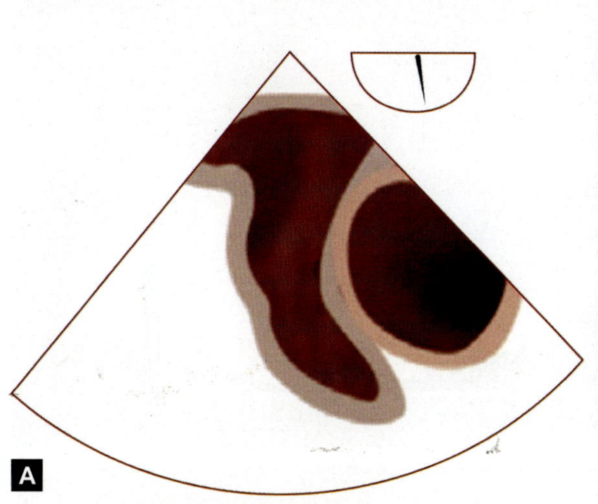

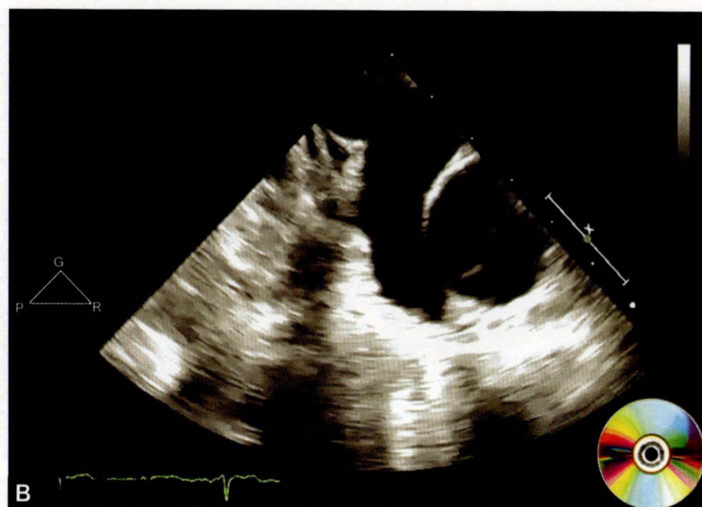

Figures 13A and B (VIDEO 12)

UE right and left PV view

Anatomy Imaged

- Pulmonary vein (upper and lower)
- Pulmonary artery

Clinical Utility

- At a transducer angle of 90 to 110, imaging of either the right or left pulmonary veins can be performed.
- From the ME bicaval view turning the probe to the left (counterclockwise) takes the imaging through the entire heart (past the left atrium) to the ME left pulmonary vein view.
- The left superior vein is to the right of the display, and typically inflow is parallel to the insonation beam, allowing accurate spectral Doppler assessment.

TRANSGASTRIC BASAL SHORT AXIS VIEW (FIGS 14A to F)

Multiplane Angle Range

- 0 to 20°
- *Sector depth*: ~ 12 cm

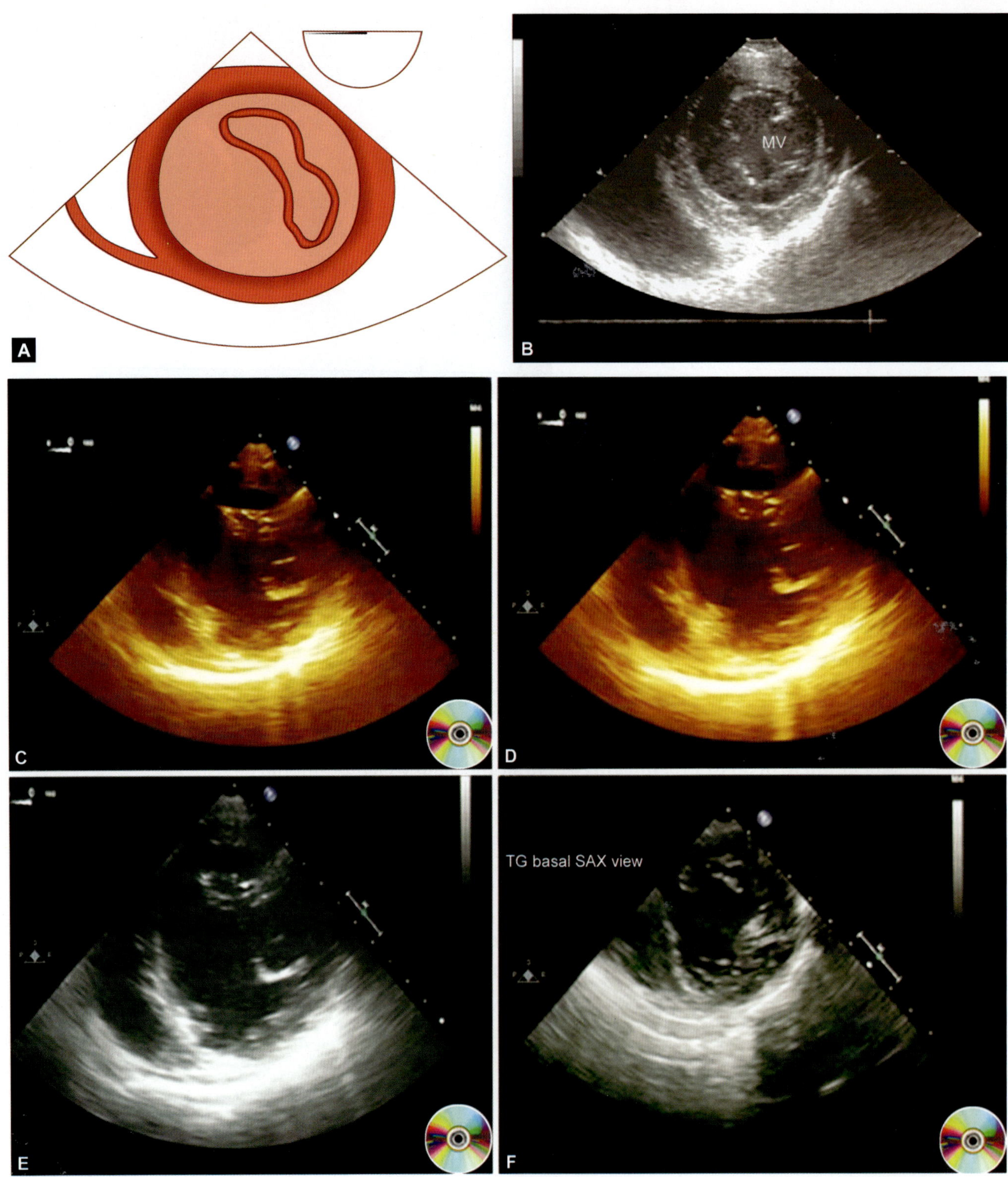

Figures 14A to F (VIDEOS 13 to 16)

TG basal SAX

Anatomy Imaged Left and Right Ventricle

- Mitral valve
- Tricuspid valve

Clinical Utility

- *Mitral valve evaluation (fish-mouth view):* Pathology, pathophysiology
- *Tricuspid valve evaluation:* Pathology, pathophysiology
- Basal left ventricular regional function
- Basal right ventricular regional function

TRANSGASTRIC MID PAPILLARY SHORT AXIS VIEW (FIGS 15A to E)

Multiplane Angle Range

- 0 to 20°
- *Sector depth:* ~ 12 cm

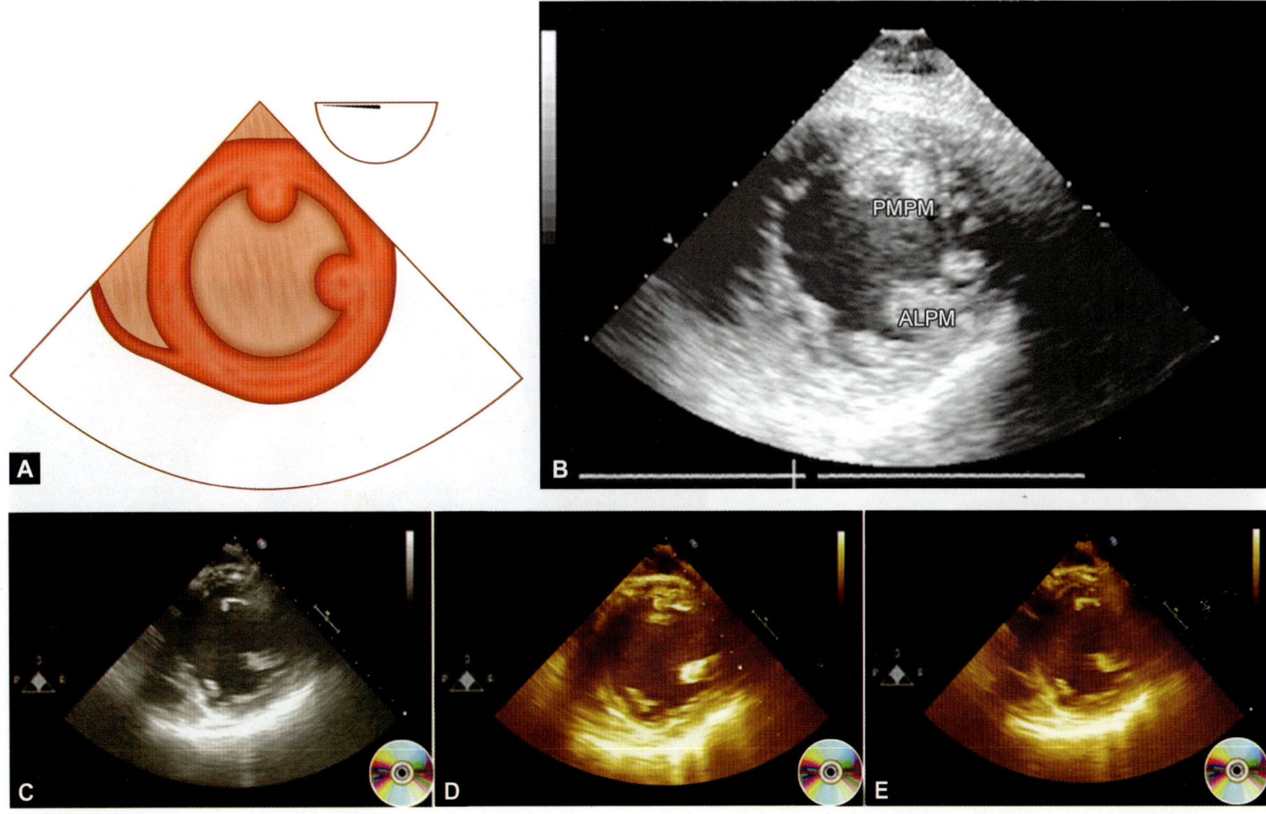

Figures 15A to E (VIDEOS 17 to 19)

TG midpapillary SAX view

Anatomy Imaged

- Left and right ventricles
- Papillary muscles

Clinical Utility

- Mid-left and right ventricular regional and global function
- Intracardiac volume status

TRANSGASTRIC APICAL SHORT AXIS VIEW (FIGS 16A AND B)

Transducer Angle

- 0 to 20°
- Transgastric

Anatomy Imaged

- Left ventricle (apex)
- Right ventricle (apex)

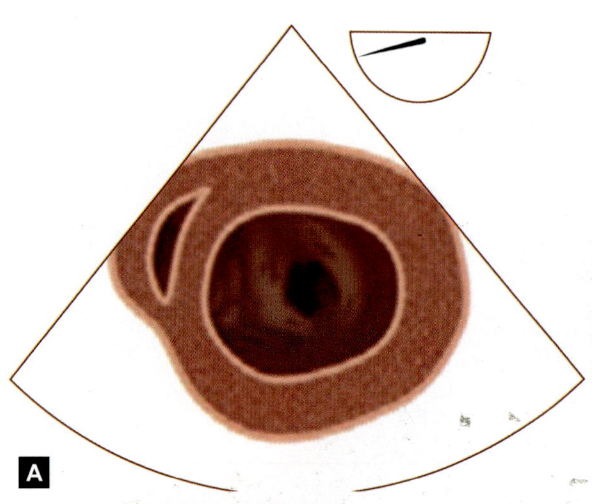

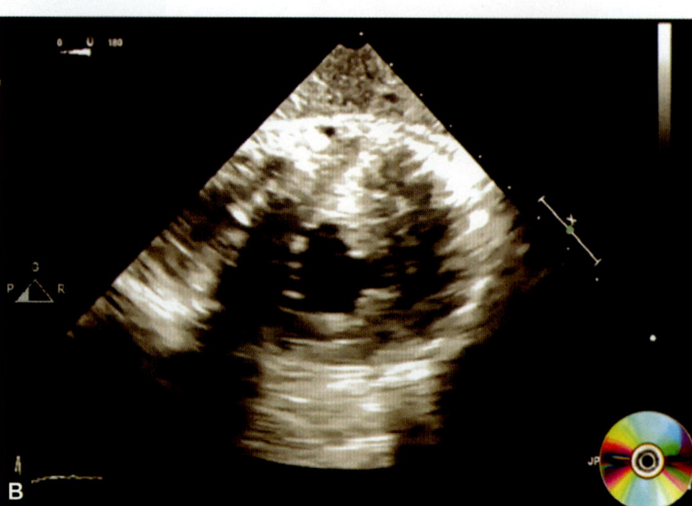

Figures 16A and B (VIDEO 20)

TG apical SAX view

Clinical Utility

- From the TG midpapillary SAX view (0–20), the probe is advanced while maintaining contact with the gastric wall, to obtain the TG apical SAX view.
- The RV apex is imaged from this view by turning to the right (clockwise). This view allows evaluation of the apical segments of the left and right ventricles.

TRANSGASTRIC RIGHT VENTRICULAR BASAL VIEW (FIGS 17A AND B)

Transducer Angle

- 0 to 20°
- Transgastric

Anatomy Imaged

- Left ventricle (mid)
- Right ventricle (mid)
- Right ventricular outflow tract
- Tricuspid valve (SAX)
- Pulmonary valve.

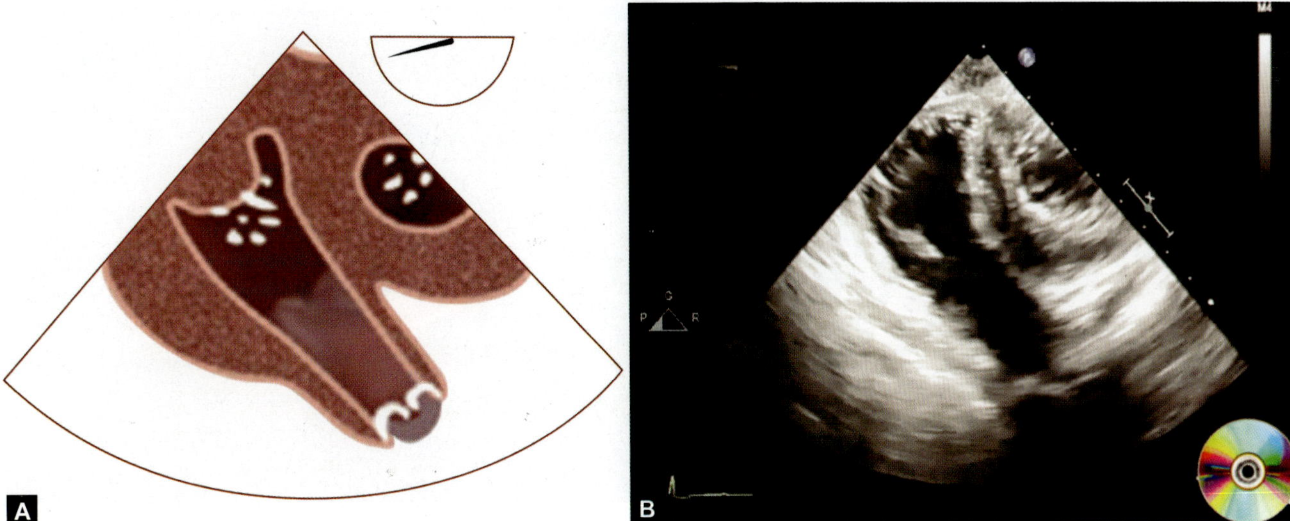

Figures 17A and B (VIDEO 21)

TG RV basal view

Clinical Utility

Returning to the TG basal SAX view (anteflexed, at a transducer angle of approximately 0 to 20) by turning the probe toward the patient's right (clockwise), the TG basal RV view can be seen.

TRANSGASTRIC RIGHT INFLOW-OUTFLOW VIEW (FIGS 18A AND B)

Transducer Angle

- 0 to 20°
- Transgastric

Anatomy Imaged

- Right atrium
- Right ventricle
- Right ventricular outflow tract
- Pulmonary valve
- Tricuspid valve

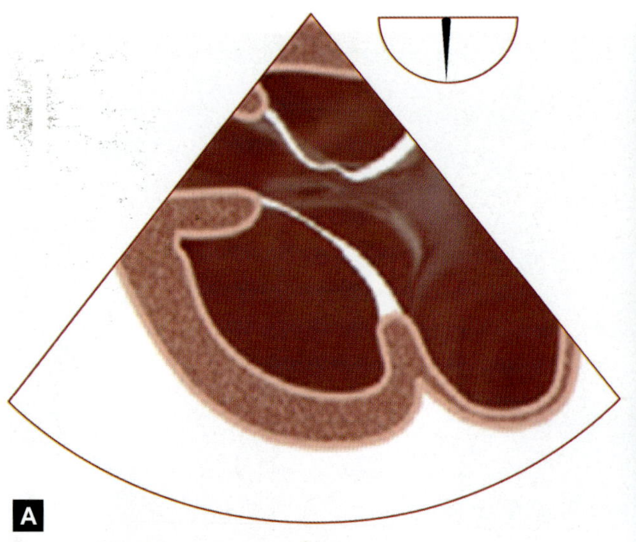

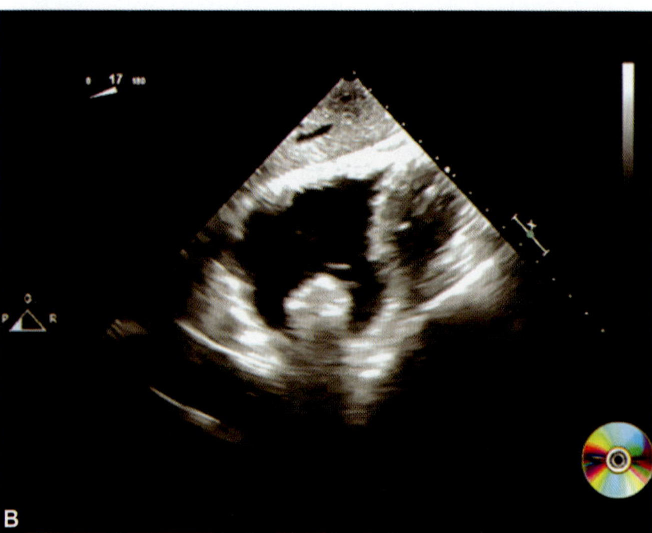

Figures 18A and B (VIDEO 22)

TG RV inflow view

Clinical Utility

- From the TG basal RV view (transducer angle of 0 to 20), maximal right flexion results in the TG RV inflow-outflow view.
- In this view, typically the anterior and posterior leaflets of the TV are imaged, as well as the left and right cusps of the PV.

DEEP TRANSGASTRIC 5-CHAMBER VIEW (FIGS 19A AND B)

Transducer Angle

- 0 to 20°
- Transgastric

Anatomy Imaged

- Left ventricle
- Left ventricular outflow tract
- Right ventricle
- Aortic valve
- Aortic root
- Mitral valve

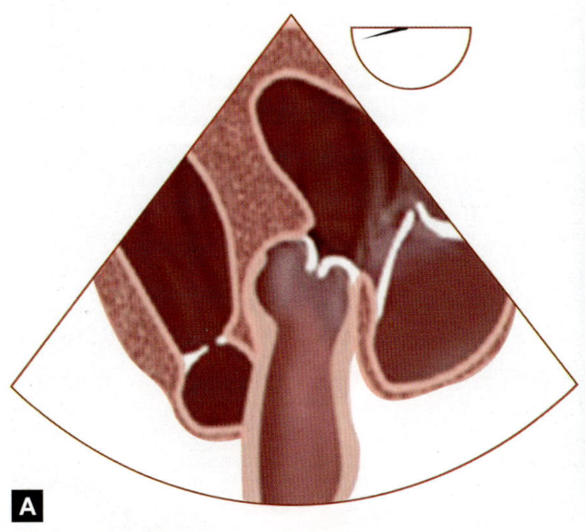

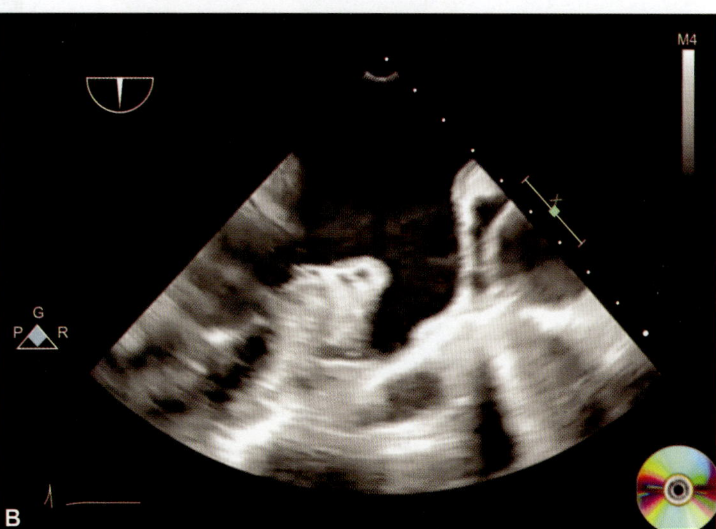

Figures 19A and B (VIDEO 23)

Deep TG 5-chamber view

Clinical Utility

- From the TG RV inflow-outflow view (transducer angle of 0 to 20), advancing the probe to the deep TG level, with anteflexion and often with left flexion, results in the deep TG five-chamber view.
- Because of parallel Doppler beam alignment with the LV outflow tract, AV, and proximal aortic root, color and spectral Doppler interrogation of the LV outflow tract and AV is possible.

TRANSGASTRIC RIGHT VENTRICULAR INFLOW VIEW (FIGS 20A TO D)

Multiplane Angle Range

- 100 to 120°
- *Sector depth:* ~ 12 cm

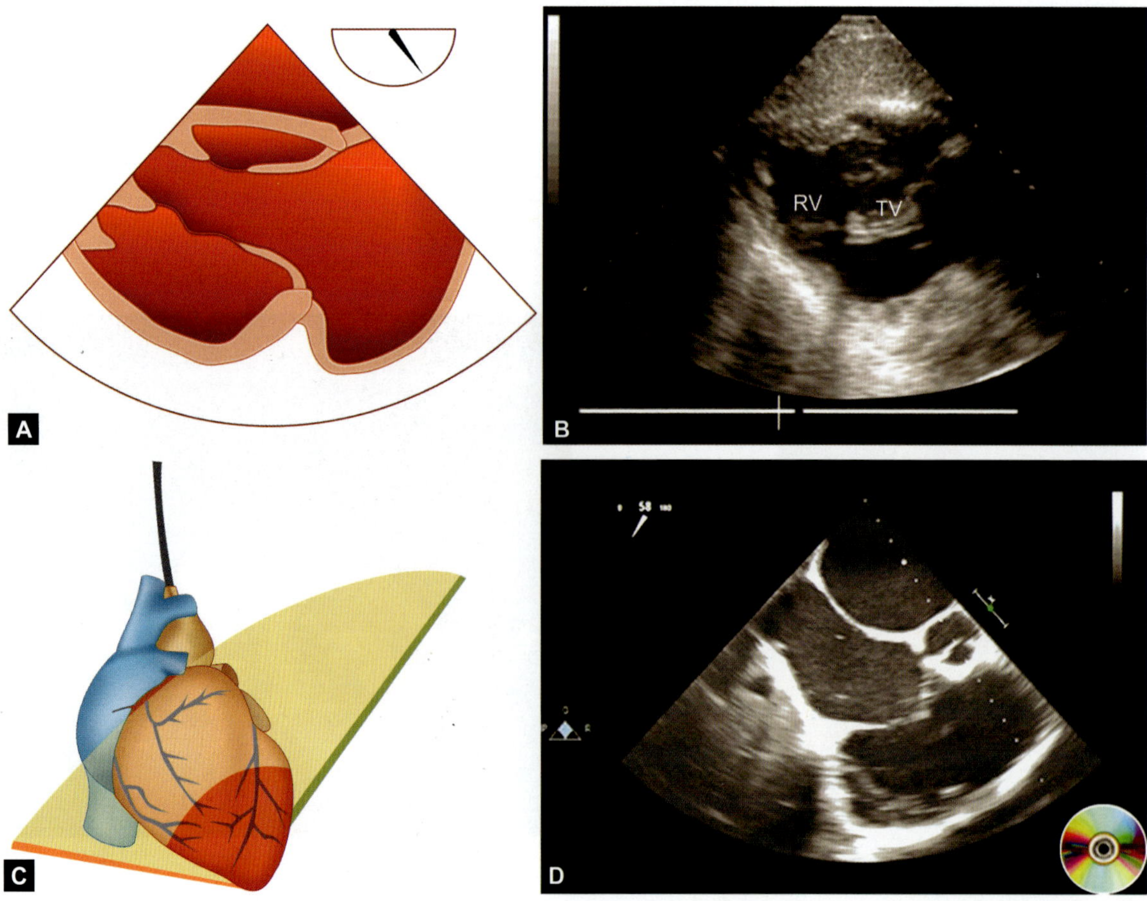

Figures 20A to D (VIDEO 24)

TG RV inflow

Anatomy Imaged

- Right ventricle and atrium
- *Tricuspid valve:* Chordae and papillary muscles

Clinical Utility

- Right ventricular regional and global function
- *Right ventricular and atrium masses:* Thrombus, embolus, tumor, foreign bodies
- *Tricuspid valve:* Pathology and pathophysiology

Probe Tip Depth Deep Transgastric (45–50 cm)

UPPER-ESOPHAGEAL AORTIC ARCH: SHORT AXIS VIEW (FIGS 21A TO C)

Multiplane Angle Range

- 90°
- *Sector depth:* ~ 10 cm

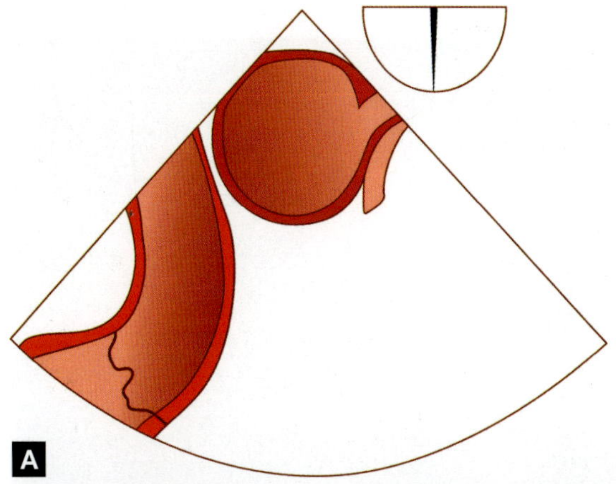

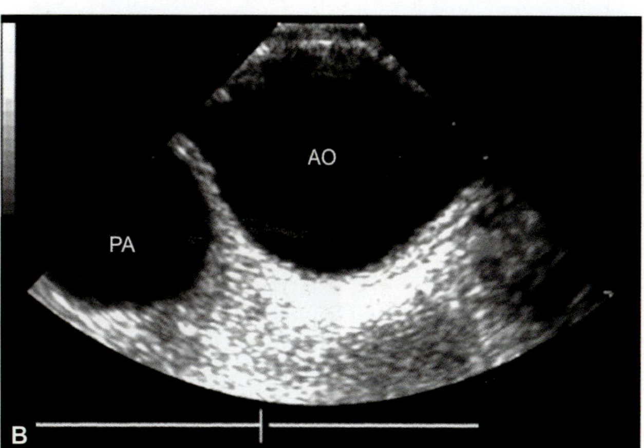

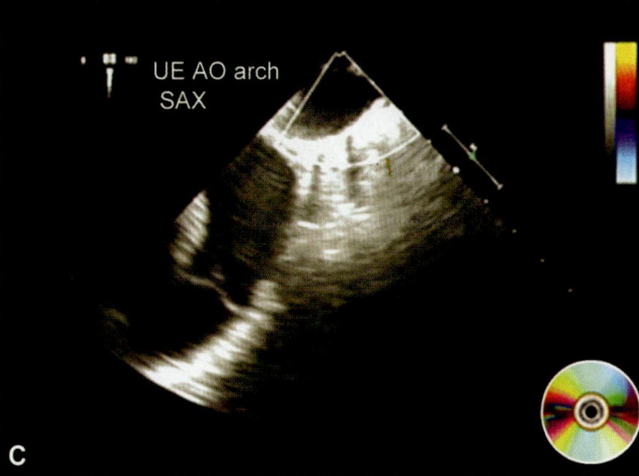

Figures 21A to C (VIDEO 25)

UE aortic arch SAX

Structures Imaged

Aortic arch; left brachiocephalic vein; left subclavian and carotid arteries; right brachiocephalic artery; main pulmonary artery and pulmonic valve.

Clinical Utility

Ascending aorta and arch pathology: atherosclerosis, aneurysms and dissections; pulmonary embolus; pulmonary valve evaluation (insufficiency, stenosis, Ross procedure); pulmonary artery catheter placement.

Image Settings

- Angle ~ 110°
- *Sector depth:* ~ 8 to 10 cm

TRANSESOPHAGEAL ECHOCARDIOGRAPHY VIEWS TO ASSESS PULMONARY VALVE

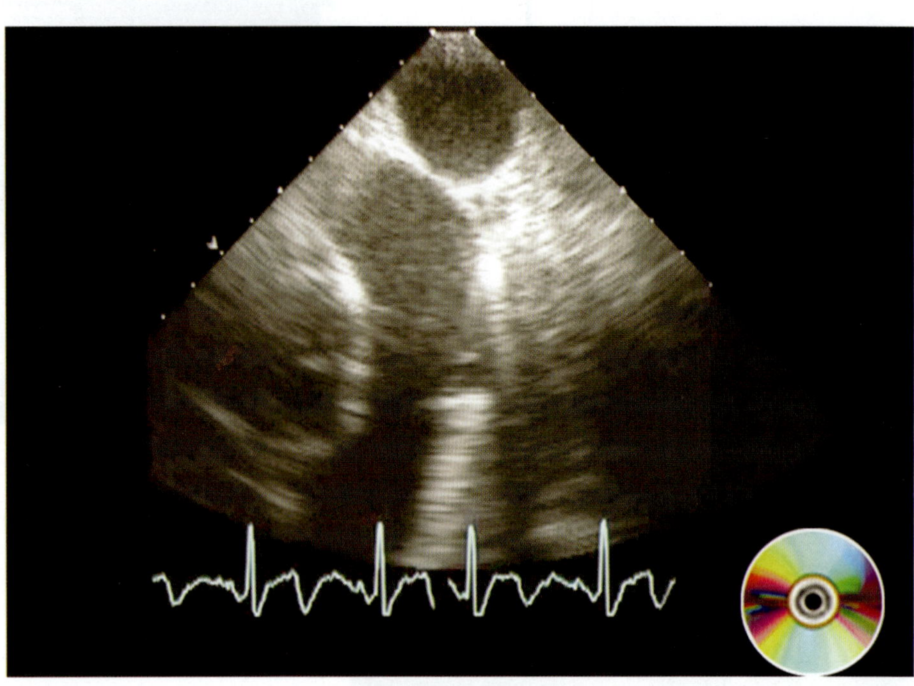

Figure 22 (VIDEO 26)

Pulmonic valve and RVOT 70–110

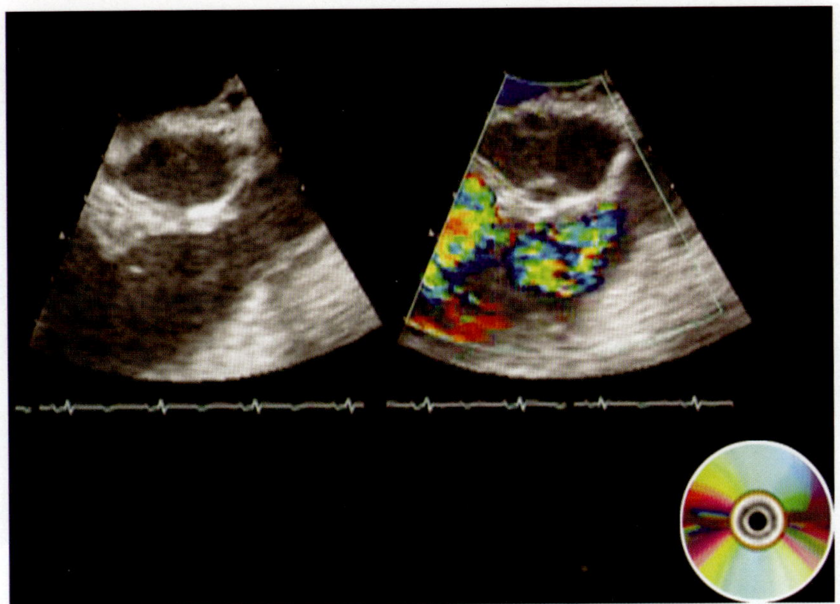

Figure 23 (VIDEO 27)

Tricuspid inflow and pulmonic regurgitation in diastole

ASE/SCA 2013 GUIDELINES FOR TRICUSPID VALVE 3D TEE

TV 3D TEE

Three-dimensional TEE of the TV allows visualization of all aspects of the TV from a single full-volume data set or a focused examination on a particular TV aspect using a narrower imaging acquisition mode with higher resolution. Acquisition is from a 0 to a 30 view, with the TV centered in the image **(Table 2)**.

3D Color Flow Doppler

Color flow Doppler should be added to the multiple-beat acquisition in patients with tricuspid regurgitation and/or stenosis. Similar to the technique for acquiring noncolor Doppler multiple-beat imaging, obtaining a 3D color flow Doppler data set initially requires the identification of a region of interest in the orthogonal planes. The size of the region of interest should be limited to the tricuspid apparatus and color flow Doppler jet to optimize frame rate. In addition, although a high line density may be desirable, a lower line density will permit a larger sector to be displayed. Finally, the largest number of individually gated component subvolumes (4–6 beats) should always be attempted when electrocardiographic gating and reasonable acquisition times can be achieved.

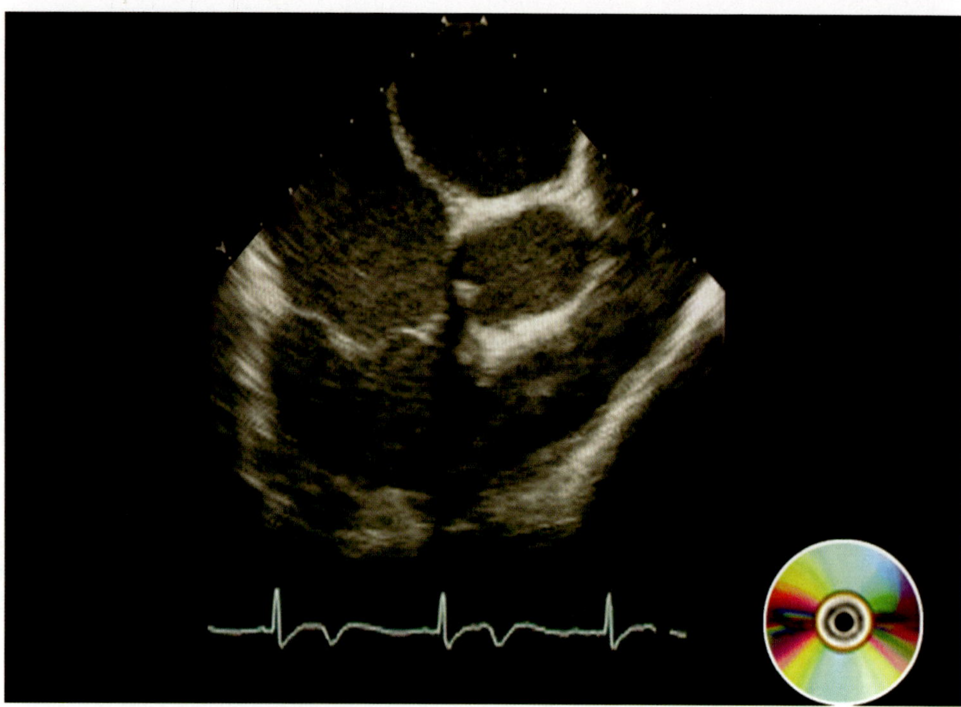

Figure 24 (VIDEO 28)

Pulmonary valve in RT sided inflow-outflow view

Narrow-Angle 3D Mode

Once the TV image is optimized with 2D echocardiography, a narrow-angle single-beat acquisition can be performed. When displaying the TV en face, the septal leaflet should be located in the 6 o'clock position, irrespective of perspective. These en face views may be especially helpful in localizing leaflet disease such as leaflet prolapse, perforation, or vegetation, as well as localizing the origin of regurgitation jets, or performing planimetry of the tricuspid regurgitant orifice area to assess the severity of tricuspid stenosis.

In addition to standard views, the cropping plane can be adjusted to visualize a particular section of the TV.

Wide-Angle 3D Mode

Wide-angle acquisition mode allows visualization of the tricuspid apparatus from the annulus to the papillary muscle tips. Enlarging the region of interest excessively will result in a further detrimental decrease of temporal resolution. This can be ameliorated using multiple-beat mode, which increases spatial resolution, permitting detailed diagnosis of complex pathologies **(Fig. 25)** with high temporal resolution (>30 Hz), which is desirable when diagnosing mechanisms of abnormal tricuspid leaflet motion.

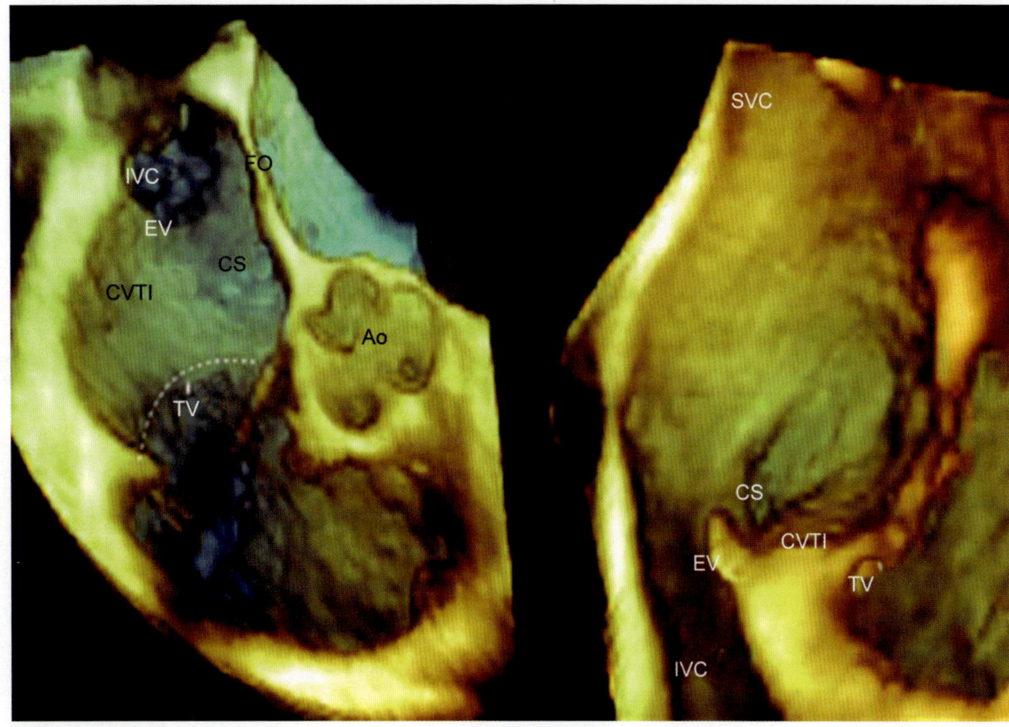

Figure 25

Wide-angle acquisition mode allows visualization of the tricuspid apparatus from the annulus to the papillary muscle tips, as well as the right atrium and associated structures. *Abbreviations*: Ao, aorta; CS, coronary sinus; CVTI, cavotricuspid isthmus; EV, eustachian valve; FO, fossa ovale; IVC, inferior vena cava; SVC, superior vena cava; TV, tricuspid valve

PULMONARY VALVE 3D TEE

PV 3D TEE

When imaging the PV in three dimensions, the transesophageal echocardiographic probe can be positioned at either the UE aortic arch SAX view position at 70 to 90 **(Figs 22 and 23)** or by obtaining a three-chamber LV–aortic root view at 120 and then turning the probe to the left (counterclockwise) to bring the PV into view **(Table 2) (Fig. 24)**. Typically, acquisition is difficult because there is signal dropout from the thin leaflets.

Narrow-Angle 3D Mode

Once the valve is optimally visualized, the PV can be acquired using single-beat, narrow-angle acquisition mode for rapid assessment. The narrow-angle, multiple-beat mode allows visualization of the PV leaflets. The image set can be cropped and rotated to display the valve in an en face view from either the PA or the right ventricle. When displayed in this en face view, the anterior leaflet should be located superiorly in the 12 o'clock position irrespective of perspective.

Wide-Angle 3D Mode

The wide-angle acquisition mode of the PV also permits examination of the main PA and the RVOT. Once the pyramidal volume is captured, cropped and rotated, the en face view of the valve can be displayed. As well, the cropping plane can be used

Table 2: Summary of 3D transesophageal echocardiographic acquisition views for TV and PV

Protocol for three-dimensional transesophageal echocardiography image acquisition		
Right ventricle	• Obtain a view of the right ventricle from the 0° mid-esophageal position with the right ventricle tilted so that it is in the center of the image • Acquire using wide-angle, multi-beat mode	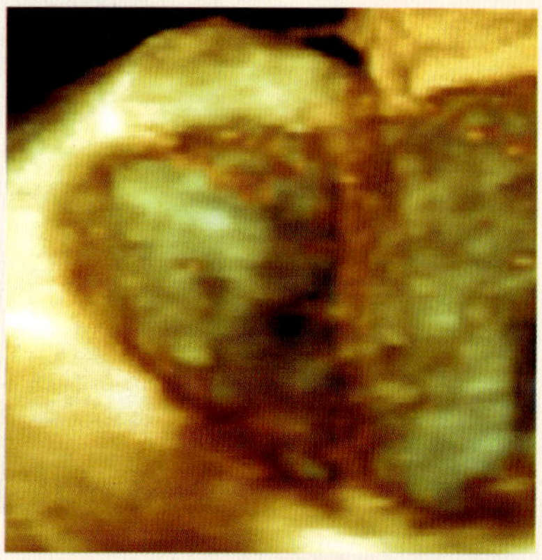
Pulmonic valve	• Obtain a view of the pulmonic valve from either the 90° high-esophageal view or the 120° mid-esophageal, 3-chamber view rotated to center the pulmonic valve • Acquire using narrow-angle, single-beat mode	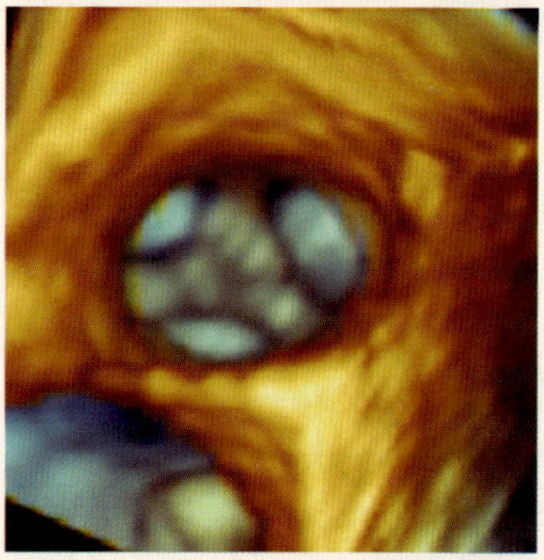
Tricuspid valve	• Obtain a view of the tricuspid valve from either the 0° to 30° mid-esophageal, 4-chamber view tilted so that the valve is centered in the imaging plane or the 40° transgastric view with anteflexion • Acquire using a narrow-angle, single-beat mode	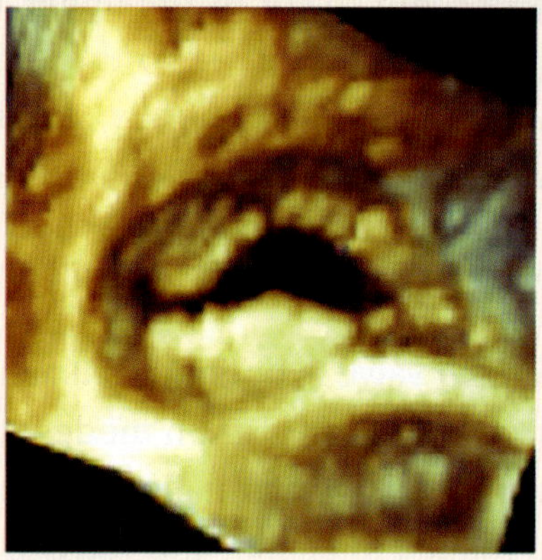

to assess the dimensions of the main PA and the RVOT. Last, the cropping plane can be used to show the RVOT, PV, and main PA in a single image.

3D Color Flow Doppler

In patients with pulmonary regurgitation or stenosis, color flow Doppler should be added to the narrow-angle, multiple-beat acquisition. The size of the region of interest should be limited to the PV and the color flow Doppler jet to optimize frame rate. As mentioned previously, the largest number of individually gated component slabs should always be attempted when electrocardiographic gating and brief acquisition times are possible. Once acquired, the pyramidal volume can first be viewed as originally obtained and then rotated to view the PV from the PA and right ventricle to identify the site of jet origin. Further cropping and the use of the black-and-white suppress can be used to identify effective orifice area, regurgitant orifice area, 3D proximal isovelocity surface areas, and vena contracta.

BIBLIOGRAPHY

1. ACCF/ASE/AHA/ASNC/HFSA/HRS/SCAI/SCCM/SCCT/SCMR 2011 Appropriate Use Criteria for Echocardiography. J Am Soc Echocardiogr. 2011;24:229-67.
2. ASE/SCA Guidelines. J Am Soc Echocardiogr. 2013;26:921-64.
3. Stoddard MF, Liddell NE, Vogel RL, Longaker RA, Dawkins PR. Comparison of cardiac dimensions by transesophageal and transthoracic echocardiography. Am Heart J. 1992;124:675-8.

3 Doppler Examination Across Tricuspid and Pulmonary Valves

Poonam Malhotra Kapoor, Sameer Taneja, Mahesh Vakamudi

- Estimation of Intracardiac Pressures
  - Right Ventricular Systolic Pressure
  - Pulmonary Artery Systolic Pressure
  - Mean Pulmonary Artery Pressure
  - Pulmonary Artery and Right Ventricular
  - Right Atrial Pressure
- Shunt Fractions

Evaluation of flow through the tricuspid valve (TV) and pulmonary valve (PV) is performed using spectral Doppler techniques. Analysis of tricuspid flow is optimally performed using the modified bicaval view, the ME RV inflow-outflow view, or the ME 4-C view **(Figs 1 to 3)**, depending on which view provides the best alignment of flow with the ultrasound beam.

The sample volume should be placed between the TV leaflet tips during diastole to assess diastolic filling patterns. Analogous to transmitral flow, characteristic early (E) wave and atrial (A) wave Doppler peaks correspond, respectively, to early ventricular filling and late diastolic filling from atrial contraction. From these recordings, E velocity, A velocity, E/A velocity ratio, and E-wave deceleration time may be measured or calculated. Typical pathologic patterns of diastolic dysfunction include impaired relaxation (E < and restriction (E>> A) of RV filling. It is important to note that tricuspid inflow patterns have lower absolute velocities than the corresponding mitral inflow velocities owing to the larger cross-sectional area of the TV. Useful information concerning TV and right ventricle (RV) function may often be obtained by the analysis of hepatic venous flow patterns. Normal venous flow in the hepatic veins is similar to pulmonary venous flow, with antegrade systolic (S) and diastolic (D) waves, and a retrograde atrial (A) wave resulting from atrial contraction. At times, an additional small retrograde wave appears at end systole and is termed a V-wave. This additional retrograde wave likely results from

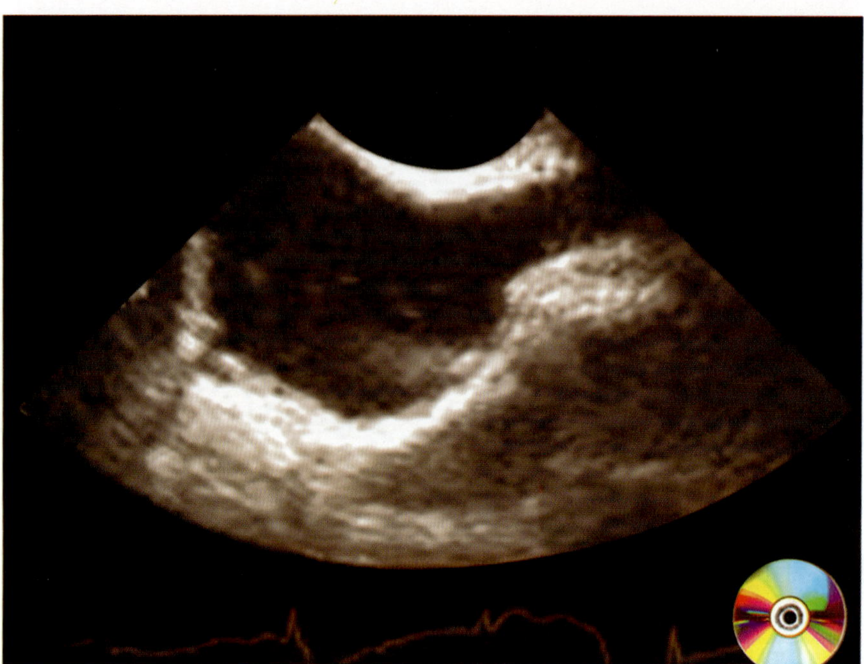

Figure 1 (VIDEO 1)

Bicaval view

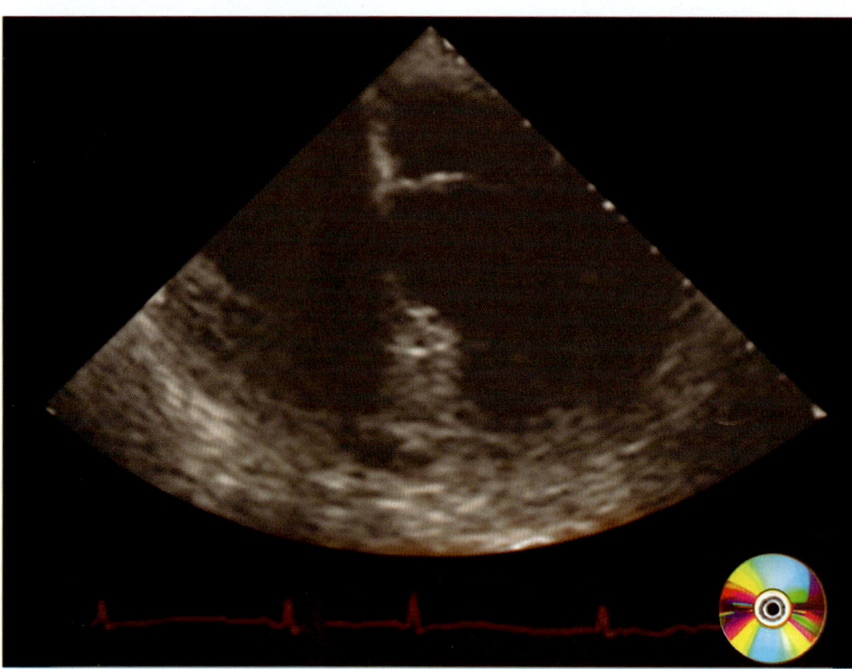

Figure 2 (VIDEO 2)

Midesophageal (ME) four-chamber view

tricuspid annular recoil motion toward the base of the heart at end systole. When right atrial pressure is increased, the S-wave and the S/D ratio decrease while the A-wave increases. Severe TR eliminates the normal antegrade S-wave and produces a reversed flow signal during systole. In patients with atrial fibrillation, no A-wave is

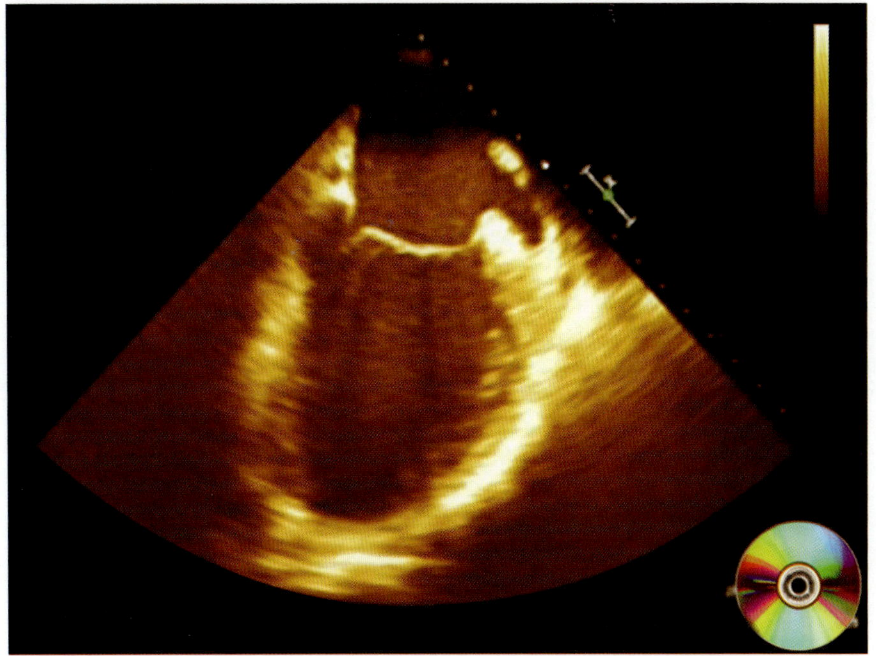

Figure 3 (VIDEO 3)

Midesophageal right ventricle (ME RV) inflow outflow view

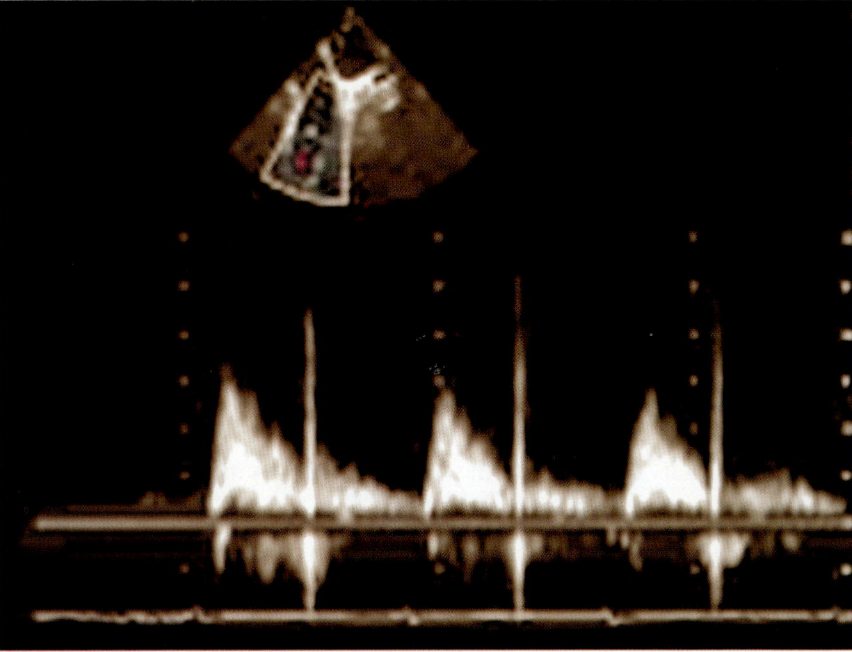

Figure 4

Spectral Doppler interrogation of the PV in the TG view of RVOT

seen in the hepatic venous or TV inflow patterns. Spectral Doppler assessment of the TV may provide a great deal of pertinent hemodynamic information. As mentioned earlier, PAs pressure may be estimated by measuring the peak velocity of the TR jet, using the simplified Bernoulli equation to estimate the transvalvular gradient, and

Table 1: Formulas useful for assessing the TV, PV and PA blood flow
PAs (RVSP) = 4 V^2 + CVP
V = Peak systolic velocity of the tricuspid regurgitant jet
PAd = 4V^2 + RVDP or CVP
V = End-diastolic velocity of the pulmonary regurgitant jet
PAm = 0.61 x PAs + 2 mm Hg
RV SV = PV area x VTI_{pv}
RV SV = 0.785 x (PV diameter)^2 x VTI_{pv}
Abbreviations: RV, right ventricle; PA, pulmonary artery; V, velocity; RVSP, right ventricle systolic pressure; PAs, pulmonary artery systolic pressure; CVP, central venous pressure; PAd, pulmonary artery diastolic pressure; RVDP, right ventricle diastolic pressure; SV, stroke volume; PAm, pulmonary artery mean pressure; VTI, velocity time integral; PV, pulmonic valve.

adding an estimate of RA pressure to derive RV (or PA) systolic pressure **(Fig. 4; Table 1)**.[1]

ESTIMATION OF INTRACARDIAC PRESSURES

Right Ventricular Systolic Pressure

The peak tricuspid regurgitant (TR) velocity reflects the peak pressure gradient between the RV and the right atrium (RA). Therefore, the right ventricular systolic pressure (RVSP) can be estimated with the continuous-wave Doppler by the following equation:[9]

$$RVSP = 4(V_{TR})^2 + RAP$$

where RVSP is the right ventricular systolic pressure (in mm Hg); VTR is the peak tricuspid regurgitant velocity, (in m/s); and RAP is the measured or estimated right atrial pressure (in mm Hg) **(Fig. 5)**.

The peak systolic velocity obtained across a ventricular septal defect reflects the peak pressure gradient between the LV and RV. In the absence of left ventricular outflow obstruction (i.e. subvalvular, valvular, or supravalvular aortic stenosis), the peak left ventricular systolic pressure can be approximated by the systolic aortic pressure, and secondarily by the arm systolic blood pressure. Therefore, in the following equation:[9]

$$RVSP = sBP - 4(V_{VSD})^2$$

where RVSP is the right ventricular systolic pressure (in mm Hg); VySO is the peak VSD velocity, (in m/s); and sBP is the systolic arm blood pressure (in mm Hg).

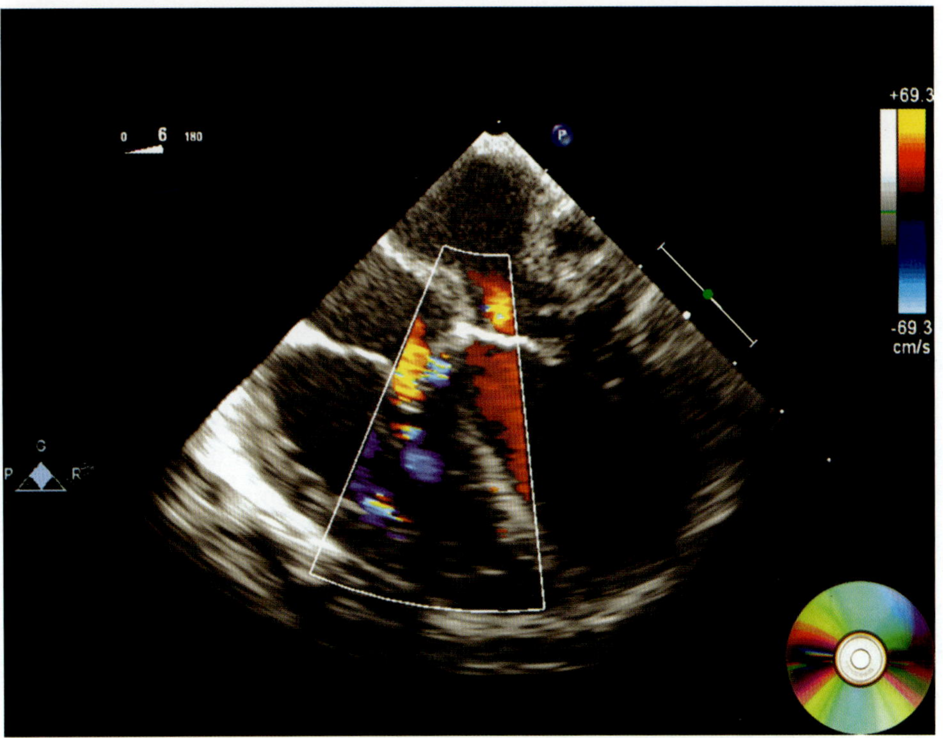

Figure 5 (VIDEO 4)

TV septal leaflet which straddles the VSD and this point measures the gradient across the VSD

Pulmonary Artery Systolic Pressure

Unless there is a right ventricular outflow obstruction (such as pulmonic stenosis), the PASP should be equal to the RSVP. In this setting, we can, therefore rewrite the two preceding equations as follows:[2]

$$PASP = 4(V_{TR})^2 = RAP$$

$$PASP = sBP - 4(V_{VSD})^2$$

In the presence of a patent ductus arteriosus (PDA) (between the thoracic aorta and the pulmonary artery), the peak velocity reflects the peak pressure gradient between the aortic and pulmonary artery pressure[3] as given in the following equation:

$$PVSP = sBP - 4(V_{PDA})^2$$

where PASP is the pulmonary artery systolic pressure (in mm Hg); V_{PDA} is the peak PDA velocity (in m/s); and sBP is the systolic arm blood pressure (in mm Hg).

Mean Pulmonary Artery Pressure

The pulmonary regurgitant velocity represents the instantaneous pressure gradient between the main pulmonary artery and the RV during diastole. The mean pulmonary artery pressure was shown to be correlated to the peak pulmonary regurgitant velocity in protodiastole:

$$MPAP = 4(V_{E\text{-}PR})^2$$

where MPAP is the mean pulmonary artery pressure (in mm Hg) and $V_{E\text{-}PR}$ is the early peak pulmonary regurgitant velocity (in m/s).

The mean pulmonary artery pressure has also been estimated by several authors using the right ventricular acceleration time, from the onset of the ejection to the peak pulmonic velocity. The Mahan and Kitabake equations are:

$$\text{Mahan MPAP} = 79 - (0.45 \times RV_{accel}\text{Time})$$

$$\text{Kitabake MPAP} = 90 - (0.62 \times RV_{accel}\text{Time})$$

where MPAP is the mean pulmonary artery pressure (in mm Hg) and RV_{accel}Time is the right ventricular acceleration time (in ms).

The MPAP estimated by the Mahan equation was studied in patients with a heart rate of 60 to 100 bpm. Also, the right ventricular acceleration time may not be shortened as much, despite high pulmonary pressures, when the right ventricular cardiac output is increased with left-to-right shunt.[4-6]

Pulmonary Artery and Right Ventricular

End-diastolic Pressure

At the end of diastole, the right atrial pressure and the right ventricular pressure should have equalized, assuming there is no evidence of tricuspid valve stenosis. Therefore, the following equation can be rewritten as:

$$PAEDP = 4(V_{PR\text{-}EO})2 + RVEDP$$

$$PAEDP = 4(V_{PR\text{-}EO})2 + RAP$$

where PAEDP is the pulmonary artery end-diastolic pressure (in mm Hg);[7,8] $V_{PR\text{-}EO}$ is the end-diastolic pulmonary regurgitant velocity (in m/s); RVEDP is the right ventricular end-diastolic pressure (in mm Hg); and RAP is the measured or estimated right atrial pressure (in mm Hg).

Right Atrial Pressure

Several methods have been proposed to estimate the right atrial pressure used in the preceding equations to measure right-sided intracardiac pressures. The jugular venous pressure estimated by physical examination or an empirical value of 10 was evaluated and compared with other regression equations.

A normal-sized inferior vena cava (IVC) collapses with a rapid negative intrathoracic pressure during a sudden inspiration ("sniffing" maneuver). When the right atrial pressure increases, there is decreased venous return and compensatory increase in the IVC diameter which serves as a capacitance reservoir for the RA.

Moreover, during sniffing, the decrease in IVC diameter is either blunted or absent with high right atrial (RA) pressure.

Correlation studies with catheterization have also shown that combined information from the IVC diameter and the hepatic venous Doppler profile can be used to assess RAP.[10]

The preceding estimate of RAP was however not prospectively validated in patients on positive pressure mechanical ventilation.

SHUNT FRACTIONS

According to the principle of conservation of mass (volume), the volumetric flow through the right heart should be equal to that through the left heart. However, in the presence of an intracardiac shunt, the SV will be greater on the side receiving the additional shunt volumetric flow. Because the left-sided intracardiac pressures are usually greater than on the right, intracardiac shunts are most often from left to right, and the pulmonary blood flow will be greater than the systemic blood flow. The magnitude of systemic-to-pulmonary intracardiac shunt can be quantitated by determining the ratio of pulmonary blood:

$$\frac{Qp}{Qs} = \frac{\text{SV pulmonary}}{\text{SV systemic}}$$

where Qp is the pulmonary blood flow, including the added left-to-right shunt flow; Qs is the systemic blood flow; and SV is the stroke volume by the hydraulic formula" ($= 0.785d^2 \times \text{TVI}$).

To reflect the magnitude of the shunt adequately, the pulmonary blood flow must be measured at a site distal to the shunt inflow while the systemic blood flow should be measured at a site distal to the shunt outflow. The location of the shunt will determine where respective Qp and Qs measurements will be made.

In the case of left-to-right shunts at the atrial level, the pulmonary volumetric flow can be obtained at the TV annulus, the RVOT or the main pulmonary artery trunk. The systemic volumetric flow can be measured at the mitral valve annulus, the LVOT or the ascending aorta.

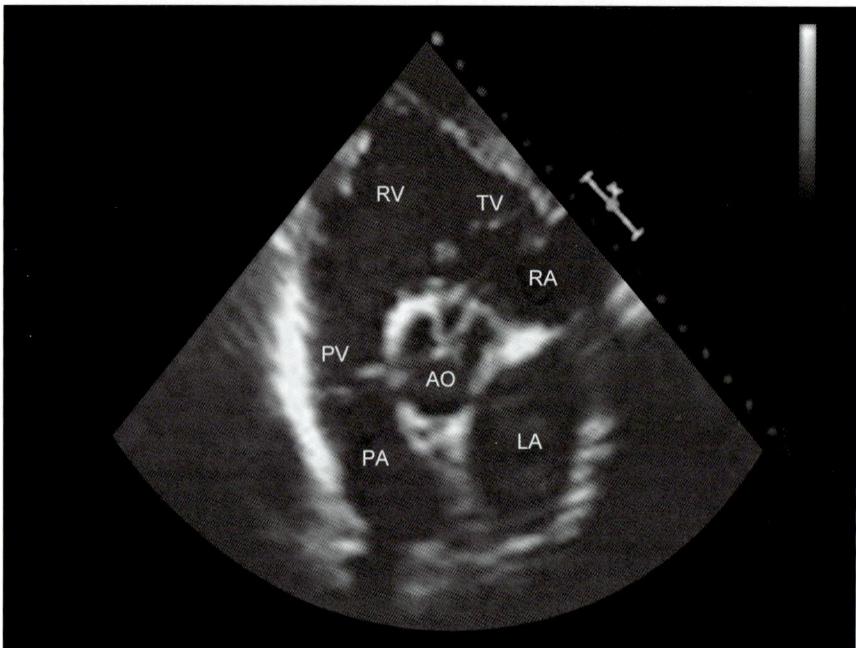

Figure 6

Transesophageal echocardiographic (TEE) view of a TG RV outflow view with focus on the RVOT and PV. Note the intimate relationship between the two semilunar valves. *Abbreviations:* RA, right atrium; LA, left atrium; RV, right ventricle; AO, aortic valve; TV, tricuspid valve; RV, right ventricular; PV, pulmonary valve; PA, pulmonary artery

For left-to-right shunts at the ventricular level, the pulmonary volumetric flow can be obtained at the RVOT, the main pulmonary artery trunk or the mitral valve annulus, while the systemic volumetric flow is measured at the LVOT, the ascending aorta or the TV annulus.

For left-to-right shunts from aorta to pulmonary artery, such as in patent ductus arteriosus, the pulmonary blood flow is obtained at the mitral valve annulus, the LVOT or the ascending aorta while the systemic blood flow is taken from the TV annulus, the RVOT or the main pulmonary artery trunk.

For technical reasons, the preferred site of SV measurements appears to be at the LVOT or RVOT where the cross-sectional area diameter is best seen at the base of the semilunar cusps and the TVI outer edge is easily traced (as opposed to modal velocity in atrioventricular valves).

In spontaneously breathing patients, RA pressure can be estimated by measuring the size and respiratory variation in IVC dimensions **(Table 1)**. For accurate results, quantitative spectral Doppler measurements must be made carefully, assuring that the ultrasound beam is parallel to the flow vector. Misinterpretation may result when the TR Doppler signal is contaminated by a high velocity jet of mitral regurgitation or aortic stenosis and not differentiated from these other high velocity signals. The TR jet may be distinguished by identifying the accompanying low-velocity antegrade diastolic flow signal that results from flow through the TV. Contrast enhancement of the TR jet with agitated saline injection may also help make the signal envelope more visible.

Spectral Doppler assessment of PV flow usually follows CFD assessment of PR and PS and is best accomplished in the UE aortic arch short-axis view or the TG view of the RVOT and the PV or the TG RV outflow view **(Figs 4 and 6)**.[15]

Color flow doppler (CFD) is helpful to define the direction of flow and assist in alignment of the Doppler beam for PW and CW techniques. Because flow through the PV is roughly perpendicular to that through the AV, the two are rarely confused. Normal blood flow through the PV is directed in an anterior-to-posterior direction and slightly right-to-left direction with respect to the patient.

Pulmonary stenosis (PS) is considered mild when the peak gradient across the PV is less than 30 mm Hg, moderate when the gradient is 30 to 50 mm Hg, and severe when the gradient is greater than 50 mm Hg.[11] It is important to remember that Doppler techniques measure peak instantaneous gradients, while catheter-based techniques measure peak-to-peak gradients and that variables such as different hemodynamic states, viscous forces, and flow acceleration effects affect these measurements differently. Correlation studies on patients with different degrees of severity of pulmonary stenosis have shown that mean Doppler and catheter-based gradients correlate better than peak gradients.[12]

Doppler patterns of regurgitant flow may also be used to estimate PA pressures. In the absence of PS, PAs pressure equals RV systolic pressure. The RV systolic pressure can be obtained from measuring the pressure gradient between the RV and RA from the TR jet peak velocity using the simplified Bernoulli equation, and then adding the RA pressure. The diastolic PA (PAd) pressure can be calculated from the end-diastolic PR jet velocity as follows: at end-diastole, the RV pressure equals RA pressure. Since, the gradient between the PA and the RV at end diastole may be calculated using the end-diastolic PR jet velocity, the PAd can then be deduced **(see Table 1)**. Several different formulas are available for the calculation of mean PA (PAm) pressure. In addition to the standard calculation of mean pressure as 2/3 of the diastolic pressure plus 1/3 of the systolic pressure, PAm pressure can also be derived from measurement of RV acceleration time, which becomes proportionally shorter as pulmonary pressures increase.[13] Of the other formulas available, the one derived by Chemla et al. and confirmed by others appears to be the most accurate and simple to use **(see Table 1)**.[14] PW Doppler can be used to assess RV stroke volume, and to calculate regurgitant and shunt fractions **(see Table 1)**.[15,16]

REFERENCES

1. Murphy DJ Jr, Ludomirsky A, Huhta Je. Continuous-wave Doppler in children with ventricular septal defect: noninvasive estimation of interventricular pressure gradient. Am J Cardiol. 1986;57:428-32.
2. Ge Z, Zhang Y, Kang W, et al. Noninvasive evaluation of right ventricular and pulmonary artery systolic pressures in patients with ventricular septal defects: simultaneous study of Doppler and catheterization data. Am Heart J. 1993;125:1073-81.
3. Ge Z, Zhang Y, Fan D, et al. Simultaneous measurement of pulmonary artery diastolic pressure by Doppler echocardiography and catheterization in patients with patent ductus arteriosus. Am Heart J. 1993;125:263-6.
4. Masuyama T, Kodama K, Kitabatake A, et al. Continuous- wave Doppler echocardiographic detection of pulmonary regurgitation and its application to noninvasive estimation of pulmonary artery pressure. Circulation. 1986;74:484-92.
5. Mahan G, Dabestani A, Gardin JM, Allfie A, Bum C, Henry WL. Estimation of pulmonary artery pressure by pulsed Doppler echocardiography. Circulation. 1983;68(suppl III):367.
6. Dabestani A, Mahan G, Gardin JM, et al. Evaluation of pulmonary artery pressure and resistance by pulsed Doppler echocardiography. Am J Cardiol. 1987;59:662-8.
7. Kitabatake A, Inoue M, Asao M, et al. Noninvasive evaluation of pulmonary hypertension by a pulsed Doppler technique. Circulation. 1983;68:302-9.
8. Otto CM, Pearlman AS. Textbook of Clinical Echocardiography. Philadelphia: WB Saunders, 1995.
9. Currie PJ, Seward JB, Chan KL, et al. Continuous wave Doppler determination of right ventricular pressure: a simultaneous Doppler-catheterizarion study in 127 patients. J Am Coll Cardiol. 1985;6:750-6.
10. Ommen SR, Nishimura RA, Hurrell DG, Klarich KW. Assessment of right atrial pressure with 2-dimensional and Doppler echocardiography: a simultaneous catheterization and echocardiographic study. Mayo Clin Proc. 2000;75:24-9.
11. Warnes CA, Williams RG, Bashore TM, et al. ACC/AHA 2008 guidelines for the management of adults with congenital heart disease: a report of the American College of Cardiology/American Heart Association Task Force on Practice Guidelines (Writing Committee to Develop Guidelines on the Management of Adults with Congenital Heart Disease). Developed in Collaboration With the American Society of Echocardiography, Heart Rhythm Society, International Society for Adult Congenital Heart Disease, Society for Cardiovascular Angiography and Interventions, and Society of Thoracic Surgeons. J Am Coll Cardiol. 2008;52:e1-e121.
12. Silvilairat S, Cabalka AK, Cetta F, et al. Echocardiographic assessment of isolated pulmonary valve stenosis: which outpatient Doppler gradient has the most clinical validity? J Am Soc Echocardiogr. 2005;18:1137-42.
13. Kitabatake A, Inoue M, Asao M, et al. Noninvasive evaluation of pulmonary hypertension by a pulsed Doppler technique. Circulation. 1983;68:302-9.
14. Chemla D, Castelain V, Provencher S, et al. Evaluation of various empirical formulas for estimating mean pulmonary artery pressure by using systolic pulmonary artery pressure in adults. Chest. 2008;135:760-8.
15. Maslow A, Comunale ME, Haering JM, et al. Pulsed wave Doppler measurement of cardiac output from the right ventricular outflow tract. Anesth Analg. 1996;83:466-71.
16. Goodman DJ, Harrison DC, Popp RL. Echocardiographic features of primary pulmonary hypertension. Am J Cardiol. 1974;33:438-43.

4 Tricuspid Regurgitation

Poonam Malhotra Kapoor, Dharmesh Aggarwal

- Severity of Tricuspid Regurgitation
- Etiology of Tricuspid Regurgitation
- Functional Tricuspid Regurgitation
- Pathogensis of Tricuspid Regurgitation in Mitral Valve Disease
- Leaflet Tethering of Functional Tricuspid Regurgitation
- TEE Views of Tricuspid Regurgitation
- Tricuspid Regurgitation Due to Infective Endocarditis
- Miscellaneous Etiologies
- Intraoperative Post-cardiopulmonary Bypass Laminar Tricuspid Regurgitation
- Atrioventricular Canal Defect Causing Tricuspid Regurgitation
- Tricuspid Regurgitation with TOF
- Double Chambered Right Ventricle
- Chronic Constrictive Pericarditis
- Tricuspid Regurgitation due to Ebstein's Anomaly
- Absent Pulmonary Valve
- 2D Echocardiography
- Color Flow Doppler
- Continuous Wave Doppler for Tricuspid Valve
- Pulse Wave Doppler
- Measurement of the Vena Contracta
- Moderate Tricuspid Regurgitation during Mitral Valve Surgery
- Endocardial Lead Induced Tricuspid Regurgitation
- Tricuspid Valve Anatomy on Real Time 3D Echocardiography
- Traumatic Tricuspid Regurgitation on 3D TEE
- Usefulness of Live 3D Echocardiography in Tricuspid Regurgitation
- Tricuspid Regurgitation 3D Color Flow Doppler

INTRODUCTION

Many patients have a small degree of tricuspid insufficiency, especially with increasing age. Athletes have significantly more tricuspid regurgitation (TR) than sedentary individuals. Patients with a PA catheter or pacemaker may have slightly more tricuspid regurgitation.

The TR may be primary when the disease process primarily involves the TV or secondary when the native valve is structurally normal but the regurgitation is due to TV annulus dilatation or right ventricular enlargement and dysfunction. Right ventricular enlargement results in displacement of the TV coaptation point into the right ventricle. This results in TR because of reduced or improper leaflet coaptation in systole. A common cause of secondary TR is pulmonary hypertension.

Tricuspid regurgitation is a common insufficiency. Since it is mostly asymptomatic and not easily audible on physical examination, it is frequently only diagnosed by echocardiography performed for another indication. Although a mild degree of tricuspid regurgitation is frequent and benign, moderate and severe tricuspid regurgitation are associated with poor prognosis.

The most common cause of tricuspid regurgitation is not a primary tricuspid valve disease but rather an impaired valve coaptation caused by a dilation of the right ventricle and/or of the tricuspid annulus.[1] A variety of primary disease processes can affect the tricuspid valve complex directly and lead to valve incompetence: infective endocarditis, congenital disease like Ebstein anomaly or atrioventricular canal, rheumatic fever, carcinoid syndrome, endomyocardial fibrosis, myxomatous degeneration of the tricuspid valve leading to prolapse, penetrating and nonpenetrating trauma, and iatrogenic damages during cardiac surgery, biopsies, catheter placement in right heart chambers **(Figs 1A to F)**.[2-8]

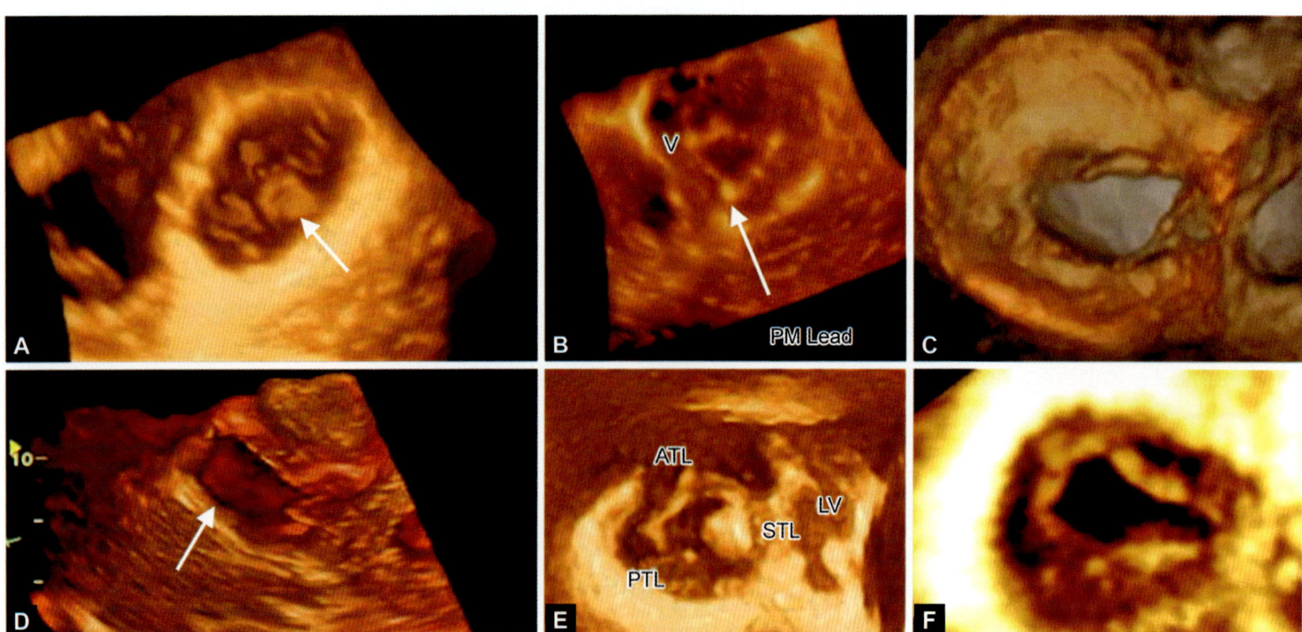

Figures 1A to F

Three-dimensional assessment of the mechanism of regurgitation in various tricuspid valve disease: anterior tricuspid leaflet prolapse with ruptured chordae (A, right atrial 'surgical' view); pacemaker lead interference causing immobilization of the septal leaflet (B, right atrial view); carcinoid tricuspid valvulopathy with adhesion of the valve leaflets to right ventricular walls that prevent the valve to close during systole (C, right ventricular view. *Courtesy:* Andreas Hagendorff, Leipzig, Germany); nearly complete detachment of the posterior tricuspid leaflet during biopsy in a heart transplant patient (D, right ventricular view); functional tricuspid regurgitation, dilated annulus, and tenting of the three leaflets with loss of systolic coaptation (E, right ventricular view); rheumatic tricuspid valve steno-insufficiency (F, right ventricular view)

The above methods provide only a semi quantitative estimate of TR severity. For exact quantitation of TR the proximal isovelocity surface area (PISA) method has been recommended. Using this technique an effective regurgitant orifice area (EROA) of 40 mm^2 or more and/or a PISA-derived regurgitant volume of 45 mL or more indicates severe TR.[9] This method requires measurement of the PISA or flow acceleration area which is done assuming the PISA to be hemispherical in shape. However, TR PISA is not hemispherical in most cases. Therefore, quantitation of TR using this technique is not reliable or accurate. A more direct and less cumbersome method for quantitating TR severity would be to measure the area of TR vena contracta (which essentially represents the "hole" in the leaflets through which regurgitation occurs) but this also requires an assumption regarding its shape. This is because it is difficult to accurately view the vena contracta en face using 2DE precluding measurement of area. In most cases the TR vena contracta, similar to vena contract as of regurgitation from other valves, is irregular in shape and does not conform to any geometrical configuration. Thus calculating the area of vena contracta from one or two measurements using 2DE and assuming its shape to be circular or elliptical would not provide a reliable estimate of TR volume. This problem is obviated by live/real time 3DE. Using this modality, the TR vena contracta can be accurately viewed en face and its shape reliable assessed. TR volume is then calculated by multiplying the vena contracta area with the velocity time integral (VTI) of the TR jet obtained by continuous wave Doppler. Thus, calculation of TR volume would be expected to be more accurate by 3DE since no assumption regarding the shape of vena contracta is necessary. Velayudhan et al. found a TR vena contracta of more than 0.75 cm^2 by 3DE indicative of severe TR with values of 1.0 cm^2 or higher denoting torrential TR.[10] Currently, the 3D technique probably represents the best echocardiographic method for quantitative estimation of TR severity **(Figs 2 to 5 and Table 1)**.

SEVERITY OF TRICUSPID REGURGITATION

Severity of tricuspid regurgitation can be assessed by:

- Jet area
- VC width
- PISA radius
- CW Doppler jet density/contour
- RA/RV/IVC size
- Hepatic vein flow

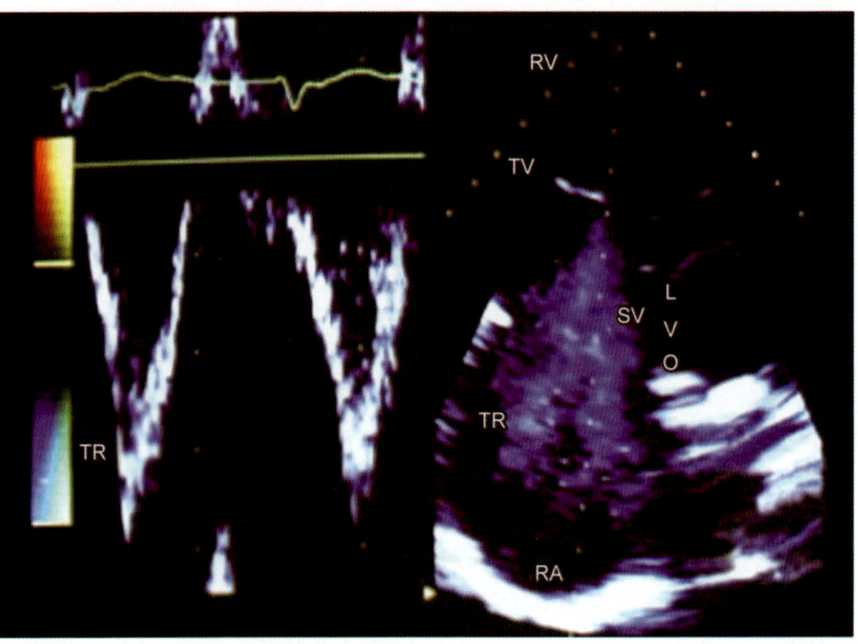

Figure 2

Torrential tricuspid regurgitation with laminar flow signals. In this patient the tricuspid valve (TV) is markedly deficient resulting in very severe tricuspid regurgitation (TR). Since the pressures are almost equal in the right atrium (RA) and right ventricle (RV) (both chambers practically act as one chamber), there is essentially no gradient across the tricuspid valve and hence the TR color Doppler signals are low velocity and laminar. Because of absence of aliased and mosaic turbulent flow signals in this patient, severe TR can be misdiagnosed as no TR. *Abbreviation:* LVO, left ventricular outflow tract

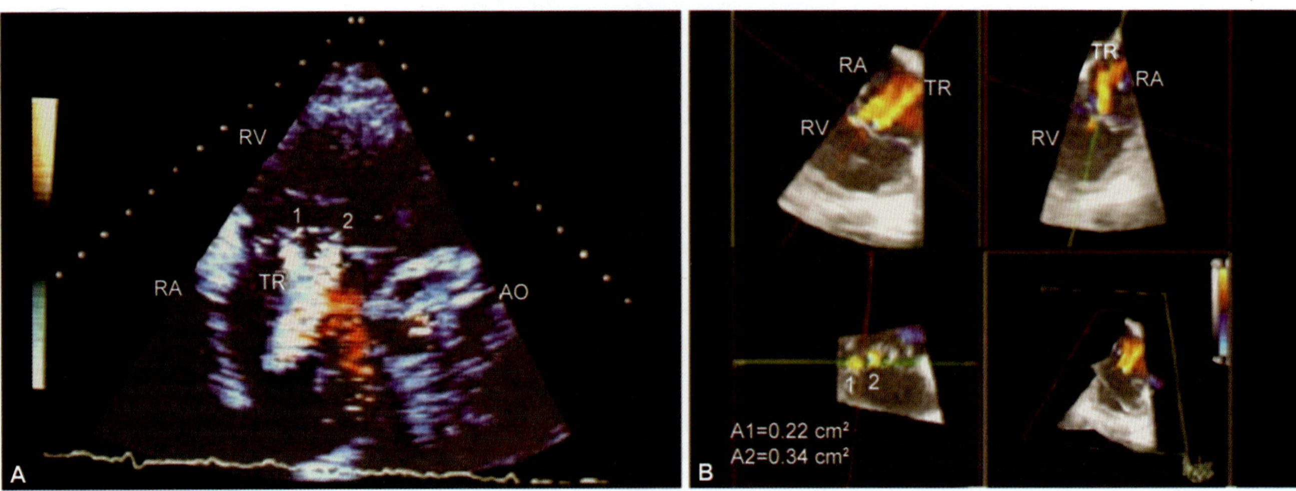

Figures 3A and B

Two jets of tricuspid regurgitation. (A) The aortic short-axis view in a 56-year-old man with scleroderma shows two distinct mosaic jets (1 and 2) of tricuspid regurgitation (TR). One of the jets originates from the septal leaflet and the other from the anterior leaflet. These two jets merge farther into right atrium (RA); (B) Quantitation of tricuspid regurgitation severity. Live/real time three-dimensional transesophageal echocardiography. The patient demonstrates two jets of tricuspid regurgitation. Both are viewed *en face* (1 and 2) and vena contracta areas (VCA) measured. VCA of jet 1 (A1) = 0.22 cm^2 and VCA of jet 2 (A2) = 0.34 cm^2

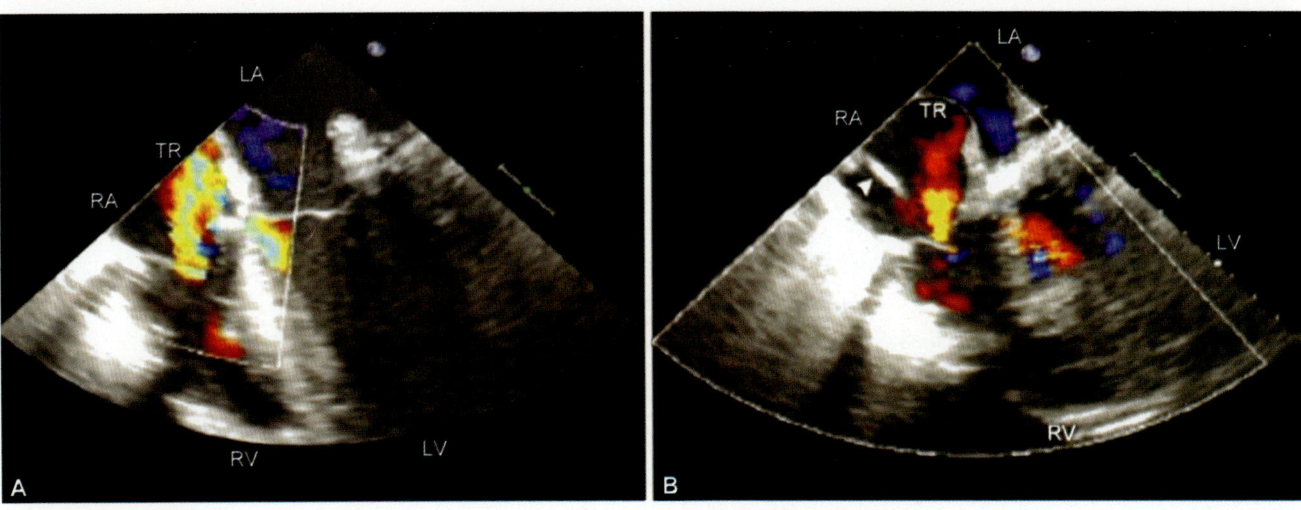

Figures 4A and B

Tricuspid regurgitation before and after annuloplasty. (A and B) Two-dimensional transesophageal echocardiography. Severe tricuspid regurgitation (TR) is noted before surgery (A). After surgery the TR is mild. Arrowhead in B points to a catheter in right atrium

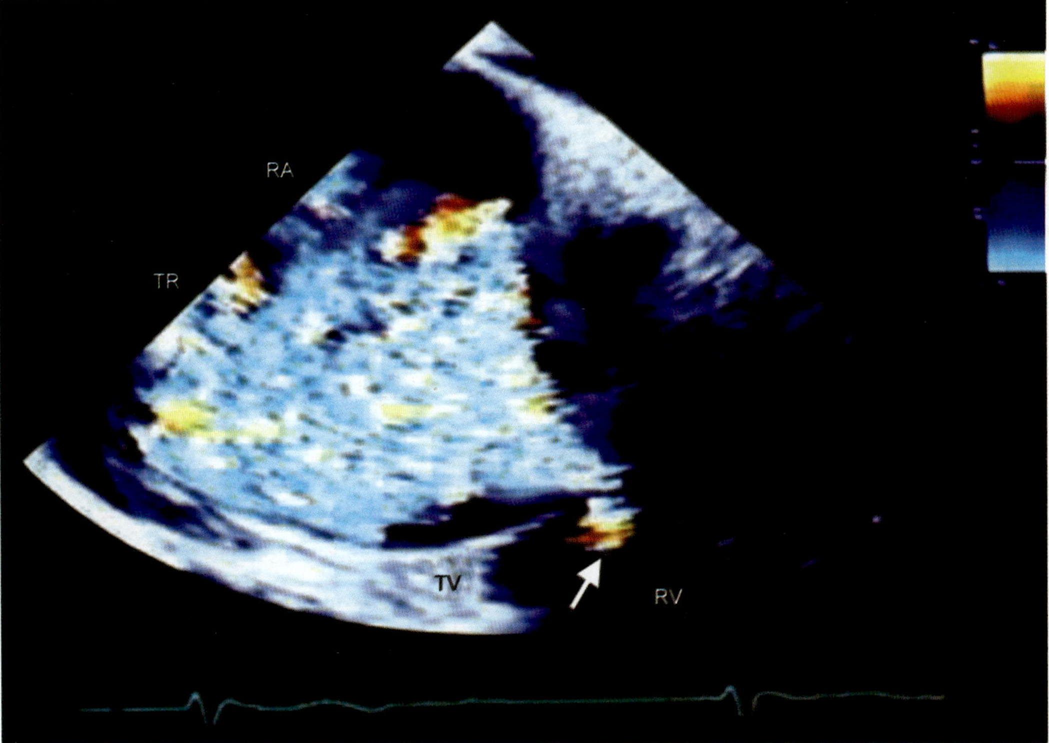

Figure 5

Severe tricuspid regurgitation. Two-dimensional transesophageal echocardiography. A large regurgitant jet is seen indicative of severe tricuspid regurgitation (TR). A relatively small zone of flow acceleration (arrow) is seen even though the patient has torrential TR, almost completely filling the massively dilated right atrium

Table 1: Echocardiography criteria for assessment of tricuspid regurgitation severity

	TR not severe	*TR severe*
Semiquantitative parameters		
Maximum TR jet area[11]	≤ 9 cm^2	≥ 9 cm^2
	< 5 cm^2 normal	> 10 cm^2
	5–10 moderate	
Maximum TR jet area/RA area in the same frame[11,12]	< 34%	> 34%
	(< 30%)	(> 30%)
Maximum TV annulus diameter in diastole	< 38 mm	≥ 38 mm
Percentage shortening of TV annulus (maximum annulus diameter-minimum diameter/maximum diameter x/w	≥ 25%	< 25%
Systolic hepatic vein flow reversal[13]	Absent	Present
Vena contracta width[12,14]	< 6.5 mm	≥ 6.5 mm
	(< 7 mm)	(> 7 mm)
TR jet intensity and contour by continuous wave Doppler	Not dense and parabolic	Dense and triangular
Quantification of TR		
PISA estimated EROA	< 40 mm^2	≥ 40 mm^2
PISA estimated regurgitant volume	< 45 mL	≥ 45 mL
D TTE vena contracta[9]	≤ 0.5 cm^2 – mild	> 0.75 cm^2
	0.5–0.75 cm^2 – moderate	(1.0 cm^2 – torrential TR)

ETIOLOGY OF TRICUSPID REGURGITATION

The most common cause of tricuspid regurgitation is not intrinsic involvement of the valve itself but dilation of the RV and of the tricuspid annulus. This is termed "Functional TR". It usually occurs in the setting of pulmonary hypertension secondary to mitral valve disease or ischemic heart disease. It can also occur after RV infarction. The leaflets are relatively normal but coaptation is inadequate. Intrinsic causes of TR include[15] each condition has characteristic findings that help the echocardiographer determine the likely etiology. *Rheumatic TR* is almost always seen in association with rheumatic mitral valve disease. It is associated with thickening and retraction of the leaflets, commissural fusion, and fusion and retraction of the chordal apparatus. The leaflets neither open, nor close normally, which leads to mixed TR and TS. *Tricupsid valve prolapse* due to myxomatous disease also usually occurs in association with mitral valve prolapse. It predominantly affects the anterior and septal leaflets. When chordae rupture, leaflet flail occurs and signs of significant TR ensue. Tricuspid prolapse may also be seen in patients with Marfan syndrome. *TV endocarditis* more commonly affects patients with history of IV drug abuse. Both right-sided valves can be affected. Friable and mobile masses are seen on the leaflet edges; destructive lesions may also occur. The presentation is usually TR along with constitutional symptoms. Endocarditic masses must be differentiated from papillary fibroelastomas. Chronic endocarditic lesions calcify and are therefore more hyperechogenic **(Table 2)**.

Fenfluramine-Phentermine valvulopathy: It is also associated with elevated serotonin levels, so the echo findings resemble those in carcinoid syndrome.[16] The leaflets thicken, shorten, and fail to coapt. The septal leaflet may be fixed to the septum. Unlike carcinoid, however, Fen-Phen valvulopathy affects the left and right-sided valves.

Classification of Tricuspid Regurgitation

Normal Valve Structure (Functional Tricuspid Regurgitation)

- Left sided valve disease
- Left ventricle dysfunction
- PA hypertension

Structural Abnormalities (Organic Tricuspid Regurgitation)

- Rheumatic
- Congenital (Ebstein, prolapse, partial atresia, clefts)
- Infective endocarditis
- Carcinoid, pergolide, cabergoline, phenfluramine
- Chest trauma, radiation
- Pacing leads

Functional Anatomy of the Tricuspid Valve Complex

The TV is the most caudally located and has the largest orifice among the four cardiac valves. Classically, the TV complex consists of three leaflets (anterior, posterior, and septal) inserted on the narrow fibrous TA and joined by chordae tendinae to their specific papillary muscles attached to the RV myocardium **(Figs 6A and B)**. Effective valve function depends on the integrity and coordination of these components.

Both the anterior and posterior (also named mural or inferior) tricuspid leaflets arise from the corresponding RV free wall. The three leaflets are unequal in size: the anterior leaflet is the largest, while the posterior leaflet is notable for the presence of multiple scallops. The septal leaflet is the smallest and arises medially directly from the TA above the membranous interventricular septum. As shown in

Table 2: Etiology of tricuspid regurgitation

Functional (morphological normal leaflets with annular dilatation)	*Structural abnormality of the tricuspid valve*	*Diseases of the tricuspid valve apparatus*
• Left heart diseases (LV dysfunction or valve diseases) resulting in pulmonary hypertension • Primary pulmonary hypertension • Secondary pulmonary hypertension (e.g. chronic lung disease, pulmonary thrombo-embolism, left-to-right shunt) • Right ventricular dysfunction from any cause (e.g. myocardial diseases, ischemic heart disease) • Atrial fibrillation • Cardiac tumors (particularly right atrial myxomas) • Mitral stenosis • Congenital heart disease • Sleep apnea • Collagen vascular disorders • Pulmonary parenchymal disease • LV dysfunction	• Rheumatic • Prolapse • Congenital – Ebstein anomaly – Tricuspid valve dysplasia – Tricuspid valve hypoplasia – Tricuspid valve cleft – Double orifice tricuspid valve – Unguarded tricuspid valve orifice • Endocarditis • Endomyocardial fibrosis • Carcinoid disease • Traumatic (blunt chest injury, laceration) • Iatrogenic – Pacemaker/defibrillator lead interference – Right ventricular biopsy – Drugs (e.g. exposure to fenfluramine-phentermine, or methysergide) – Radiation	• Rheumatic heart disease • Infective endocarditis • Trauma • Right ventricular infarction • Myxomatous disease • Right ventricular cardiomyopathy • Congenital (Ebstien's anomaly) • Radiation therapy eosinophilic myocarditis • Right ventricular cardiomyopathy • Postcardiac transplantation

Figure 6, the anatomy of the mitral and TVs displays many differences beyond the number of leaflets. The papillary muscles are different than those supporting the mitral valve, smaller, often multiple, widely separated, and carrying chordae to a single TV leaflet. Finally, there may be accessory chordal attachments to the RV free wall and to the moderator band. These complex and multiple chordal connections play an important role in the genesis of FTR, as they affect proper leaflet coaptation in the setting of RV enlargement and dysfunction. Indeed, as mitral papillary muscles each serve both leaflets, the separation of leaflets by annular enlargement is limited, while the link of one tricuspid leaflet to only one set of subvalvular support allows wide separation of leaflets with annular and cavity enlargement.

FUNCTIONAL TRICUSPID REGURGITATION

Functional TR occurs with dilatation of the annulus and poor leaflet coaptation. Any condition that results in RV dilation and dysfunction can initiate this cycle. This may be a primary disease of the RV such as cardiomyopathy or infarction. Rarely, unexplained TR and right sided heart failure is the presenting lesion in a patient with RV dysplasia or Uhl's disease, and is the result of cardiomyopathic changes

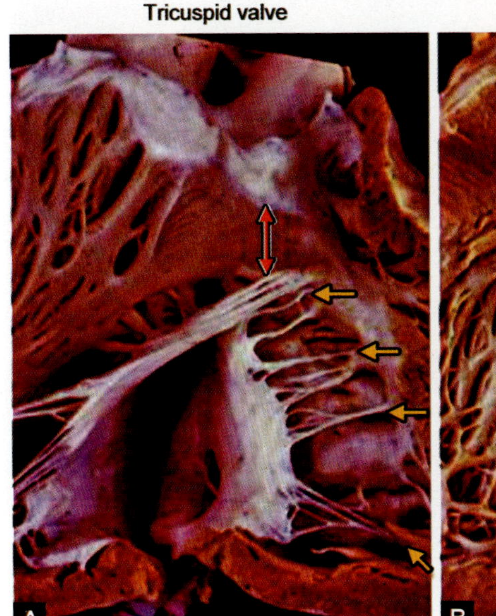

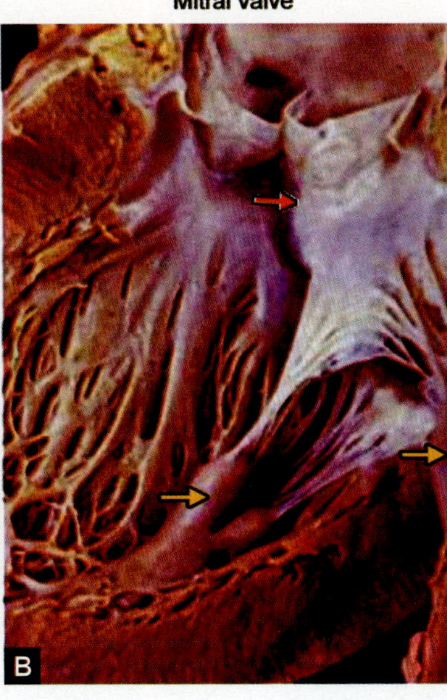

Figures 6A and B

Anatomic specimens showing tricuspid and mitral apparatus anatomy. Red arrows indicate the atrio-ventricular to semilunar valve distances. Yellow arrows indicate the specific differences between tricuspid and mitral valves. Tricuspid valve apparatus is characterized by multiple, widely separated papillary muscles which carry chordae to a single tricuspid valve leaflet. Accessory chordal attachments to the right ventricular free wall are also noted (*Courtesy:* Dr Willam Edwards, Mayo Clinic)

in the RV. Functional TR may also be secondary to pulmonary hypertension, which in turn may be primary or secondary to left-sided heart disease and lung pathology. Left-sided mitral valve lesion e.g. mitral regurgitation or mitral stenosis may lead to moderate to severe tricuspid regurgitation which should be seen in all the views before differentiate it as functional or organic tricuspid regurgitation. All these conditions can perpetuate the cycle of "TR begets TR": with progressive RV dilation, the annulus is more stretched, the leaflets tethered, thus worsening the regurgitation. In functional TR, the tricuspid leaflets and chordate themselves appear normal, while there is RV dilatation, with and without hypertrophy with tethering of chordate or poorly aligned papillary muscles. Functional TR is not necessarily only mild, as it can encompass varying degrees of severity but should always be differentiated from organic tricuspid regurgitation. It is generally associated with mitral stenosis or regurgitation **(Figs 7A to H)**.

Functional tricuspid regurgitation (FTR) is the most common type of tricuspid insufficiency and occurs approximately in 30 percent of patients with mitral valve disease. The major etiologic factor in the triggering of right ventricular dilation and thus causing functional tricuspid regurgitation is pulmonary artery hypertension secondary to mitral valve disease. Mete Gürsoy et al. aimed to analyze long-term outcomes of patients with mild tricuspid regurgitation at the time of mitral valve replacement.

In their study of 66 patients with mild tricuspid regurgitation, who underwent mitral valve replacement were divided into 2 groups and they found that a LA

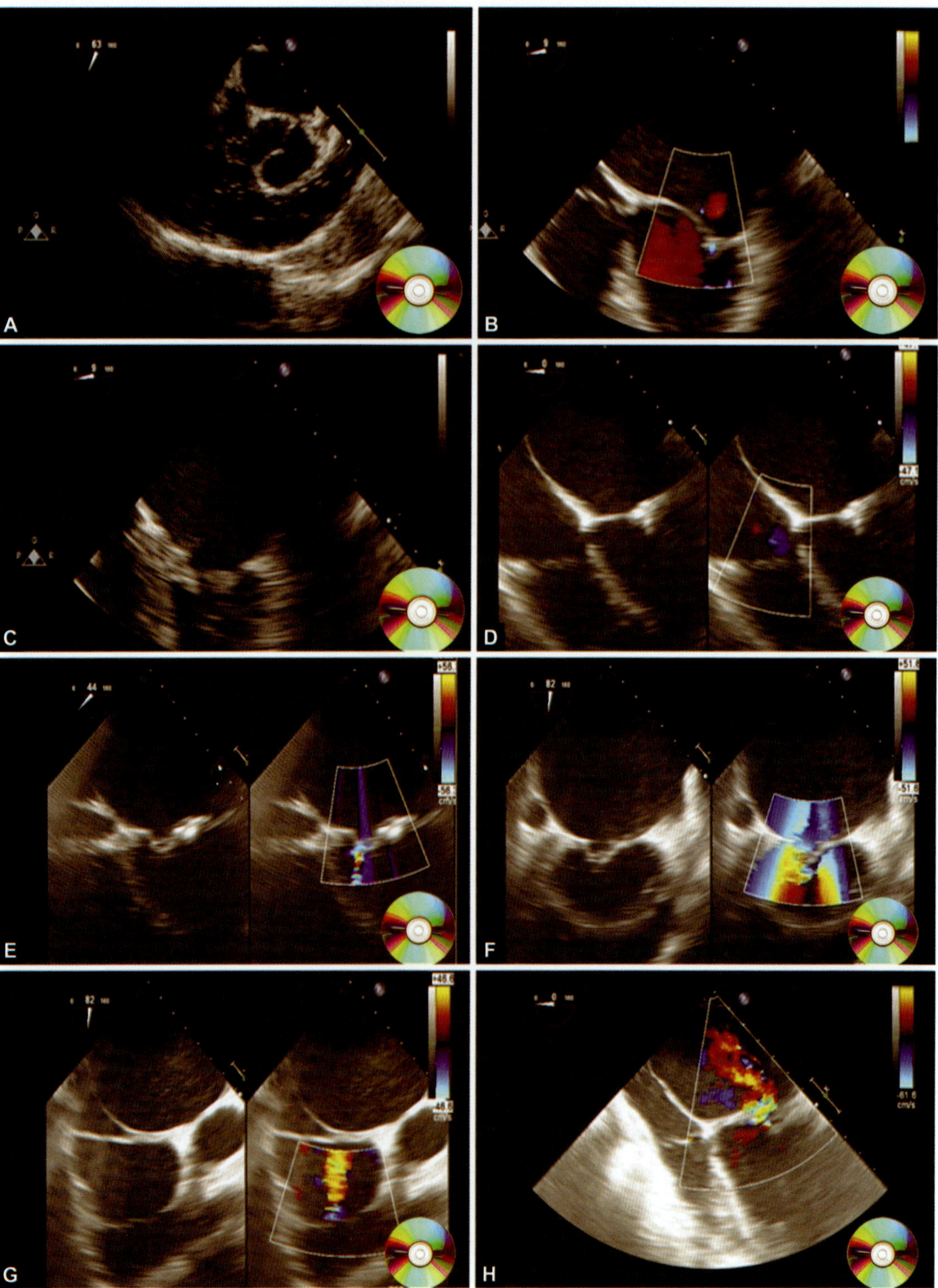

Figures 7A to H (VIDEOS 1 TO 8

Functional tricuspid regurgitation with severe mitral restenosis following a CMV done on this patient in dysphonic with mitral area of 0.6 and moderate tricuspid regurgitation. TV annulus measures 32 mm and anterior papillary muscle is tethered

diameter and female gender were found to be independent risk facors for functional tricuspid regurgitation progression and Thus surgical approach to even mild FTR should be individualized based on patient's risk assessment.[17]

PATHOGENSIS OF TRICUSPID REGURGITATION IN MITRAL VALVE DISEASE

The pathogenesis of TR in MV disease is complex and multifactorial **(Flow chart 1)**. Most often TR is functional, secondary to RV dilation. Mitral valve disease (usually rheumatic or ischemic) leads to mitral stenosis or regurgitation, which in turn leads to increased left atrial pressure and, if severe enough, to

Flow chart 1

Pathogenesis of tricuspid regurgitation in mitral valve disease

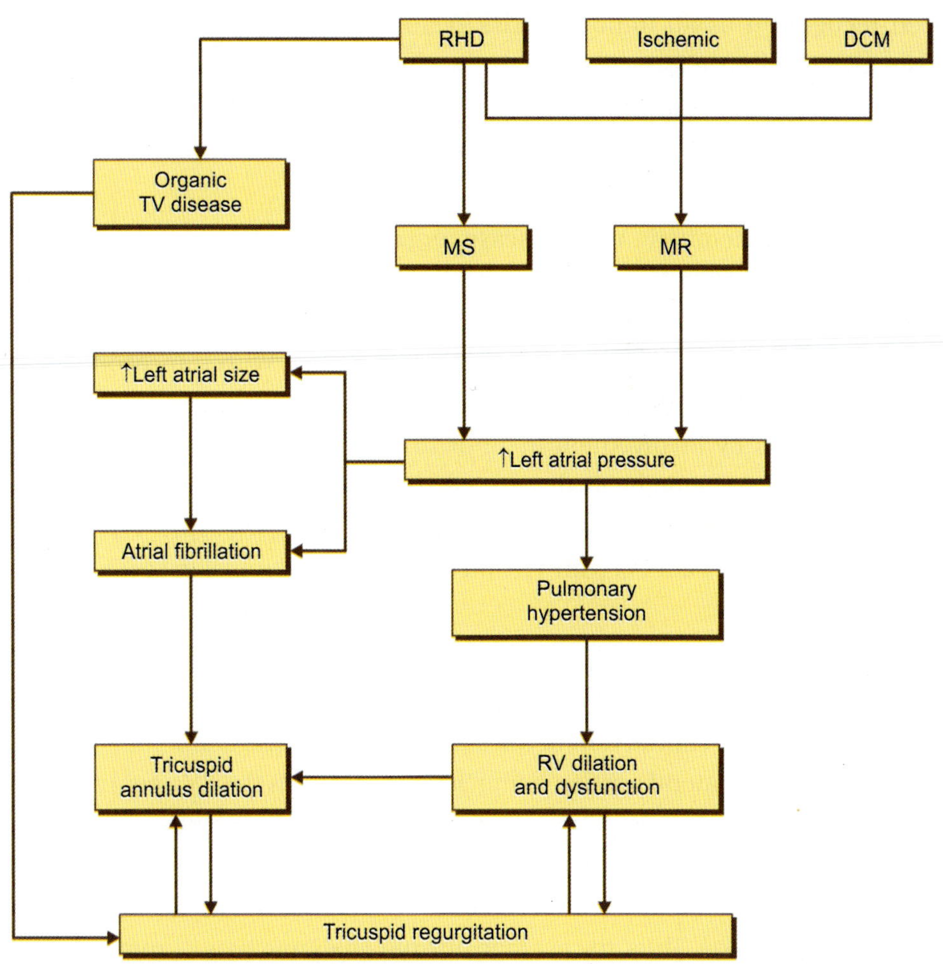

secondary pulmonary hypertension. Long-standing pulmonary hypertension might lead to RV dysfunction and remodeling, which lead to RV dysfunction and remodeling, which leads to TA dilation, papillary muscle displacement, and tethering of the TV leaflets, leading to TR.[18-21]

Tricuspid regurgitation itself leads to further RV dilation and dysfunction, more TV annular dilation and tethering, and worsening TR. With increasing TR the RV dilated and eventually fails, causing increased RV diastolic pressure and eventually fails, causing increased RV diastolic pressure and a shift of the interventricular septum toward the LV. Because of ventricular interdependence, this might compress the LV, causing restricted LV filling and increased LV diastolic and pulmonary artery pressure. This phenomenon was named "restriction dilation syndrome" by Antunes and barlow.[22]

Increased left atral size and pressure might also caused AF, which in turn causes right atrial dilation leading to further tricuspid annular dilation. Atrial fibrillation has been recognized as an important risk factor for the development of TR in patients with MV disease as well as for the persistence or occurrence of TR after MV surgery or balloon mitral valvotomy.[23,24] Furthermore, patients who have a concomitant successful Maze procedure during their MV surgery were reported to have significantly less TR at follow-up.[25]

In patients with rheumatic valve disease, organic TV involvement might also cause TR. Tricuspid valve leaflet thickening and restriction had been reported in about one-third of the patients with moderate or severe TR after MVR, but the true incidence of organic TV involvement might be higher. With transesophageal echocardiography and 3 dimensional reconstructions, Henein et al.[26] found more subtle organic TV involvement in 12 of 15 patients with isolated severe TR who had MVR for rheumatic heart disease. Scarring, leaflet thickening, and even some chordal shortening are routinely found when some tricuspid valve were resected some TVs from patients with TR and severe RV hypertension secondary to congenital heart disease.

The TA is a complex (less symmetric than the 'saddle-shaped' mitral annulus) non-planar, highly dynamic structure, which changes in shape and size during the cardiac cycle due to the contraction of the surrounding myocardium.[27] It is oval in shape, with the posterolateral portion being 'lowest' (towards the RV apex) and the anteroseptal portion the highest.[28] Tricuspid annulus diameter, circumference, and area are all larger than that of mitral annulus by about 20 percent. Although values of major TA diameter of 30 to 35 mm are described for normal adults, the orifice size is related to body size. Thus, the average normal TA diameter is 21 mm/m^2. The TA displays a ≤19% reduction in annular circumference (≤30% reduction in annular area) during atrial systole. It provides a firm and pliable base for the three-valve leaflets and it is in continuity with the aortic and mitral annuli. The septal portion of the TA is relatively fixed due to its position between the fibrous trigones. Therefore, as the RV free wall expands outwards, dilatation of the TA occurs primarily in its free wall aspect.

The diastolic opening of the valve along with corresponding expansion of the annulus provides a tricuspid orifice area of 7–9 cm^2. The systolic narrowing of the orifice provides an effective valve closure; however, a trivial or mild TR is detectable using Doppler echocardiography in 80 to 90 percent of normal subjects.[29,30]

LEAFLET TETHERING OF FUNCTIONAL TRICUSPID REGURGITATION

Though annular dilatation contributes to FTR, the tethering height of tricuspid valve leaflets may be more important as it defines the leaflet surface area of coaptation **(Figs 8A to C)**.

Fukuda et al. found a significant correlation between FTR severity and tethering height independent of annular dilatation: in the absence of FTR, the tethering height was 1.6 mm and in the presence of significant FTR, the tethering height was 6.8 mm. In another study, Sukmawan et al.[31] found that in the absence of FTR, the tethering height was 1.3 mm and in the presence of FTR, the tethering height was 5.3 mm. These studies appear to suggest that although annular dilatation and tethering of leaflets coexist in FTR, leaflet tethering plays a prominent role in the pathogenesis of FTR. Tethering of tricuspid valve leaflets is due to right ventricular dilatation and changes in right ventricular sphericity, geometry and function, with the lateral displacement of papillary muscles, leading to reduction and eventual failure of coaptation of leaflets and the development of FTR. Therefore, correction of annular dilatation alone with an annuloplasty ring may be insufficient to treat FTR

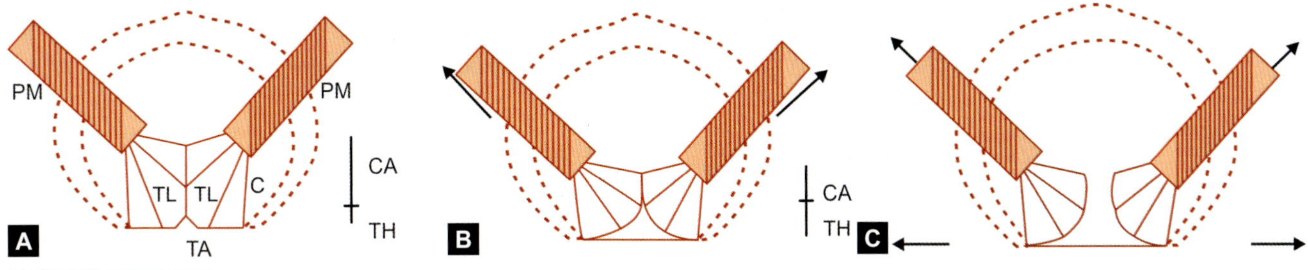

Figures 8A to C

Stages of the progression of functional tricuspid regurgitation. (A) Normal tricuspid valve; (B) Right ventricular (RV) dilatation leading to reduction in coaptation area (CA) and increase in tethering height (TH); (C) Further RV dilatation leading to failure of coaptation, further increase in TH and dilatation of the tricuspid annulus (TA). Tricuspid valve leaflets (TL), chords (C) and papillary muscles (PM)

in all cases; residual FTR after correction of annular dilatation is strongly correlated with the tethering height and the surface area of coaptation. Leaflet tenting volume (volume occupied under the tethered leaflets) has also been shown to correlate with FTR this denotes another method of measuring the tethering height, and thus implies a reduced area of coaptation. Therefore, methods to reduce the tethering height (and tenting volume) and increase the area of coaptation by augmenting the anterior leaflet with a pericardial patch have been advocated by some surgeons. Other determinants of FTR include endsystolic right ventricular eccentricity index, tricuspid valve tethering area and end-diastolic tricuspid annulus diameter.[32]

Mild-to-moderate functional tricuspid regurgitation in patients undergoing valve replacement for rheumatic mitral disease: the influence of tricuspid valve repair on clinical and echocardiographic outcomes.

In a study done in 2011 by Joon Bum Kim et al. in Korea, the decision to repair mild-to-moderate functional tricuspid regurgitation (TR) during left-side heart surgery remains controversial **(Table 3)**.[33]

Freedom from moderate-to-severe TR at 5 years was 92.962. Nine percent in the repair group and 60.866. Nine percent in the non-repair group (p<0.001 and 0.048 in crude and adjusted analyses, respectively). Postoperative moderate-tosevere TR was an independent predictor of poorer event free survival (HR¼2.90, p¼0.038). These findings support the strategy of correcting mild-to-moderate functional TR at the time of MV replacement to maintain TV function and improve clinical outcomes. The degree of TR was evaluated using the apical four-chamber view, and graded as mild, moderate or severe when the distal jet area was <5 cm^2, 5e10 cm^2 or >10 cm^2, respectively[34] **(Figs 9A and B)**.

Compared with MV replacement alone, concomitant TV repair was associated with better postoperative TV function in patients with mild-to-moderate functional TR undergoing MV replacement with mechanical prosthesis for rheumatic mitral diseases. These findings support the strategy of correcting mild-to-moderate functional TR at the time of MV replacement to maintain TV function, a strategy that may help to improve long-term clinical outcomes.

Functional tricuspid regurgitation

- **Tricuspid valve dilatation is a pre-requisite**
- **Tricuspid valve annular shape is flattened**
- **Tricuspid correlates with annular dimensions, right ventricle eccentricity and leaflet tethering**
- **Left/right ventricle interaction is not fully elucidated**
- **Pulmonary artery hypertension correlates with tricuspid regurgitation but does not presuppose it**
- **Fluid status affects the severity of tricuspid regurgitation**

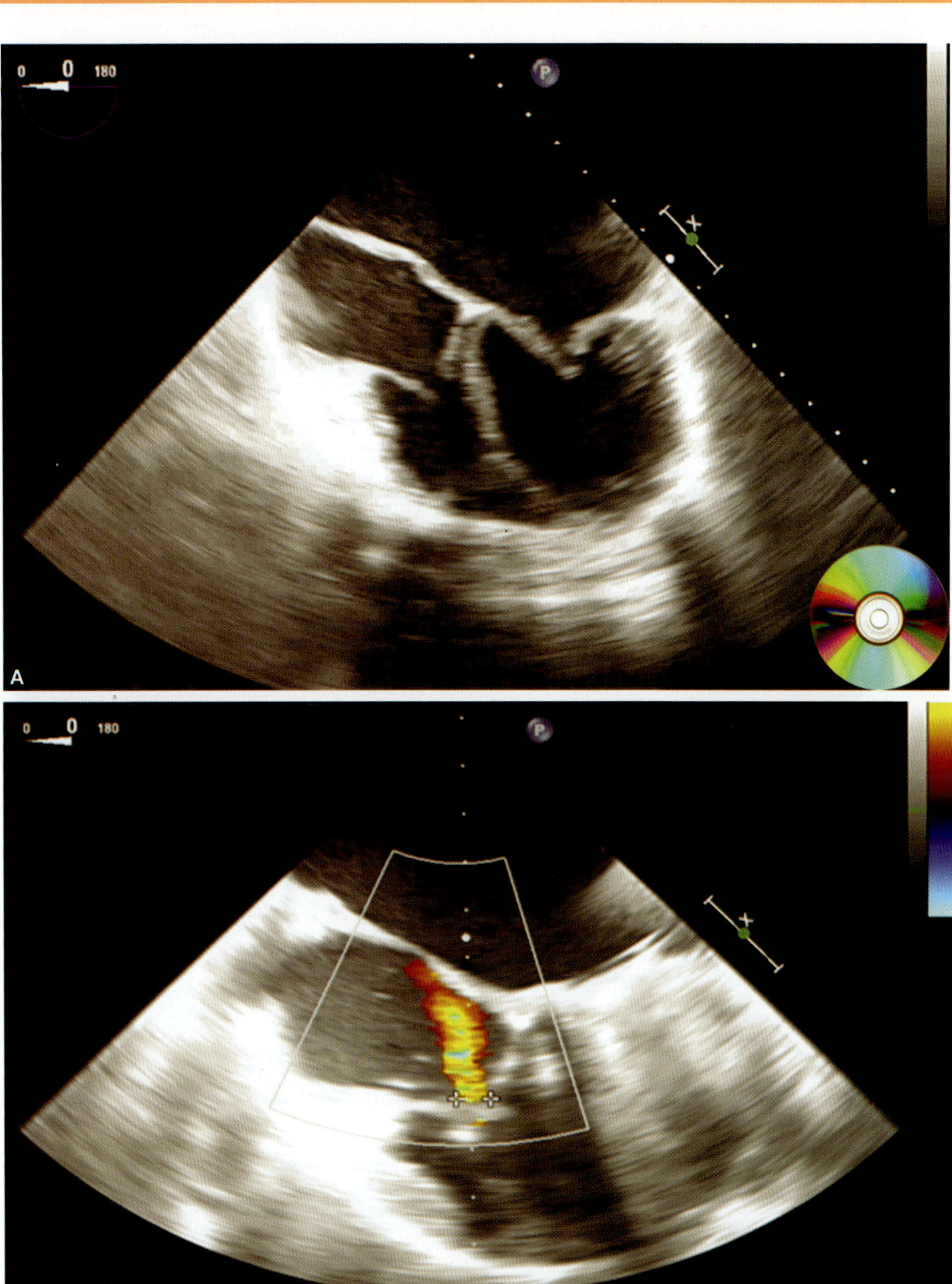

Figures 9A and B (VIDEO 9)

(A) Functional tricuspid regurgitation with mitral stenosis; (B) Mild to moderate functional tricuspid regurgitation with mitral valve stenosis

TEE VIEWS OF TRICUSPID REGURGITATION (FIGS 10 TO 16)

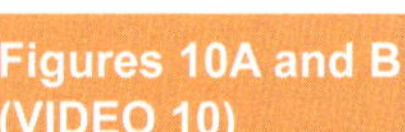

Figures 10A and B (VIDEO 10)

Tricuspid valve 4 chamber view

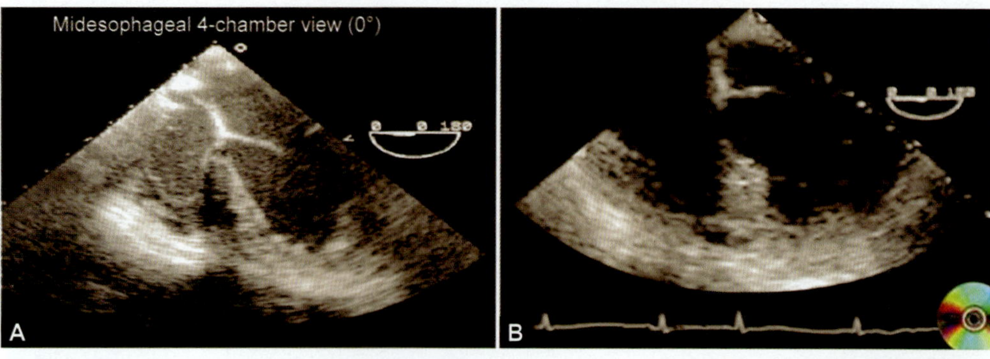

Figures 11A and B (VIDEO 11)

ME RV inflow—outflow view

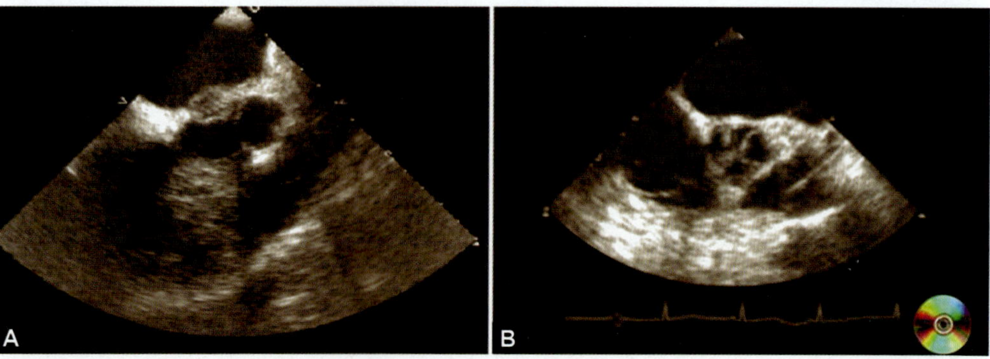

Figures 12A and B (VIDEO 12)

Mid-esophageal bicaval modified view

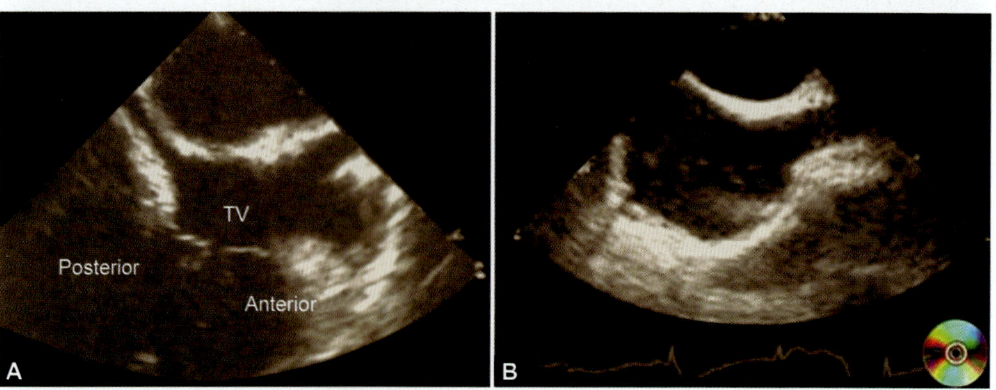

Figures 13A and B (VIDEO 13)

View of coronary sinus

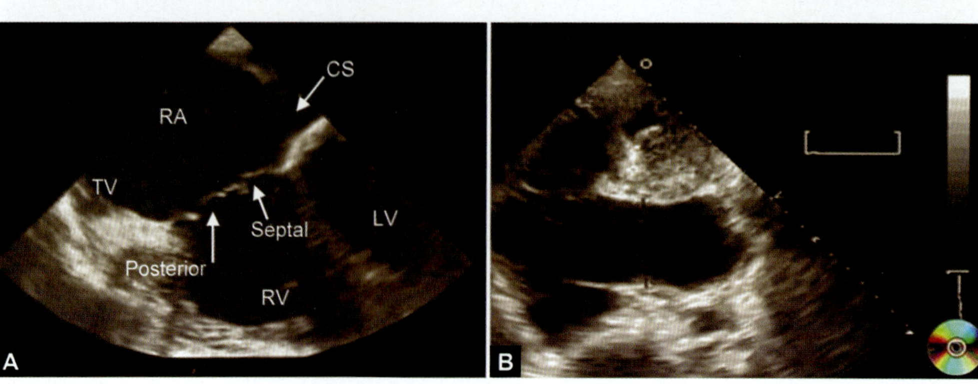

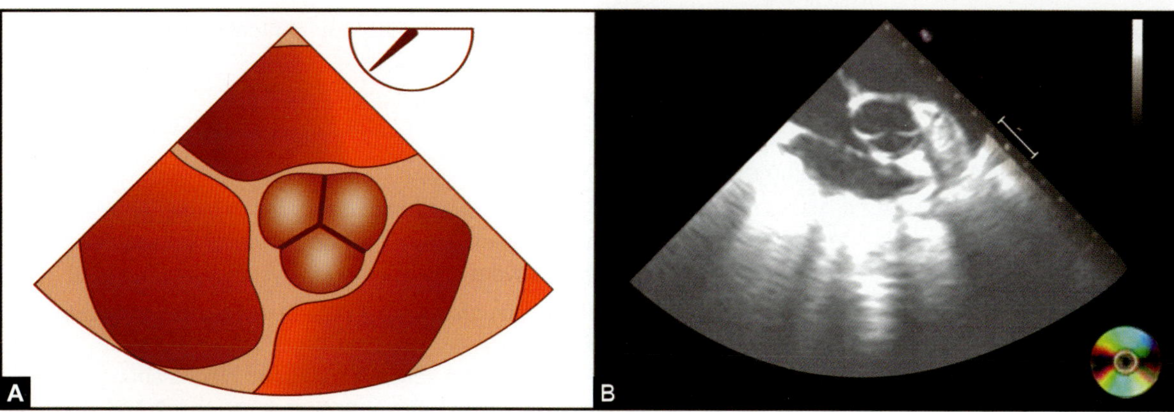

Figures 14A and B (VIDEO 14)

ME-AV SAX (Midesophageal aortic valve short axis view)

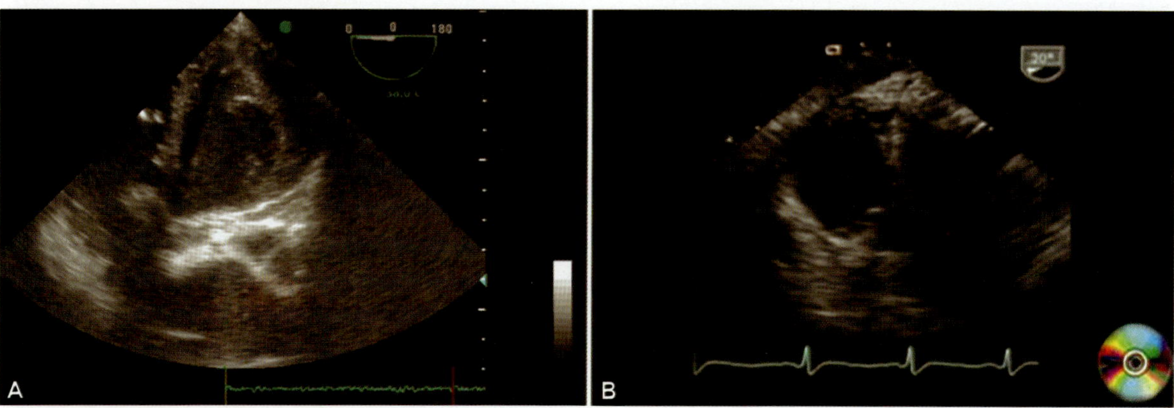

Figures 15A and B (VIDEO 15)

TG-TV SAX (Transgastric tricuspid valve short axis view)

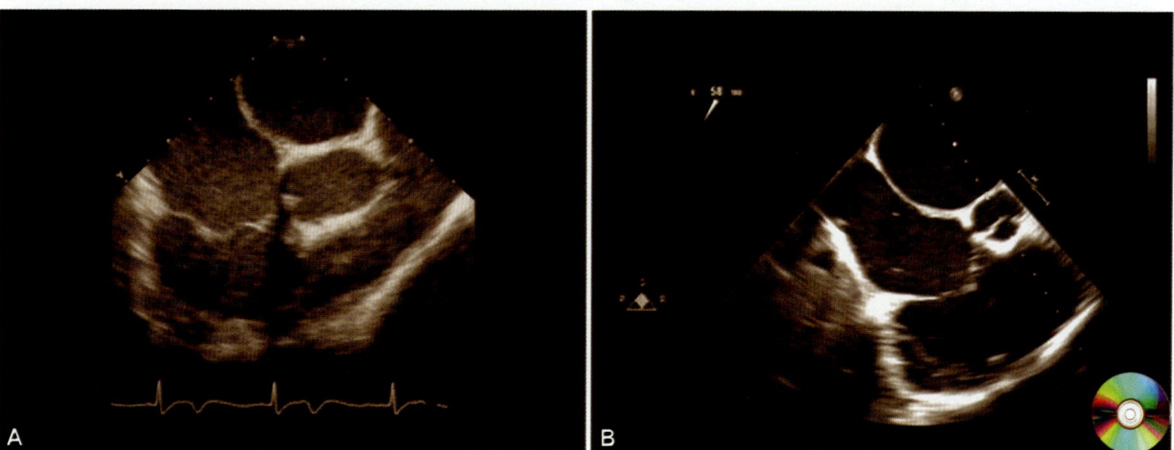

Figures 16A and B (VIDEO 16)

Transgastric-RV inflow view

- **These views were discussed in Chapter 2nd comprehensive TEE views.**

Table 3: Comparison of American College of Cardiology/European Society of Cardiology clinical guidelines for managing patients with tricuspid regurgitation

	ACC/AHA guidelines[35]	*ESC/EACTS guidelines*[36]
Class IB	TV repair is beneficial for severe TR in patients with MV disease requiring MV surgery	
Class IC		Severe TR in a patient undergoing left-sided valve surgery Severe organic TR and symptoms despite medical therapy without severe right ventricular dysfunction
Class IIaC	TV replacement or annuloplasty is reasonable for severe primary TR when symptomatic TV replacement is reasonable for severe TR secondary to diseased/abnormal TV leaflets not amenable to annuloplasty or repair	Moderate organic TR in a patient undergoing left-sided valve surgery Mild-to-moderate secondary TR with dilated annulus (0.40 mm or 21 mm/m^2) in a patient undergoing left-sided valve surgery Severe TR and symptoms, after left-sided valve surgery, in the absence of left-sided myocardial, valve, or right ventricular dysfunction and without severe pulmonary hypertension (systolic pulmonary artery pressure 0.60 mm Hg) Severe isolated TR with mild or no symptoms and progressive dilatation or deterioration of right ventricular function
Class IIbC	Tricuspid annuloplasty may be considered for less than severe TR in patients undergoing MV surgery when there is pulmonary hypertension or tricuspid annular dilatation	
Class III	TV replacement or annuloplasty is not indicated in asymptomatic patients with TR whose pulmonary artery systolic pressure is 60 mm Hg in the presence of normal MV TV replacement or annuloplasty is not indicated in patients with mild organic TR	

TRICUSPID REGURGITATION DUE TO INFECTIVE ENDOCARDITIS

Most often infective endocarditis is seen with intravenous drug abuse or indeweling catheters in the central circulation (e.g. hyperalimentation, chemotherapy, or access for hemodialysis). In immunocompromised hosts, endocarditis may be fungal in etiology, with large bulky vegetations seen on echocardiography **(Table 4)**. In developing countries, TV encocarditis is also associated with septic abortions. Rarely an infected ventricular septal defect jet may be the culprit. In patients with pacemaker lead infection, there may be incidental involvement of the valve. Most often endocarditis results in TR. Very large vegetations, however, may mimic valvular stenosis. In technically adequate studies, the transthoracic approach is usually sufficient for the detection of the majority of native tricuspid

Table 4: Pathological conditions causing tricuspid regurgitation	
•	Valve disease
•	Tricuspid valve prolapse
•	Endocarditis
•	Carcinoid syndrome
•	Ebstein's anomaly
•	AV canal defect
•	Blunt chest trauma
•	CCP
•	DCRV
•	TOF
•	Fen-Phen valvulopathy
•	Post cardiac transplant
•	Pacemaker insertion
•	Post CPB laminar TR

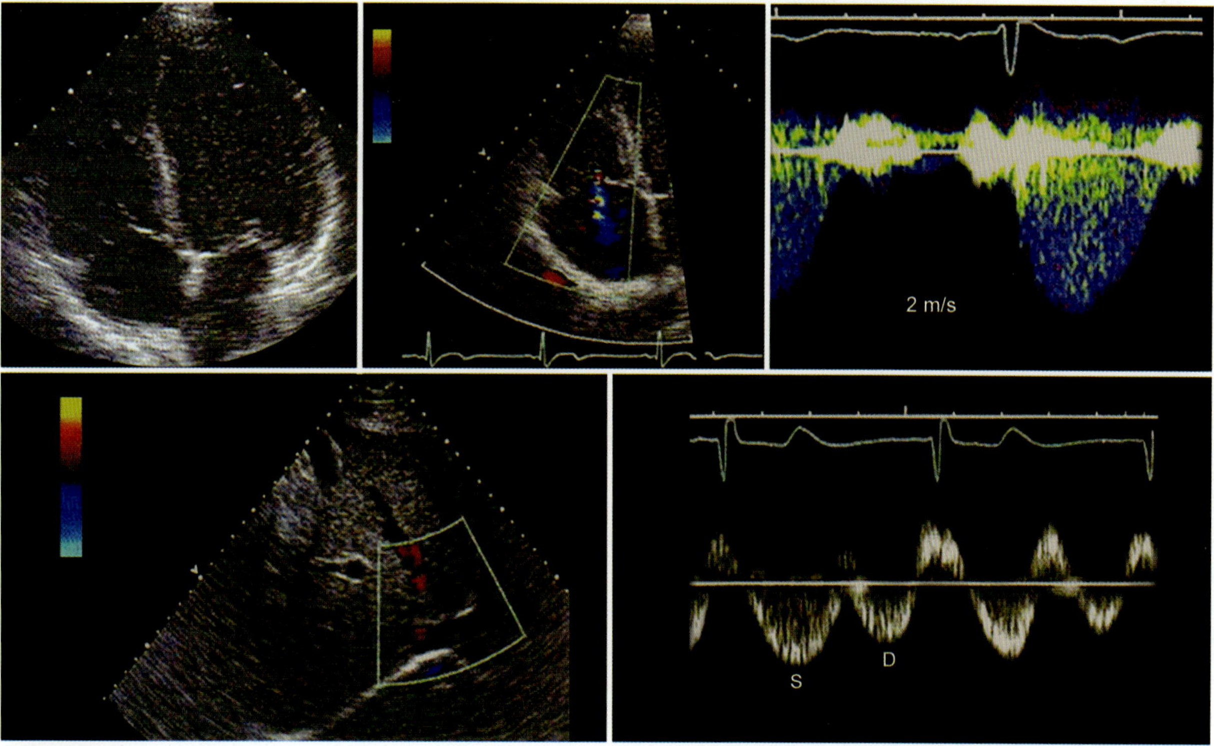

Figure 17

Mild tricuspid regurgitation in an otherwise normal individual. A very thin jet of regurgitation is seen on color Doppler, with a low velocity by continuous—wave Doppler and a round contour to the jet velocity. The hepatic veins and inferior vena cava of normal size and display a normal hepatic venous flow pattern of systolic dominant flow by pulsed Doppler

valve associated TR. Transesophageal echocardiography is reserved for technically difficult cases and where other valvular involvement is suspected or during the intraoperative period before and after TV repair **(Fig. 17)**.

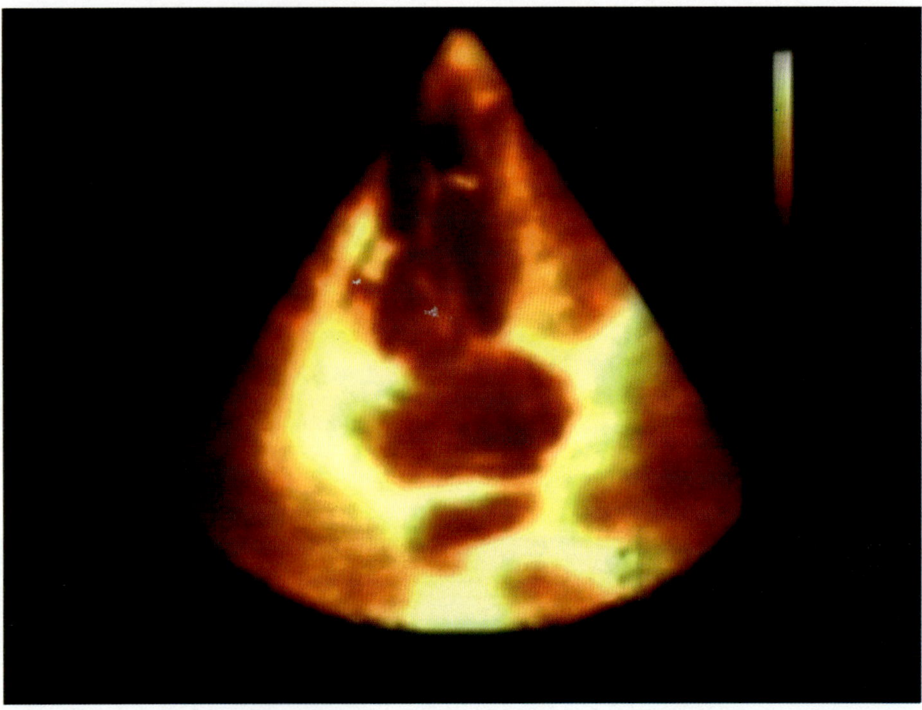

Figure 18
Flail tricuspid leaflet

MISCELLANEOUS ETIOLOGIES

Iatrogenic TR may occur in cardiac transplant patient after trauma from cardiac biopsies or after the placement of a Swan-Ganz catheter or a pacemaker. After myocardial biopsies, TR may result from damage to the valvular apparatus (papillary muscles, chordae, or leaflets). In this setting, the TR jet is often eccentric **(Fig. 18)**. External penetrating trauma can also directly injure the TV apparatus including puncture of the leaflets, rupture of the chordae or the papillary muscles **(Fig. 19)**. Rarely flail segments may be seen. On the other hand, blunt trauma may result in RV contusion which, if extensive, can lead to RV failure and functional TR **(Fig. 20)**.

INTRAOPERATIVE POST-CARDIOPULMONARY BYPASS LAMINAR TRICUSPID REGURGITATION

Post cardiopulmonary bypass (CPB) very often the systolic flow across the tricuspid valve is laminar and there is a low peak velocity of 0.9 m/s. Both hepatic venous systolic flow reversal and a dense triangular-shaped spectral Doppler tricuspid regurgitant flow pattern are noted **(Figs 21A and B)**.

When flow is laminar, the borders of a color jet can be so difficult to appreciate that even a large jet can be missed entirely. Regurgitant laminar flow in contrast

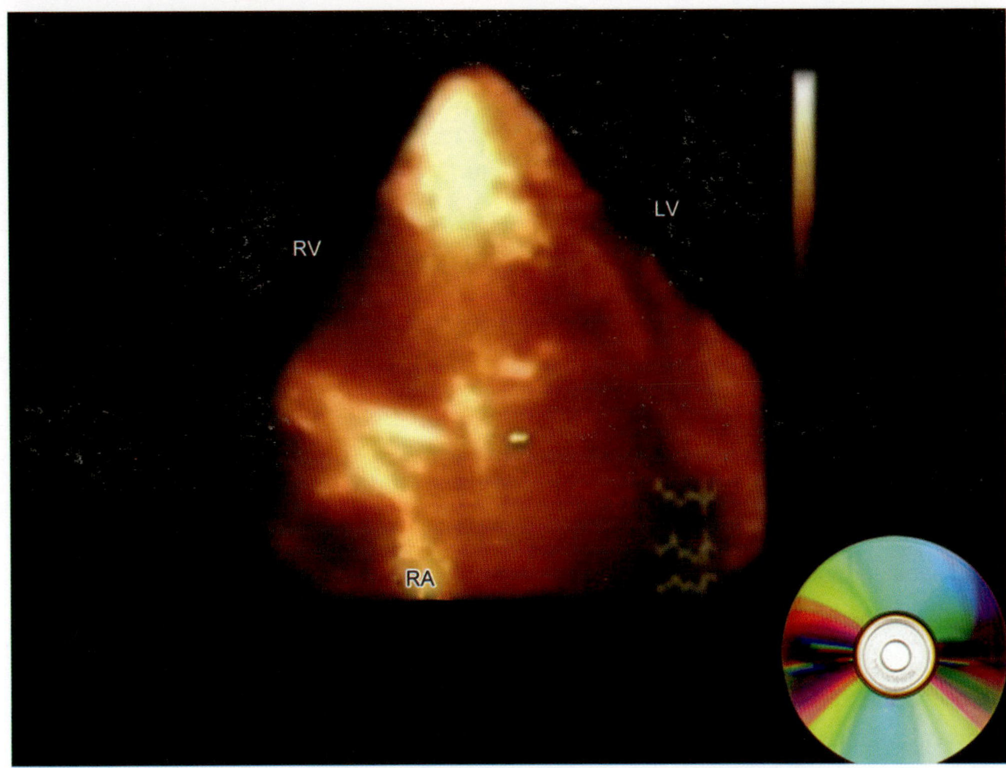

Figure 19 (VIDEO 17)

The ruptured papillary muscle

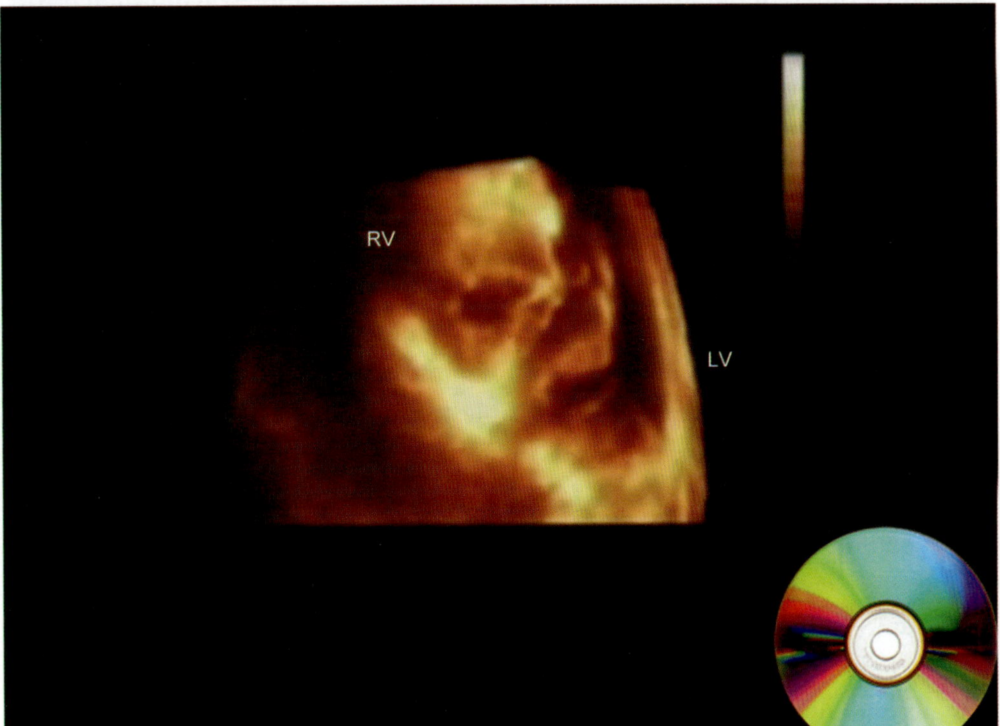

Figure 20 (VIDEO 18)

The carcinoid heart disease. The tricuspid valve seen "*enface*" with all 3 leaflet with thickened and shortened leaflets causing stenosis and/or regurgitation and ultimately right heart failure

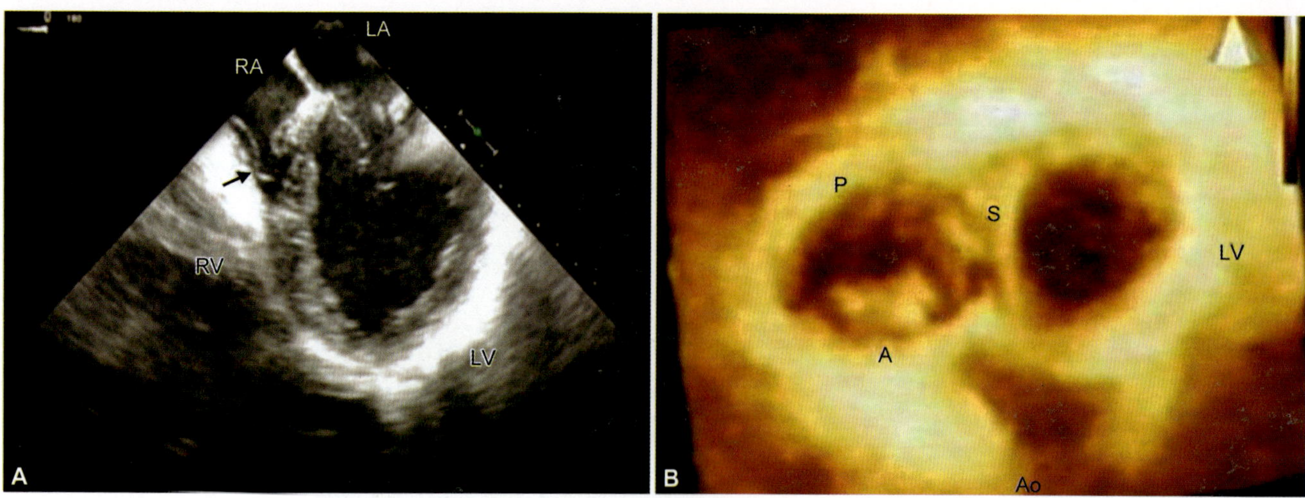

Figures 21A and B

Tricuspid valve prolapse. Transesophageal echocardiography five-chamber views showing redundancy of all the three leaflets

to flow that is turbulent allows a much greater regurgitant volume for a given transvalvular pressure gradient. The lower energy loss of laminar flow likely results in a smaller pressure drop and sustained flow. The American Society of Echocardiography (ASE) guidelines for evaluating regurgitant valve lesions suggest integrating different parameters when evaluating TR severity to avoid such errors. Right-sided anatomic changes consistent with severe TR include enlarged cardiac chambers with a dilated tricuspid annulus, a lack of leaflet coaptation, paradoxic septal motion, and a distended venous system. The morphology of the spectral tracing also may be used, with a dense triangular pattern suggestive of severe TR. A high-velocity jet does not indicate severe TR, and, indeed, laminar jets generally are associated with velocities around 2 m/s. Antegrade and retrograde spectral patterns may almost mirror each other relating to the "to-andfro" flow across the valve. Hepatic venous systolic flow reversal is a sensitive indicator of severe TR and also should be present. If most of the ASE parameters suggest moderate-tosevere TR, even in the absence of a clearly visible turbulent jet, then the presence of a significantly incompetent valve needs to be considered **(Fig. 22)**.

Tricuspid dilation may be the most important risk factor for late TR and that the valve should be repaired regardless of the regurgitant severity if significant dilation is present. New TR that is present immediately after CPB presents a different management dilemma because this may be related to myocardial stunning or coronary air embolization and may be recoverable and is seen as laminar TR, post CPB. Its organic nature needs to elucidated later.

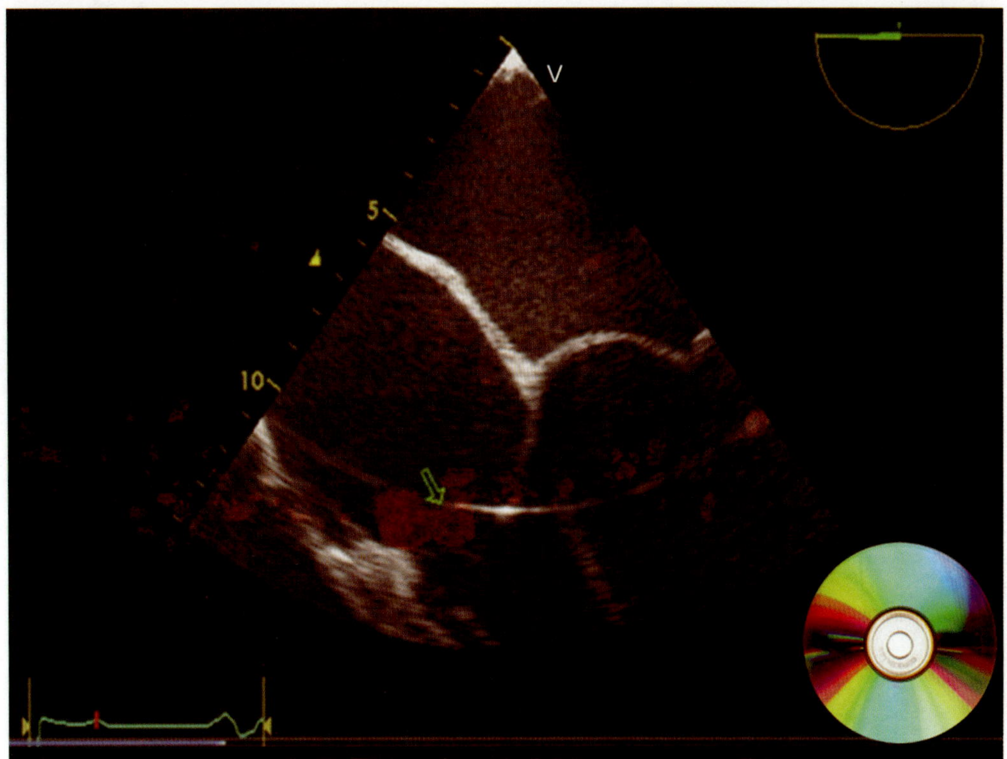

Figure 22 (VIDEO 19)

Laminar tricuspid regurgitation in transthoracic view

ATRIOVENTRICULAR CANAL DEFECT CAUSING TRICUSPID REGURGITATION

Improperly formed mitral and/or tricuspid valves: The valves that separate the upper heart chambers (atria) from the lower heart chambers (ventricles) are improperly formed. Specifically, there is an abnormality in the left-sided valve (the mitral valve): it has three cusps rather than the two cusps that normally form the valve. One of the normal cusps is divided into two cusps. This division between these two cusps is called the cleft (or a cut in the mitral valve). The abnormal mitral and tricuspid valves with clefts are associated with AV canal defects. *AV canal defects* may be associated with TR since the septal leaflet and the anterior mitral leaflet both are derived from the endocardial cushions.

TRICUSPID REGURGITATION WITH TOF

Tricuspid valve regurgitation occurs frequently in postoperative TOF patients with right ventricular enlargement[37] **(Figs 23 and 24)**. In 2003, Mahle et al. investigated the factors contributing to tricuspid regurgitation and the relation between tricuspid regurgitation and right ventricular dilation.[38] They found that not only is tricuspid regurgitation is common (present in 32% of patients), but it is related to

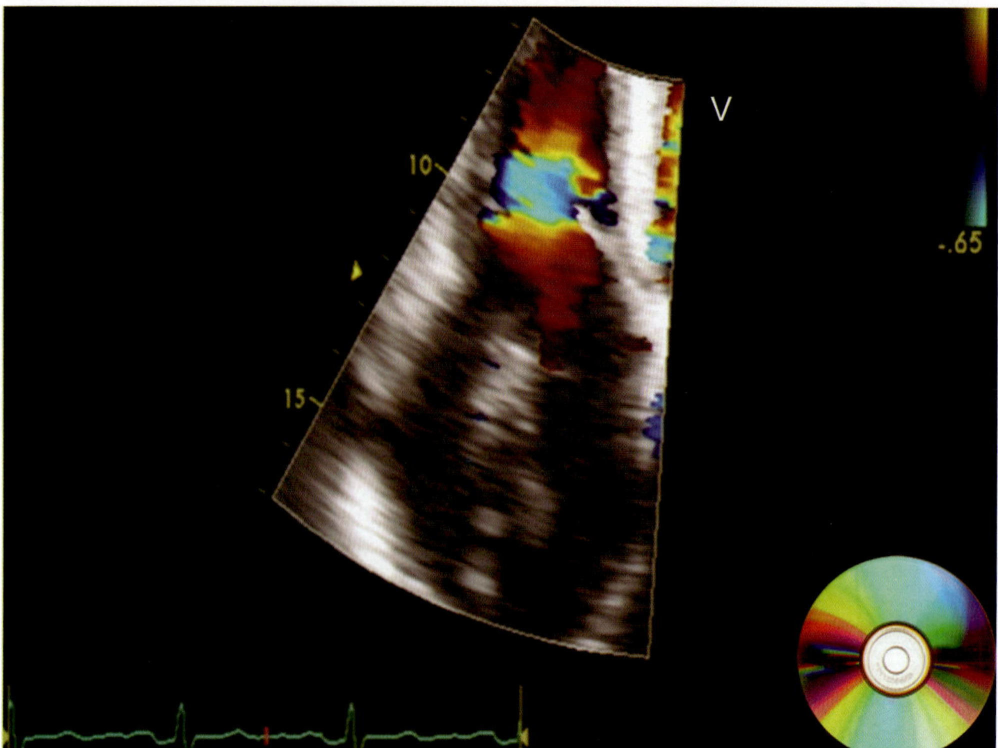

Figure 23 (VIDEO 20)

The laminar flow in tricuspid regurgitation, wherein, the regurgitant volume is much greater for a given transvalvar pressure gradient. The velocity of the jet is around 2 m/s

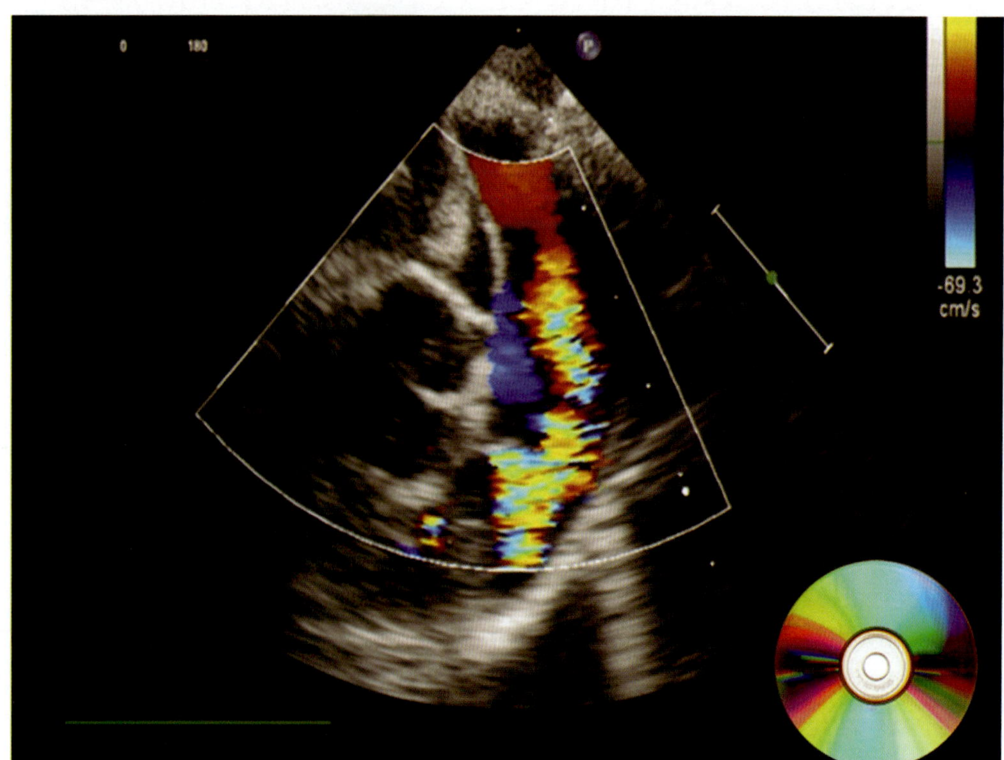

Figure 24 (VIDEO 21)

Severity of RVOT abstruction should be ruled out with Doppler. This may dilate the TV annulus and cause a TR as in this 22-year-old male

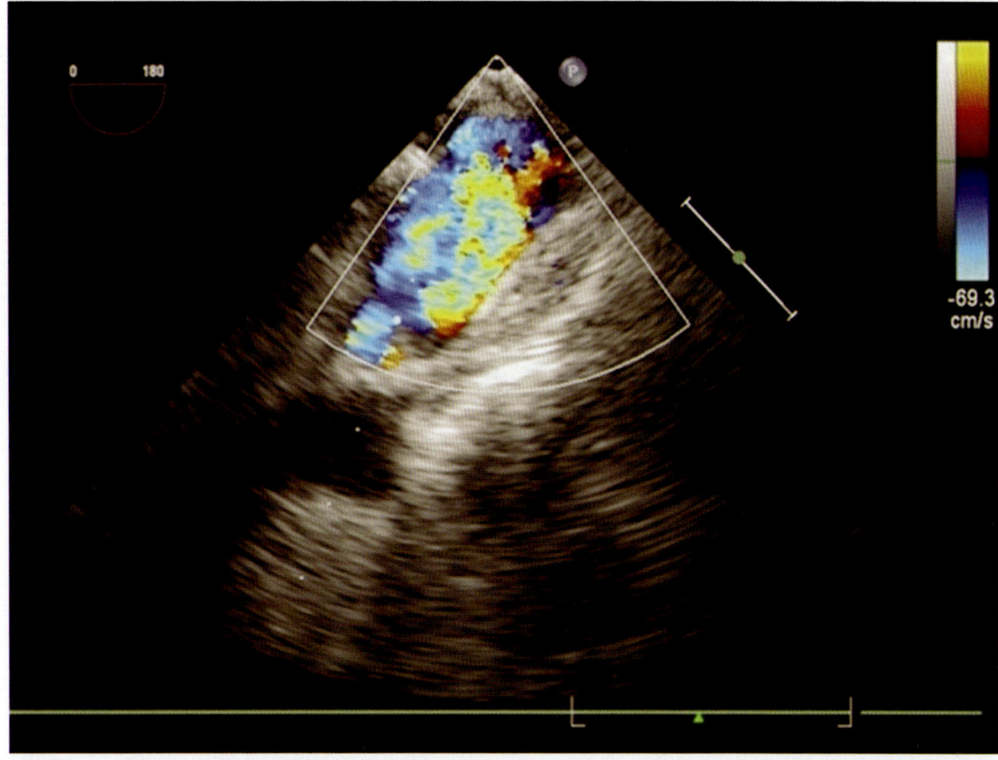

Figure 25

Twelve TR seen in a 17-year-old with TOF due to high RV end-systolic and end-dystolic pressure

structural valve abnormalities and dilatation of the tricuspid annulus (most likely related to previous surgery). Furthermore, tricuspid regurgitation was significantly correlated with right ventricular volume, suggesting that tricuspid regurgitation may also contribute significantly to right ventricular dilatation in postoperative TOF patients **(Fig. 25)**. These results are in agreement with the study by Kobayashi et al. who found that tricuspid regurgitation is significantly associated with pulmonary regurgitation, residual VSD, and right ventricular end-systolic and end-diastolic pressures.[39]

DOUBLE CHAMBERED RIGHT VENTRICLE

Double chambered right ventricle (DCRV) is usually associated with VSD ready with TR. Isolated DCRV is very rare and is another variety of obstruction to right ventricular outflow tract (RVOT). It is characterized by aberrant hypertrophied muscular bands that divide the RV cavity into a proximal high pressure chamber and distal low pressure chamber located beyond the hypertrophied muscle bands **(Figs 26A and B)**. These muscle bundles may be formed by hypertrophied moderator band or markedly hypertrophied trabacula septomarginalis. The fibromuscular diaphragm causes double chambered right ventricle and the obstruction caused is sometimes progressive and very severe. The echocardiography not only shows the dense echoes by the hypertrophied bands but also the gradient across the

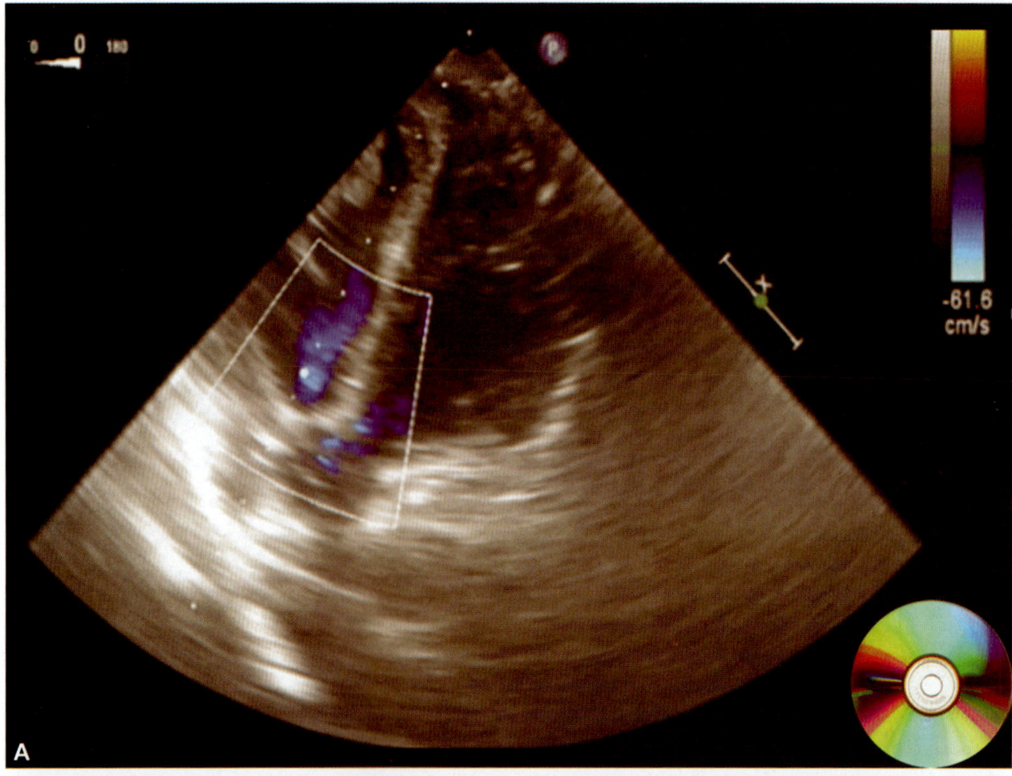

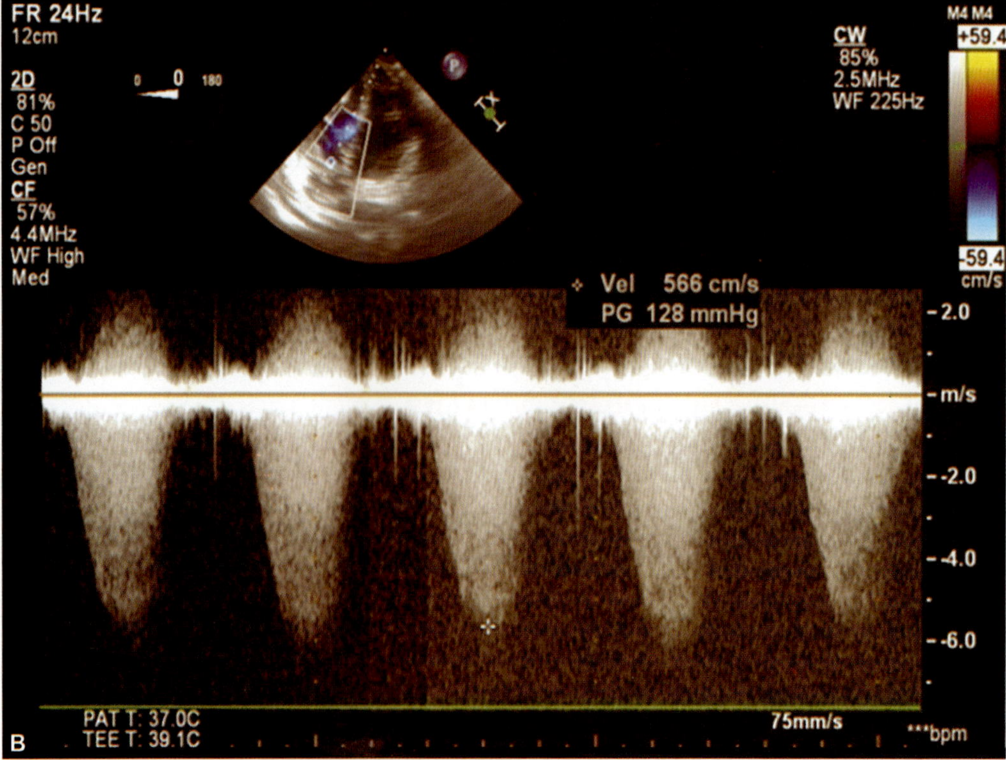

Figures 26A and B (VIDEO 22)

(A) TR coexisted with PS in this 24-year-old patient who underwent a DCRV repair with a diverge repair for the TV; (B) Double chamber right ventricle with pulmonary stenosis

chambers can be assessed, focus on ventricular—morphology, ventriculo-arterial connections and associated congenital malformations like ASD, VSD, PAPVC, TAPVC, CTGV, PS, pulmonary atresia.

CHRONIC CONSTRICTIVE PERICARDITIS

Severe tricuspid regurgitation, constrictive pericarditis and restrictive cardiomyopathy can all present with signs and symptoms of right heart failure and similar hemodynamic findings of elevation and equalization of diastolic pressures at catheterization **(Figs 27 and 28)**.

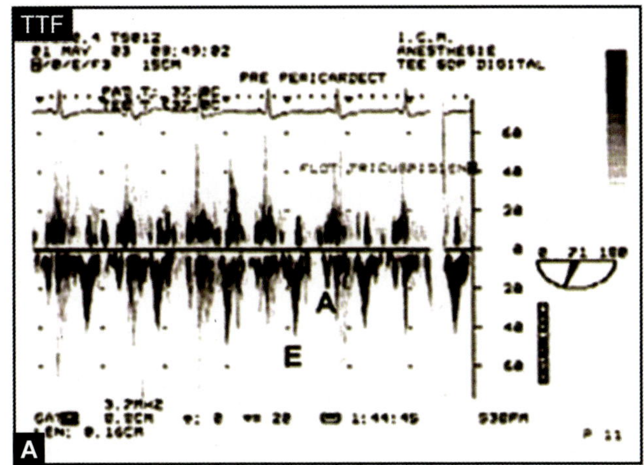

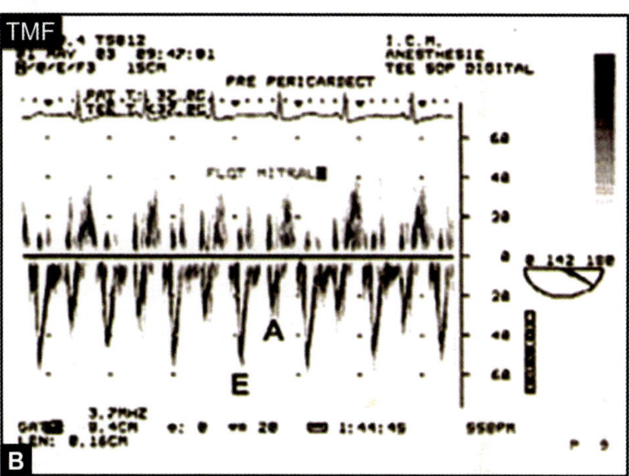

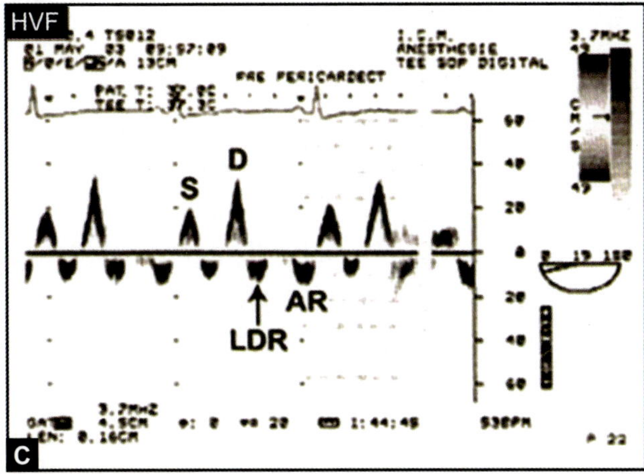

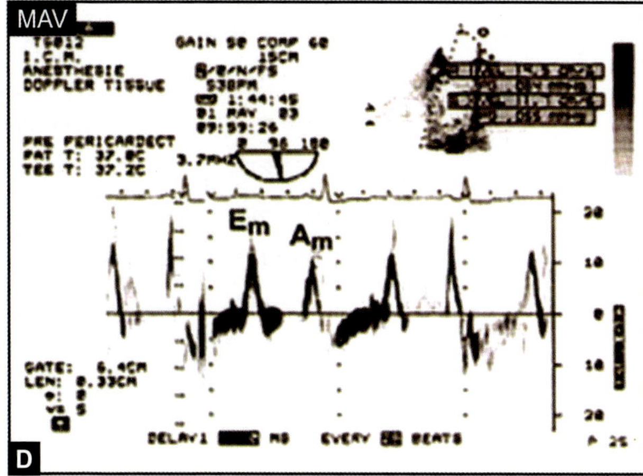

Figures 27A to D

(A) The transtricuspid flow velocity tracing displays respiratory variation. On both the Doppler TTF and transmitral flow, (B) there is predominance of the early E diastolic velocities. (C) On the hepatic venous flow Doppler tracing, there is abnormal systolic or S flow blunting with diastolic or D flow predominance and even late diastolic reversal flow. (D) Mitral annular velocity shows norma E_m velocities, which argues against the presence of restrictive cardiomyopathy

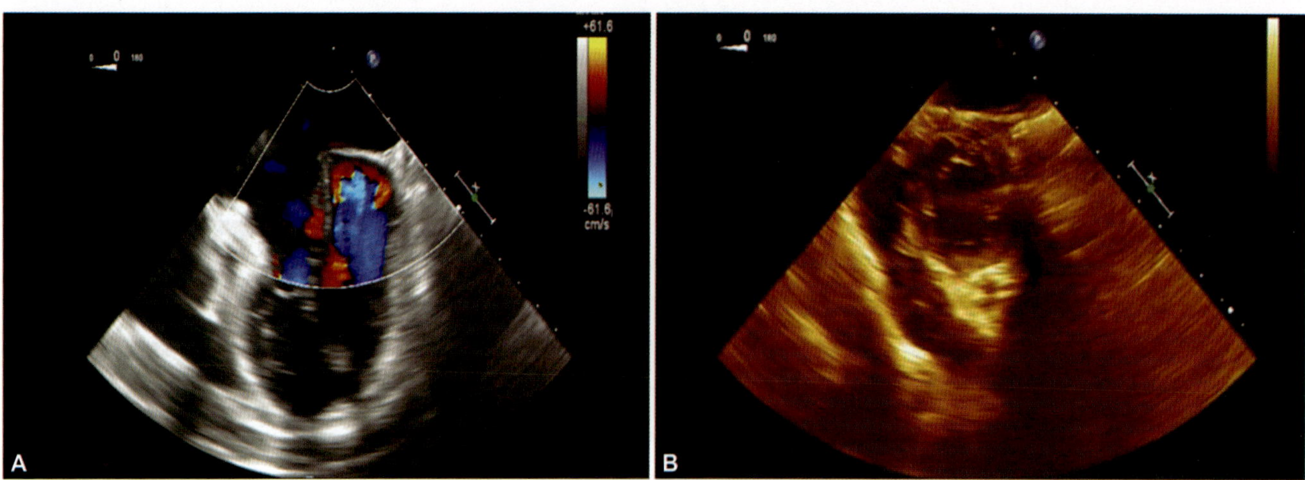

Figures 28A and B

Increased pericardial thickening and the presence of a septal bounce with dilation of TV annulus giving rise to TR

Associated findings in constrictive pericarditis peritoneal fluid from right sided failure in a 68-year-old man scheduled for pericardiectomy. Pericardial calcifications are seen on the chest X-ray and computed tomography.

Jong Won Ha, et al.[40] have showed that E′ velocity is well preserved in patients with isolated CP even when there is no characteristic respiratory variation of E velocity. Thus, when the respiratory variation in Doppler E velocity is blunted or absent during the evaluation of suspected CP in patients with restrictive mitral inflow velocity, preserved E′ velocity shown by DTE should support the diagnosis of CP over a primary myocardial disease.

The septal bounce (SB), a brief rapid motion of the ventricular septum toward the right ventricle in early diastole, is considered a reliable echocardiographic sign of pericardial constriction, but its genesis remains uncertain. There is a belief that the SB is due to the unique pathophysiology of pericardial constriction is based on two postulates: (1) the ventricles are completely enclosed by the thick constricting pericardium, (2) in early diastole the left ventricular free wall, after very early initial expansion, can expand no further, whereas, the ventricular septum is not constricted and is the only part of the left ventricle that can yield to the filling forces. This septal

Differentiate constrictive pericarditis from restrictive cardiomyopathy. TEE findings in CCP

- **Increased pericardial thickness**
- **Abnormal ventricular septal bounce**
- **Inspiratory TMF and PVF velocity variation >20%**
- **Normal or increased Vp on color M-Mode**
- **Correlate with pericardial calcification on PA view of chest X-ray and computed tomography (CT) scan**

yielding motion manifests on the 2-D echo as a typical SB, and on M-mode echo as an early diastolic brief anterior rightward motion or 'notch'.

On TTE, septal bounce, vena cava plethora, and pericardial adhesions are three 2-D echocardiographic signs that are useful in differentiating pericardial constriction from hemodynamically insignificant pericardial thickening or restrictive cardiomyopathy.[41]

Two-dimensional and M-mode echocardiographies with findings of pericardial thickening, septal bounce, and systemic venous congestion, are routinely used for the diagnosis of CCP. However, Doppler flow velocity measurements across the mitral valve have excellent sensitivity and specificity for diagnosing and distinguishing CCP from other cardiomyopathies.[42]

Typically on TEE, the signs are of a patient being in a pseudonormal stage of diastolic dysfunction with an E/A ratio 1 to 1.5 and DT > 240 ms, or in a restrictive-like stage with an E/A ratio of > 1.5 and DT < 160 ms. They show an increase in mitral E velocity greater than or equal to a 25 percent during expiration, as explained earlier. Tissue Doppler with mitral annulus velocity (E') has also been used for the measurement of diastolic dysfunction with good effects.[43]

Taguchi et al. reported in 2013 of marked increase in tricuspid regurgitation after pericardiectomy for constrictive pericarditis **(Fig. 29)**. This was thought to be due to dilatation of the right chambers and the annulus of the TV. Tricuspid

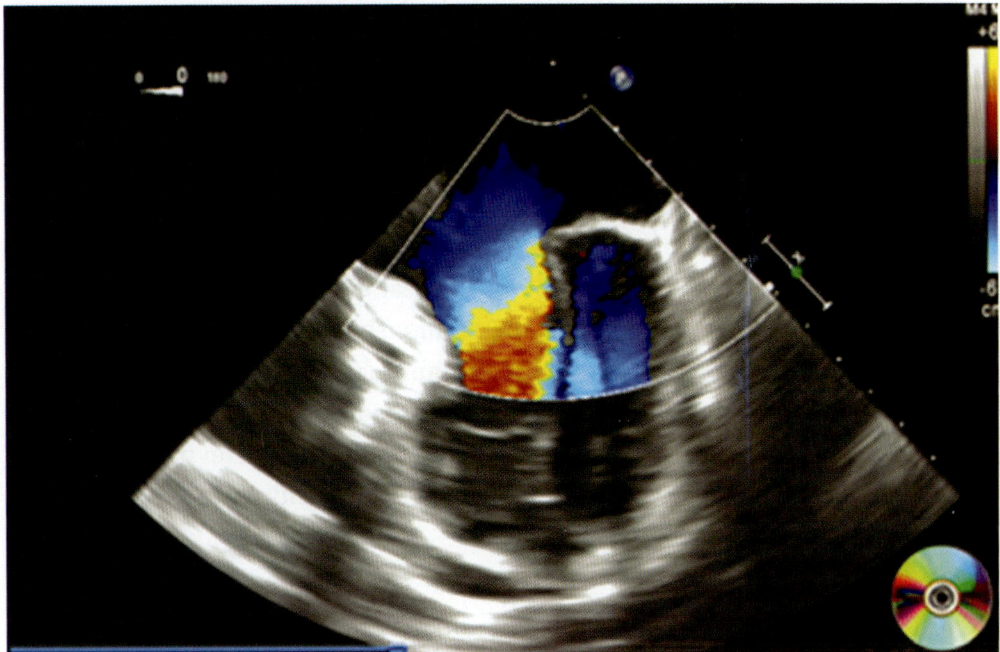

Figure 29 (VIDEO 23)

Tricuspid regurgitation in a patient with chronic constrictive pericarditis

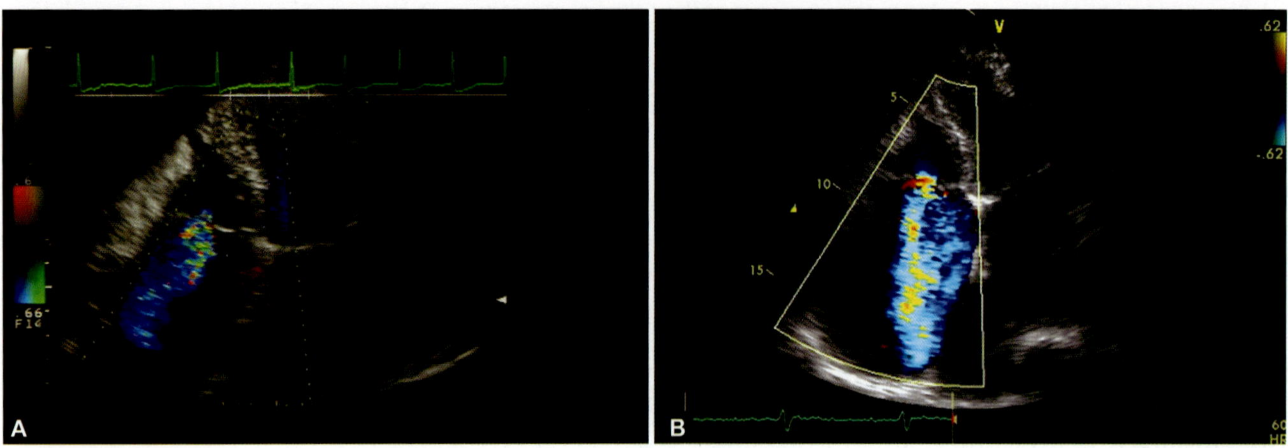

Figures 30A and B

(A) Preoperative color Doppler echocardiography showing mild-to-moderate tricuspid regurgitation (TR); (B) Postoperative color Doppler echocardiography showing severe TR

annuloplasty was performed and the authors concluded that in treating contrictive pericarditis, care must be taken to evaluate tricuspid regurgitation, even if it is mild. Even if tricuspid regurgitation deteriorates to a severe level, it may regress due to compensation **(Figs 30A and B)**.

In the case of tricuspid regurgitation as well as the hypotheses of change in RV has been reported by others for the mitral valve[44] the change in the left ventricular geometry and shift of the papillary muscles[45] increased mobility of the lateral wall, and increased the left ventricular volume,[46] was the hypotheses for the cause of MR. In the case of TR in CCP, the same hypotheses may be applied to the right ventricle.

Double Outlet Right Ventricle and Tricuspid Regurgitation

When both the great arteries arise from the right ventricle, the left ventricular stroke volume is then ejected through the VSD into both aorta and pulmonary artery, it is termed DORV. The 2-D echo provides the diagnostic information like (i) the origin and the spatial relationships of great arteries, (ii) the presence and position of infundibular septum, (iii) the relationships of the VSD to aortic and pulmonic valves, (iv) mitral to aortic discontinuity, (v) the absence or presence of pulmonic stenosis, and (vi) the association of subaortic stenosis, COS, PDA, and subpulmonic VSD **(Fig. 31A)**. The aorta and pulmonary artery run parallel and are separated by a prominent conus septum and are related entirely or predominantly to the morphologic right ventricle.

In the short axis at the cardiac base, the great arteries appear as double circles, with aorta to the right of the pulmonary trunk. The pulmonary trunk is confirmed as such by its bifurcation into right and left branches, and the aorta by

its brachiocephalic committed. There could be 16 types of DORV, depending on combination and permutation of four types of position of great arteries and four type of commitment of VSD **(Fig. 31B)**. The DORV with subpulmonic VSD is called "Taussig-Bing anomaly". TR with DORV happens due to the two great vessels arising from the RV and causing TV annular dilator.

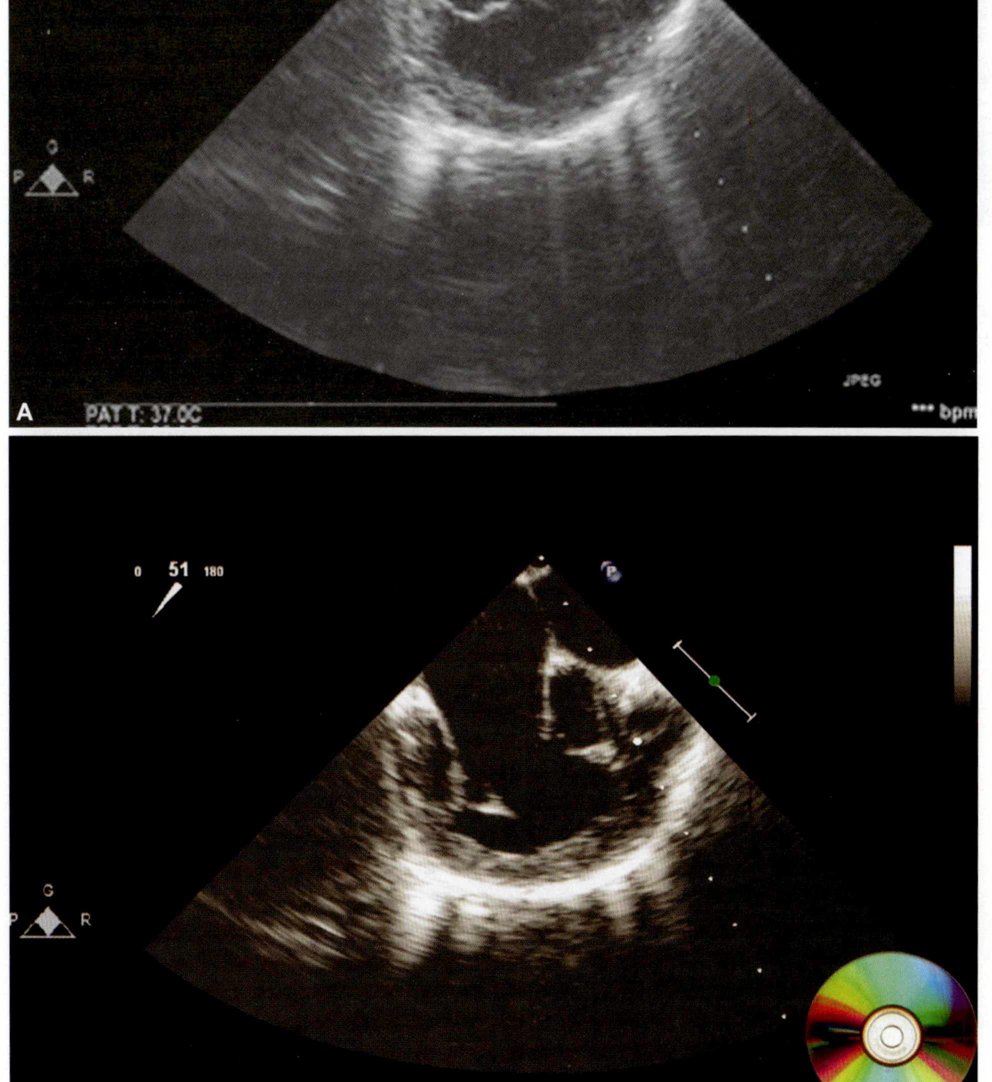

Figures 31A and B (VIDEO 24)

(A) Double outlet right ventricle with ventricle septal defect; (B) Double outlet right ventricle with ventricle septal defect with mitral stenosis

TRICUSPID REGURGITATION DUE TO EBSTEIN'S ANOMALY

The marked distortion of right ventricular and right atrial geometry occurs in Ebstein's anomaly. The approximate position of the mitral annulus is noted by the broad arrow at the lower right **(Figs 32A to C)**.

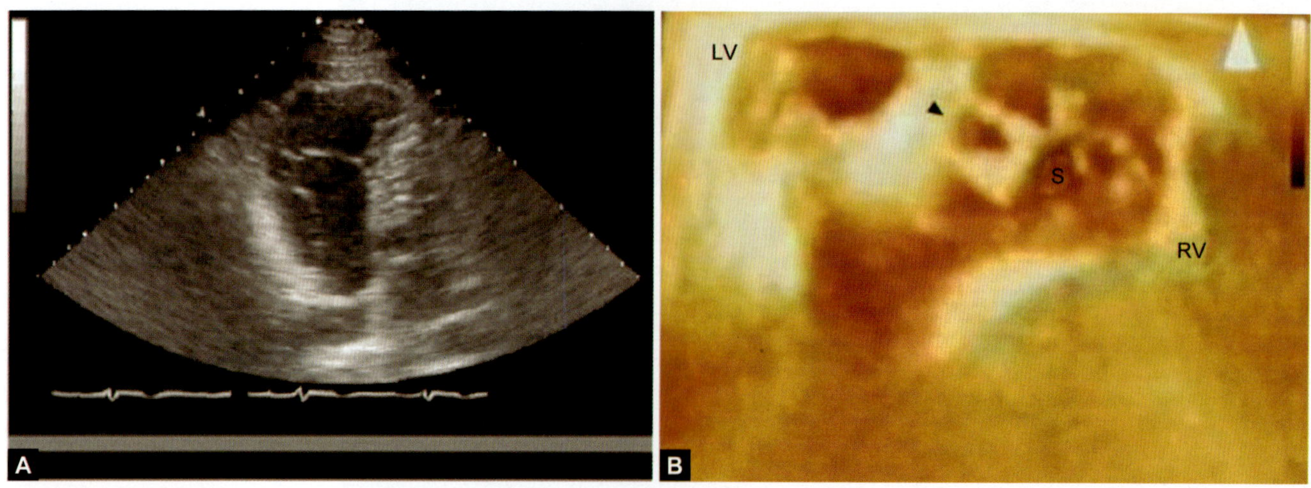

Figures 32A and B

(A) Ebstein's anomaly of tricuspid valve; (B) The arrowhead shows a bubble-like appearance resulting from tethering of the septal leaflet (S) of the tricuspid valve to the ventricular septum

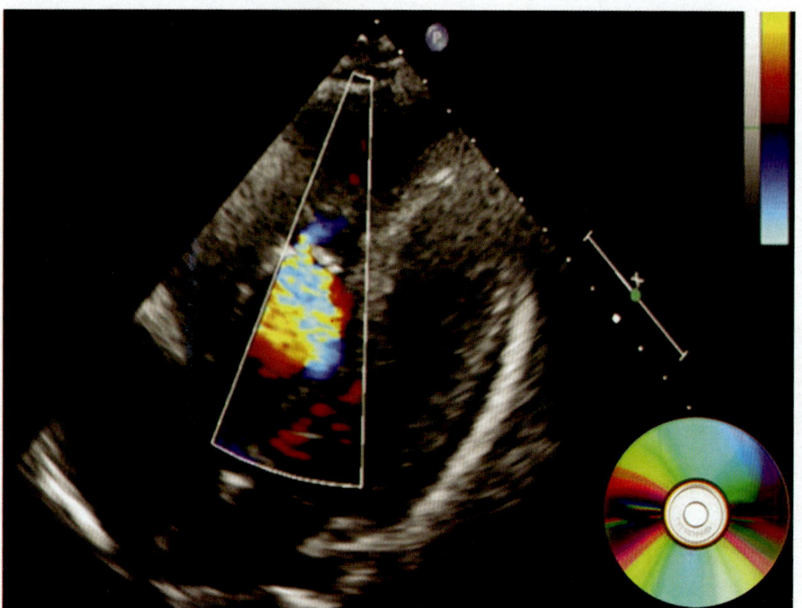

Figure 32C (VIDEO 25)

Ebstein anomaly of the tricuspid valve

"Anomaly" means a difference or irregularity. In a child born with Ebstein's anomaly, the tricuspid valve did not form properly during fetal development. One or two of its three leaflets may be "stuck" to the walls of the right ventricle or the septum (the muscular wall between the heart's left and right ventricles). The valve may be severely malformed and found lower than in a normal heart. As a result the right atrium may be larger and the right ventricle smaller than normal.

Ebstein's Anomaly in TTE

The basic anatomic feature of Ebstein's anomaly is a remarkable displacement of septal—tricuspid leaflet leading to three morphological components in the right side of the heart. These components are: (i) right atrium proper, (ii) the functional right ventricle, and (iii) intervening zone that is anatomically ventricular but functionally right atrium (atrialized right ventricle). The displacement of septal tricuspid leaflet is measured as the distance from the anatomic annulus to the distal attachment of the septal leaflet. For the diagnosis of Ebstein's anomaly, the displacement index to body surface area of 8 mm/m^2 is significant **(Figs 33A and B)**.

Two dimension (2D) echo is uniquely equipped for studying and establishing the diagnosis of Ebstein's anomaly. M-Mode imaging reveals an increased

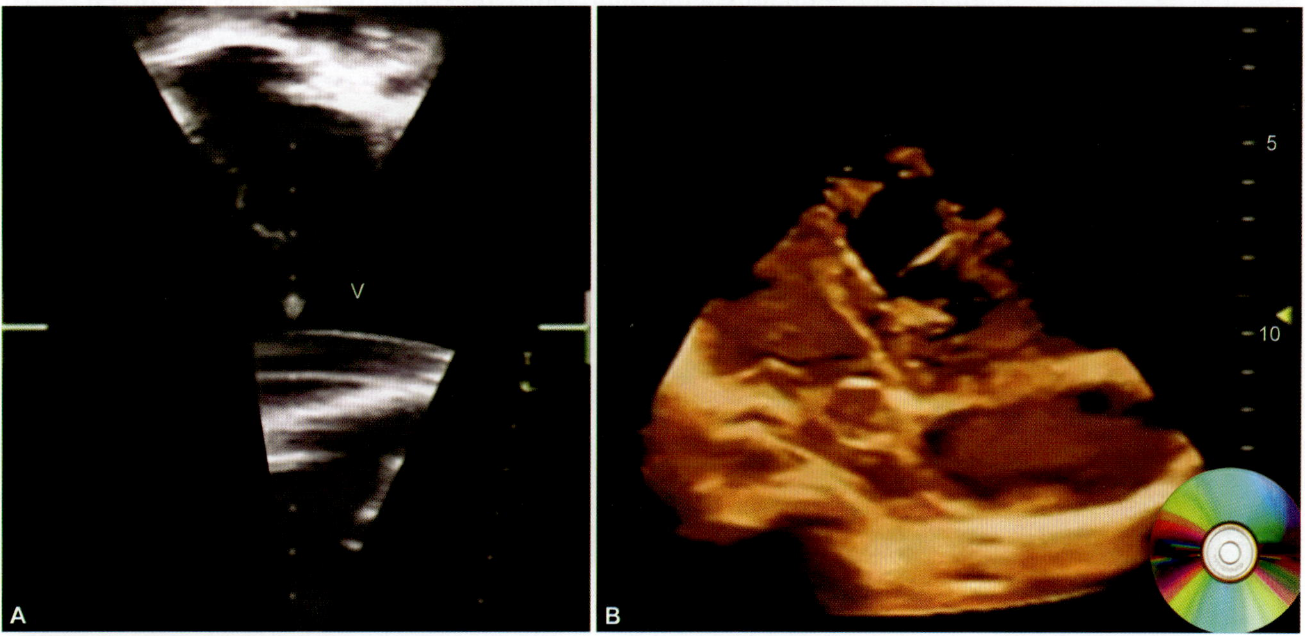

Figures 33A and B (VIDEO 26)

Three dimension (3D) echo cardiogram of Ebsteins' anomaly of tricuspid valve regurgitation

excursion of the anterior tricuspid leaflet and delayed closure of the tricuspid valve. An exception to this useful sign is the closure of tricuspid valve earlier than closure of mitral valve in response to pre-excitation of the right ventricle (WPW syndrome).

In apical four chamber view displacement of the septal tricuspid leaflet is measured as the distance from the anatomic annulus to the distal attachment of the septal leaflet, the atrialized right ventricle is identified in the same view as the distance between the anatomic tricuspid annulus and the functional annulus, defined as the leading edge of the displaced septal leaflet.

The functional right ventricle occupies the area distal to the displaced leaflet and the large atrialized RV and the large atrium is proximal to the anatomic annulus. The tethered septal leaflet is in contrast to the "whip like" or "sail like" motion and the diastolic doming of the large, elongated anterior leaflet seen in real time.

The parasternal long axis view and apical four chamber view shows septal tricuspid leaflet adherent to IVS. The echo in and cavity size caused by diastolic displacement of the atrialized ventricular septum toward the left ventricular free wall leads to tricuspid regurgitation developing.

Tricuspid Atresia and TR

The atretic tricuspid valve is represented by dense band of echoes. The 2D echo is not only diagnostic of tricuspid atresia, but also establishes the position of great arteries, the condition of the inter-ventricular septum and the nature of ASD. A TR may be seen in this anomaly **(Figs 34A and B)**.

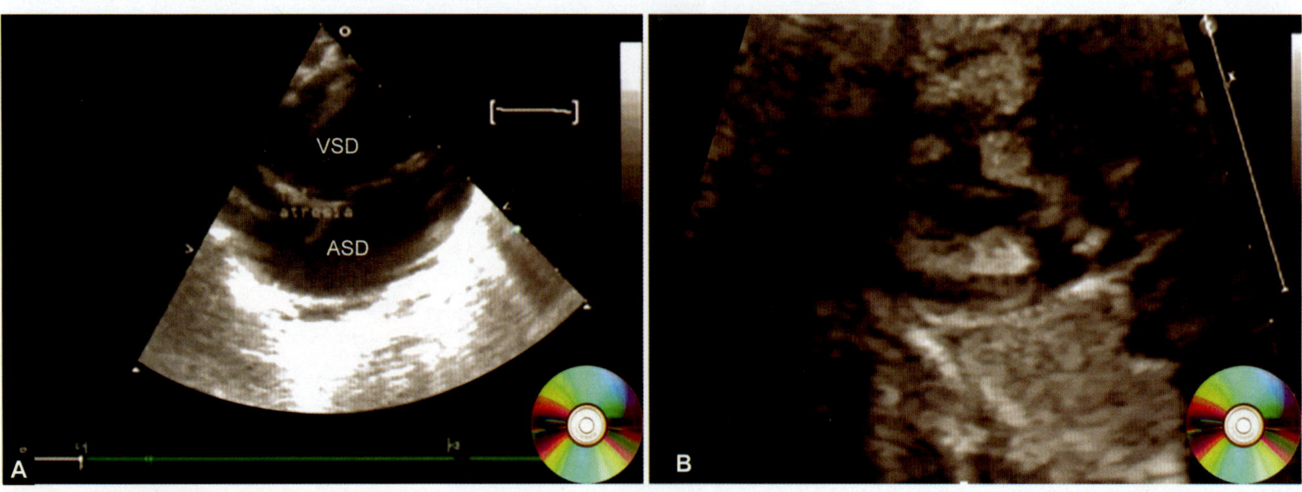

Figures 34A and B (VIDEOS 27 and 28)

(A) Tricuspid atresia with ASD and VSD; (B) 3D tricuspid atresia

- **For the diagnosis of Ebstein's anomaly, the displacement index to body surface area of 8 mm/m^2 is significant.**

The ventricular to great arterial connections are best established in parasternal and subcostal short axis views. These views along with CW Doppler study assist in identification of the presence or absence of pulmonic stenosis and collaterals.

The comparison of the relative sizes of aortic root and pulmonary trunk can also be done in the common variety of tricuspid atresia, the apical 4 chamber view identifies a dense band of echoes at the site normally occupied by the tricuspid valve. The right ventricular cavity is small, and the left ventricular cavity is only moderately enlarged.

The right atrium is increased in size and the atrial septum bulges towards the left if the interatrial communication is restrictive. When tricuspid atresia occurs with transposition of the great arteries, a large ventricular septal defect is imaged in the apical 4 chamber view and the right ventricular cavity is well developed. When pulmonary stenosis is present the echocardiogram identifies the obstruction.

ABSENT PULMONARY VALVE

TOF with Pulmonary Valve and Absent Left Pulmonary Artery and Tricuspid Regurgitation

The incidence of absent left pulmonary artery is 2.8 percent and absent right pulmonary artery is 0.7 percent. The patients with TOF with unilateral absence of pulmonary artery or valve are high-risk group for whom there is no consensus on the correct approach to management.

Usually in TOF there is RV hypertrophy, infundibular and/or pulmonary valvar stenosis with small underfilled and under developed pulmonary tree. In contrast in TOF with absent pulmonary regurgitation and though the pulmonary annulus is narrow causing stenosis, the pulmonary artery is huge and aneurysmally dilated.

Truncus Arteriosus and Tricuspid Regurgitation

The truncus arteriosus is characterized by a single great artery that arises the base of the heart and gives rise to coronary, pulmonary and systemic arteries. The pulmonary valve is absent. 2D echo in parasternal long axis view reveals large single arterial trunk overriding a large defect in the infundibular septum, with continuity between the truncus and the anterior mitral leaflet.

Quantification of tricuspid regurgitation

- **Vena contracta**
- **Hepatic vein systolic reversal**
- **Annular dimensions**
- **Pulmonary artery pressure**
- **Right ventricle function**
- **Fluid status (IVC, RA, IAS)**

The short axis reveals blunt RVOT with no pulmonary valve or pulmonary artery, but sometimes more than three cusps in truncal valve. Normally the ascending aorta does not give rise to any branches, other than coronaries. But in truncus arteriosus, direct visualization of truncal origin of the main pulmonary artery from the side of truncus (type 1), or separate right and left branches (type 2) is the major requirement for echocardiographic diagnosis. The truncal valve is usually tricuspid or quadricuspid. Direct visualization of truncal origin of the main pulmonary artery or its main branches is the major requirement for the echocardiographic diagnosis of truncus arteriosus. A TR accompanies this lesion due to annular dilation, giving rise to RV dysfunction.

M-Mode in TR

The most prominent and consistent findings on M-mode or 2D echocardiography in tricuspid regurgitation are enlargement of the right ventricle and right atrium. *Additional findings include:* The tricuspid annulus is often dilated. Septal movement may be paradoxical, reflecting the increased RV volume overloaded pattern B "bump" or "notch" indicates increased right ventricular end diastolic pressure ($\geq$ 9 mm Hg) within the right ventricle (diastolic overload). Right ventricular function may be hyperdynamic, normal or reduced, reflecting the underlying cause of the tricuspid regurgitation. Tricuspid valve motion may be normal or abnormal if there is a primary valvular abnormality such an Ebstein's anomaly, carcinoid, rheumatic valve disease, prolapse, flail leaflet, or endocarditis.[47] The presence of pulmonary hypertension can be established by abnormalities of pulmonic valve motion, especially an absence of the wave **(Figs 35 and 36)**.

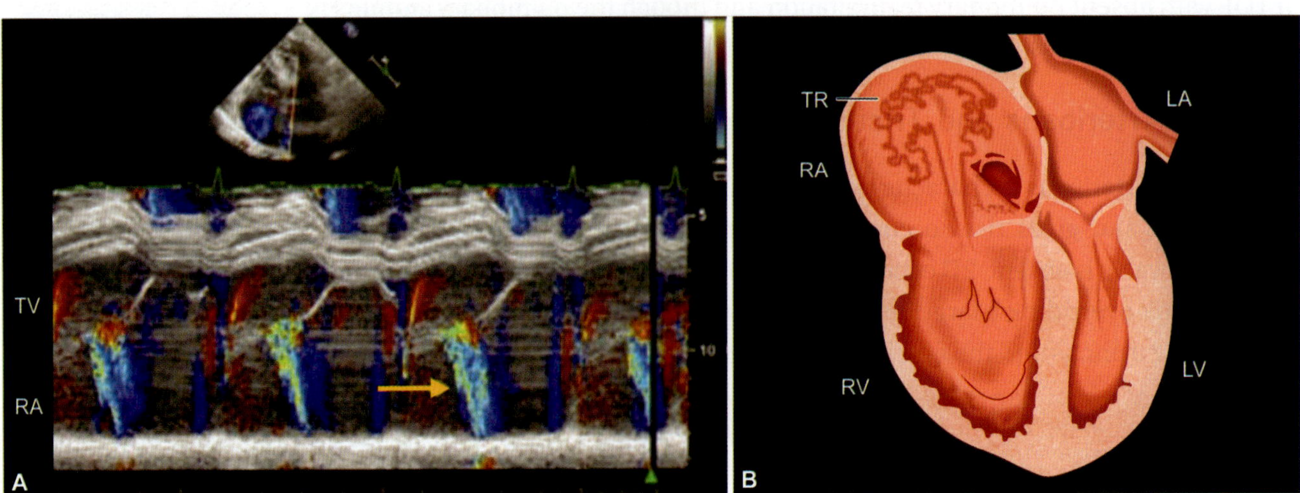

Figures 35A and B

Color M-mode examination in 40-year-old patient shows mid to late systolic TV regurgitation (arrow)

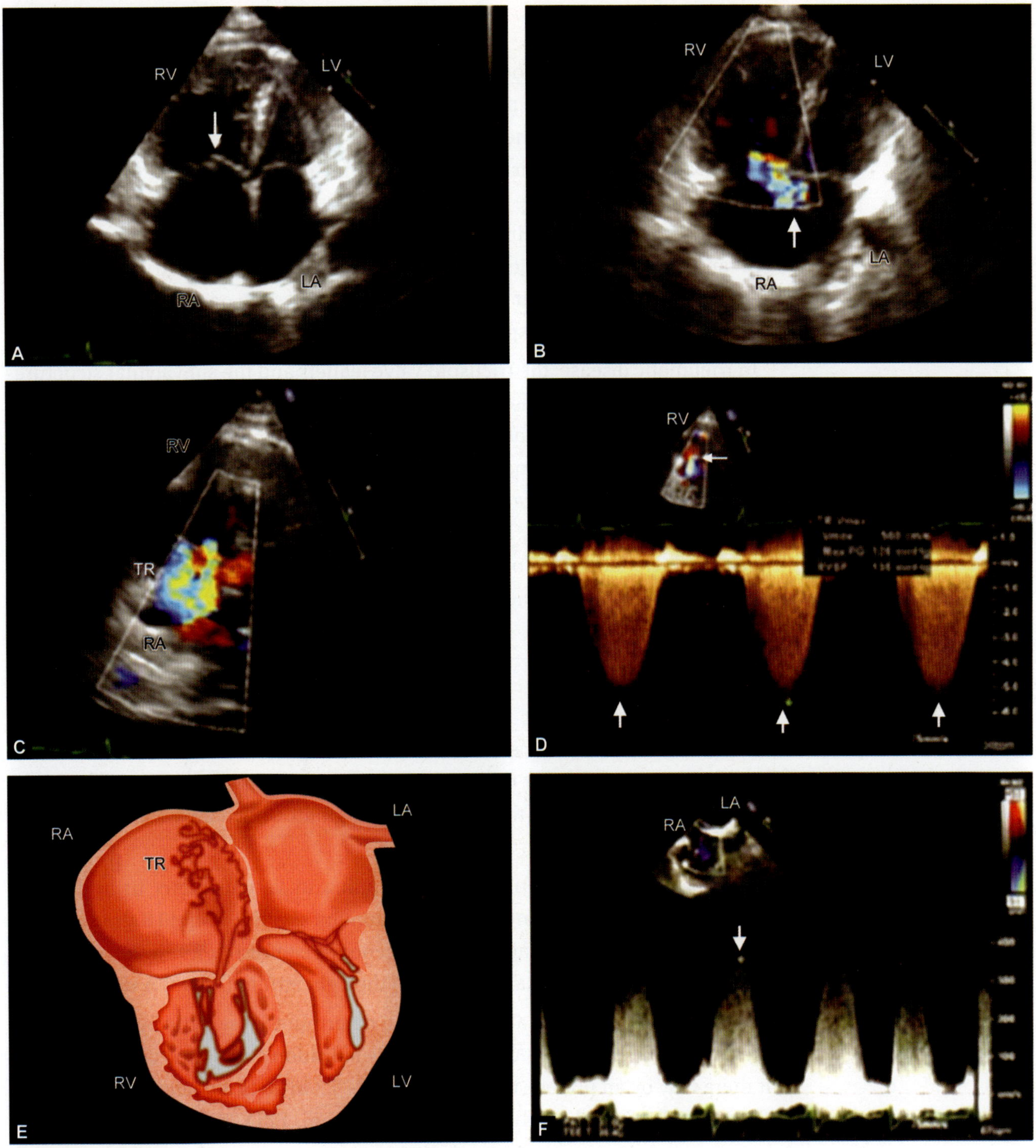

Figures 36A to F

Schematic illustrates a dilated RV and RA, an eccentrically directed TR jet and bulging of atrial septum toward the LA. Transesophageal echocardiography at 124° in a different patient. The pulmonary artery systolic pressure measured from tricuspid regurgitation jet was calculated to be 60 mm Hg (arrow)

2D ECHOCARDIOGRAPHY

Significant TR may be associated with right atrial and annular dilatation, RV dysfunction/enlargement, paradoxical ventricular septal motion, ruptured chordae or vegetations on the valve caused by endocarditis. Since the right atrium is not always completely visualized on TEE in the same view as the maximum regurgitant jet area, absolute areas have been used. Mild regurgitant is considered to be present when the maximum area is 4 cm^2, moderate when the jet area is 4 to 8 cm^2 and severe when the jet is 8 cm^2. In functional TR, secondary to pulmonary artery hypertension, annular dilatation >3.2 cm in systole or >3.4 cm in diastole is associated with severe tricuspid regurgitation.[48]

In rheumatic disease, the tricuspid valve leaflets and the subvalvular structures are often thickened, shortened and retracted, leading to incomplete coaptation. In carcinoid disease, right atrial and ventricular enlargement is present in up to 90 percent of cases.[49] In myxomatous tricuspid valve disease, billowing and prolapse of leaflets is seen. In endocarditis, friable, mobile and destructive lesions can be observed. Ebstein's anomaly is characterized by apical displacement of TV into the RV causing "arterialization" of the right ventricle. It is diagnosed when the distance from the mitral annulus to the septal leaflet exceeds at least 8 mm/m^2 body surface area.[50]

COLOR FLOW DOPPLER

The diameter of the vena contracta (VC), defined as the narrowest part of the regurgitant jet distal to the regurgitant orifice, is a simple, quantitative method which correlates well with the effective regurgitant orifice area (EROA) and the regurgitant volume.[51]

Overall, color flow Doppler (CFD) mapping in various views using jet area correlates well with clinical measures of regurgitant severity.[52] Mild TR shows a small central color jet with minimal flow convergence in contrast to severe TR, which has very large flow convergence and jet area in the right atrium **(Figs 37A to E)**.

Color flow imaging may also be used to determine TR severity by the proximal isovelocity surface area (PISA) method or visualization of the vena contracta width but there may be an underestimation of severe TR in 20 to 30 percent of patients.[53] PISA method is based on the continuity equation. PISA is the surface area of a

- **The increased RV volume overloaded pattern B "bump" or "notch" indicates increased right ventricular end diastolic pressure (≥ 9 mm Hg) within the right ventricle (diastolic overload)**
- **In functional TR, secondary to pulmonary artery hypertension, annular dilatation >3.2 cm in systole or >3.4 cm in diastole is associated with severe tricuspid regurgitation.**

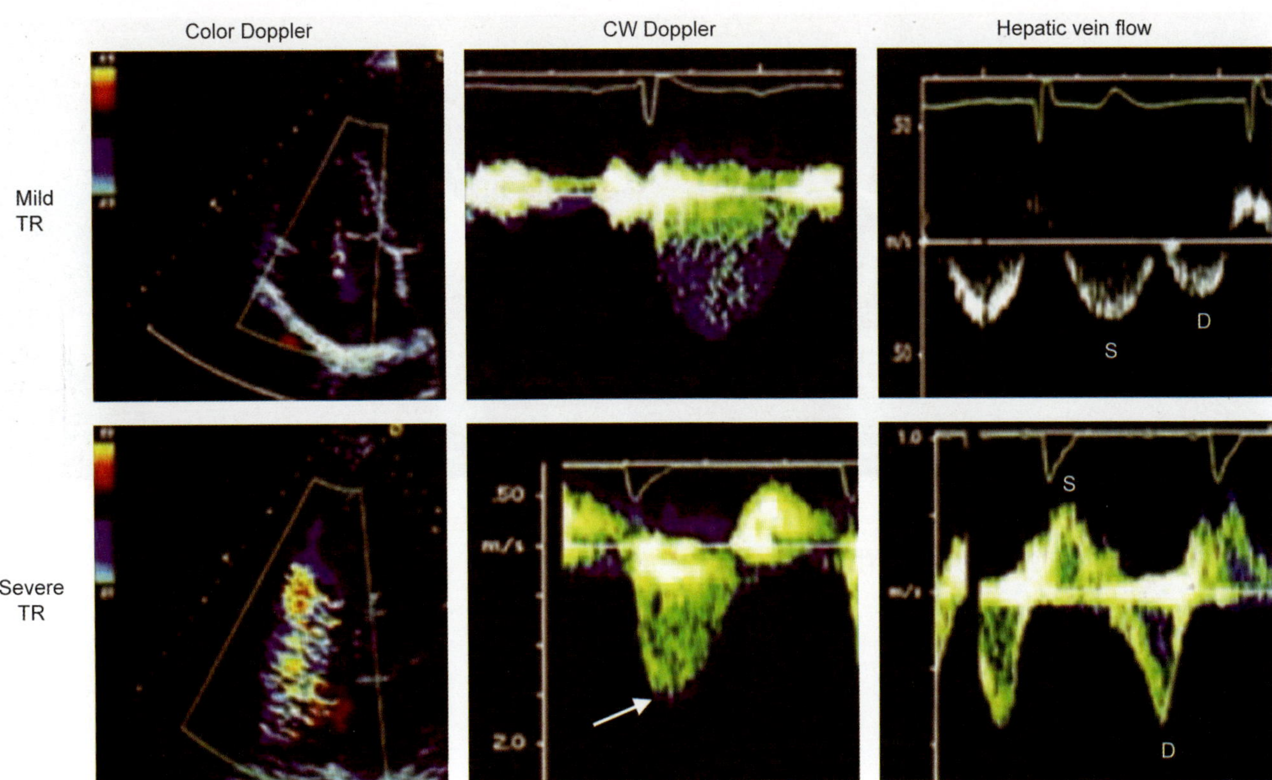

Figure 37A

Examples of jet recordings by color Doppler, continuous wave (CW) Doppler, and hepatic vein flow by pulsed Doppler in a case of mild tricuspid regurgitation (TR) and another with severe TR. The case of mild TR shows a small central color jet with minimal flow convergence in contrast to the severe TR with a very large flow convergence and jet area in the right atrium. CW Doppler recording shows a parabolic spectral display in mild TR whereas in severe TR, early peaking and triangular shape of the velocity is seen (arrow). Hepatic vein flow pattern in mild TR is normal whereas in severe TR, hepatic venous flow reversal in systole (S) is seen. (D: Diastolic hepatic venous flow)

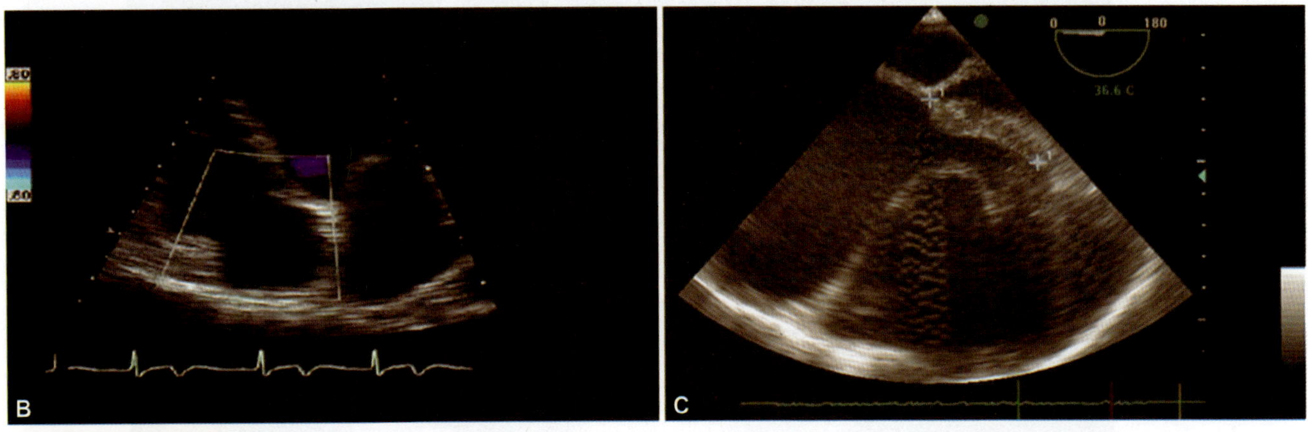

Figures 37B and C

(B) Mild tricuspid regurgitation; (C) Severe tricuspid regurgitation

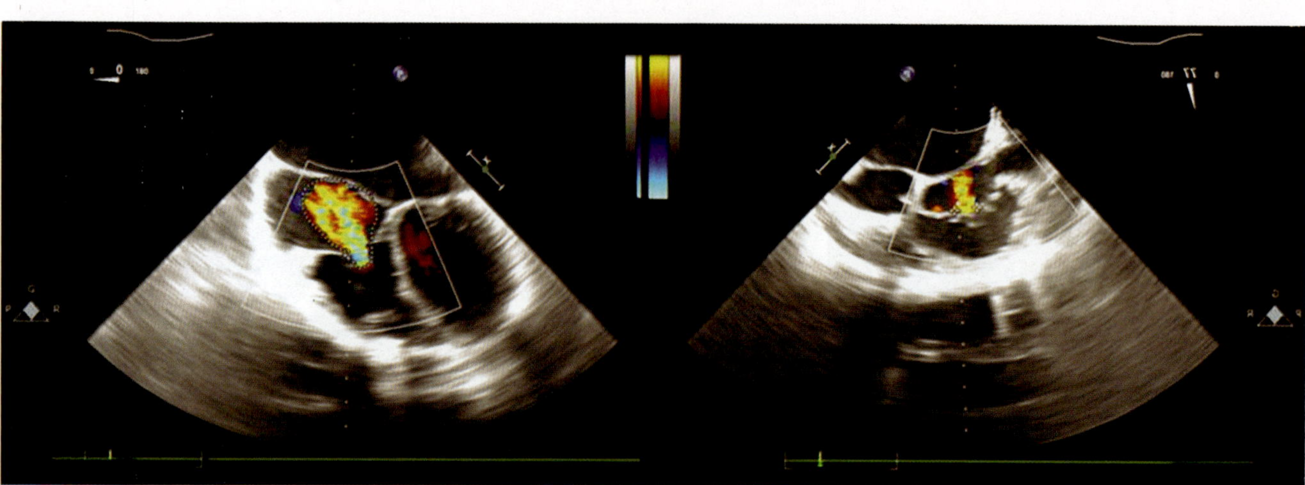

Figure 37D

Mild tricuspid regurgitation with post MVR

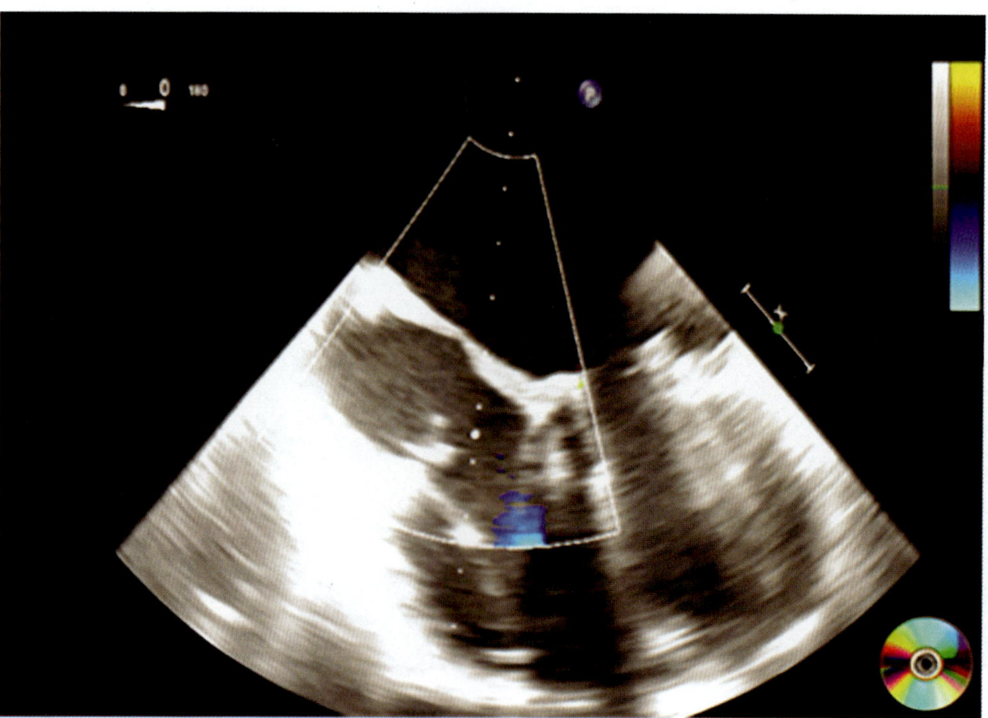

Figure 37E (VIDEO 29)

Mild tricuspid regurgitation with mitral valve repair

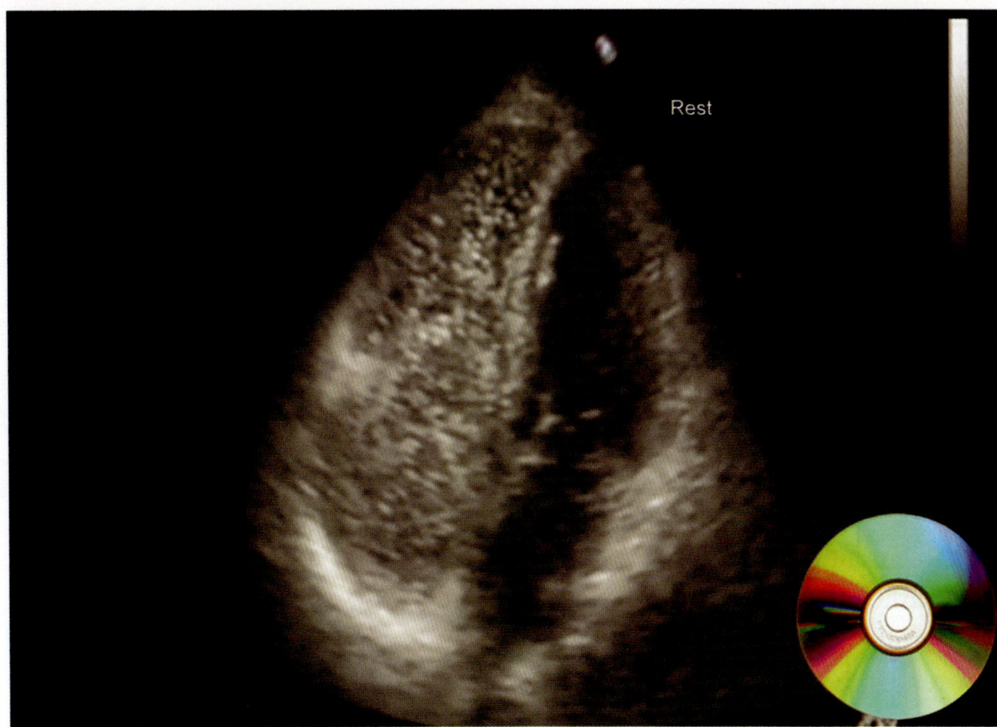

Figure 38 (VIDEO 30)

Huge tricuspid regurgitation

hemisphere at the aliasing region formed by layers of equal velocity caused by flow acceleration and convergence through a small circular orifice in a flat plate. The PISA method has been validated in small studies.[54] The vena contracta width >0.65 cm identified severe TR with a sensitivity of 89 percent and a specificity of 93 percent. Eccentric, wall-impinging jets may be underestimated **(Fig. 38)**.

CONTINUOUS WAVE DOPPLER FOR TRICUSPID VALVE

Currently, TR is diagnosed by noting reversed color Doppler flow signals moving from the right ventricle into the right atrium during systole. Similar to mitral regurgitation, its severity can be estimated by noting the size of the regurgitant jet in relation to the size of the right atrium taken in the same frame, which shows the largest area of regurgitation. Multiple examining planes should be assessed for the largest jet keeping the Nyquist limit between 40 and 50 cm/s and optimizing color gain as described in the chapter on mitral valve disease for evaluation of mitral regurgitation severity. In patients with eccentric TR, portions of the jet may no longer appear to have a mosaic pattern of colors indicative of high velocity and turbulence because of a marked reduction in the velocity of blood cells resulting from the impact of the TR jet with the adjoining leaflet or right atrial wall immediately after its exit from the TV. This Coanda effect converts a significant portion of the high velocity turbulent flow signals into low velocity laminar flow signals, which are easily recognized, because they move with the turbulent flow signals in systole. They need to be taken into account when assessing TR severity. Also, in patients with very severe TR, for example in patients with markedly deficient TV leaflet tissue, the pressure in the right atrium and right ventricle are almost equal (both the right atrium and right ventricle practically function as a single chamber), the TR jet may show no turbulence at all and the flow signals are completely laminar. Thus, torrential TR may be completely missed and misdiagnosed as no TR. Attention to these technical factors is mandatory otherwise over or underestimation of TR severity will occur. A prominent flow acceleration and a large vena contracta are useful signs of significant TR. A TR jet extending into a hepatic vein producing reversed flow in systole usually indicates severe TR but may be noted with moderate TR also and is therefore, useful in excluding mild TR. Extension of TR into the coronary sinus is generally believed to occur only with severe TR. Unlike mitral and aortic regurgitation, angiography cannot be used as a "gold standard" to test the echocardiographic findings because the angiographic catheter has to necessarily pass through the TV for the required injection into the right ventricle which by itself may render the TV incompetent.

In contrast to PW Doppler, CWD records the velocities of all the red blood cells moving along the path of the sound beam. The Doppler beam should be oriented as parallel as possible to the flow, guided by the 2D image, color flow imaging and the presence of a well-defined envelope. CWD is used to estimate the severity of tricuspid stenosis and the pulmonary artery systolic pressures (PASP). The maximal velocity of the tricuspid regurgitation (TR) jet is measured and PASP is calculated using the simplified Bernoulli equation: PASP = 4(TR jet velocity)^2 + central venous pressure CWD may be used to evaluate the antegrade flow in the setting of tricuspid stenosis or to evaluate the TR jet. Using the TR jet, one can estimate of the RV systolic pressure: RVSP = 4 (TR peak velocity)^2 + RAP. One can also assess the intensity and rate of deceleration of the TR jet to assist in the determination of TR severity. If the Doppler alignment is suboptimal, the CWD exam should be performed in other views. In contrast to PW Doppler, CWD records the velocities of all the red blood cells moving along the path of the sound beam. The Doppler beam should be oriented as parallel as possible to the flow, guided by the 2D image, color flow imaging and the presence of a well-defined envelope. CWD is used to estimate the severity of tricuspid stenosis and the pulmonary artery systolic pressures (PASP). The maximal velocity of the tricuspid regurgitation (TR) jet is measured and PASP is calculated using the simplified Bernoulli equation:

PASP = 4 (TR jet velocity)^2 + central venous pressure where PASP is the pulmonary artery systolic pressure. Care must be taken to align the beam with the maximum TR jet, which may be more difficult in TEE then TTE. If the jet is not aligning the pressure will be underestimated.

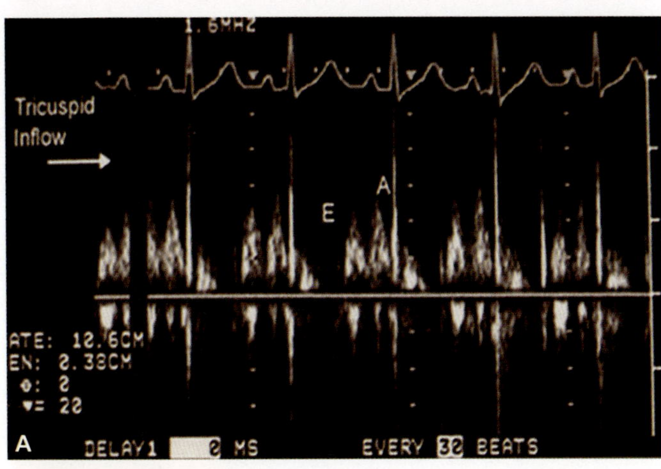

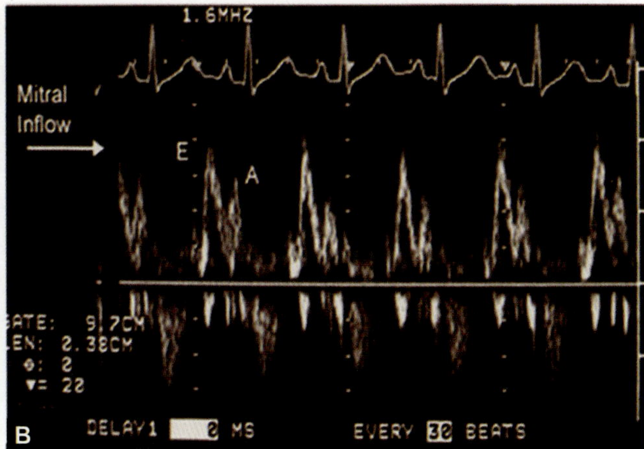

Figures 39A and B

Tricuspid and mitral valve inflow view

PULSE WAVE DOPPLER

Pulse wave Doppler is used in combination with the 2D imaging to record the flow velocity by placing the sample volume (SV) at the level of the tips of the open TV leaflets in the 4-chamber view or RV inflow-outflow view **(Figs 39A and B)**. The SV axial length is adjusted to 5 to 7 mm with low-level wall filters and the velocity is recorded over two or three respiratory cycles at a sweep speed of 50 or 100 mm/s.[55]

Peak E and A velocities and E/A ratios, velocity-time integrals and deceleration times of E wave can be determined. The TV flow velocity is about 0.3 to 0.7 m/sec. The pressure half-time method has not been as extensively validated for the calculation of tricuspid valve area as in case of the mitral valve.

PW Doppler examination of the hepatic veins can be done by advancing the probe from the bicaval view to track the inferior vena cava into the liver. The sample volume is placed 1 to 2 cm into the orifice of a central hepatic vein. The normal pattern of flow velocity consists of antegrade systolic (S wave), transient flow reversal as the TV annulus recoils at the end of systole (V wave), antegrade diastolic (D wave) and a retrograde A wave caused by atrial contraction. Both the tricuspid and hepatic flow patterns are affected by respiration **(Table 5)**. However, if the M-mode is performed without the guide by the two-dimensional image, it may miss the most adequate beam direction for the observation, resulting in underestimating severity. The influences of tricuspid regurgitation are generally seen in the flow pattern of the major veins. However, they are more sharply reflected by the flow condition in the right atrial cavity than by the flows patterns in the major veins.[56]

Table 5: Indications of severity of tricuspid Insufficiency	
Method	*Indication of severe TR*
Jet area	> 10 cm^{2}.[3]
Jet area/right atrial area	> 67%
Vena contracta width	> 6.5 cm
Hepatic vein flow profile	*Systolic flow reversal*
TR jet intensity	>65% of antegrade flow
TR jet deceleration	Rapid
TV annular dimension	>34 mm at end systole

Table 6: Grading tricuspid regurgitation			
Parameter	*Mild*	*Moderate*	*Severe*
Tricuspid valve	Usually normal	Normal or abnormal	Abnormal/flail leaflet/ poor coaptation
RV/RA/IVC size	Normal	Normal or dilated	Usually dilated
Jet area-central jets (cm^2)	<5	5–10	>10
VC width (cm)	Not defined	<0.7	>0.7
PISA radius (cm)	<0.5	0.6–0.9	>0.9
Jet density and contour—CW	Soft and parabolic	Dense, variable contour	Dense, triangular with early peaking systolic reversal
Hepatic vein flow	Systolic dominance	Systolic blunting	Systolic reversal

Severe TR will increase the early diastolic tricuspid E wave velocity (>1.0 m/s). Difficulties in measuring the TV annulus preclude the measurement of tricuspid regurgitant volume.

PW Doppler examination of the hepatic veins will show a blunting of the dominant systolic wave with increasing severity of TR and finally culminate in flow reversal with severe TR (sensitivity 80%) **(Figs 40A and B)**.[57] However, the absence of systolic flow reversal does not rule out severe TR. The hepatic vein flow patterns are also affected by abnormalities in right atrial (RA) and RV relaxation and compliance **(Table 6)**.[58]

- Severe TR will increase the early diastolic tricuspid E wave velocity (>1.0 m/s).
- PW Doppler examination of the hepatic veins show:
  - Blunting of the normally dominant systolic wave with increasing severity of TR and finally culminate in flow reversal with severe TR (sensitivity 80%).
- The hepatic vein flow patterns are also affected by:
  - Abnormalities in right atrial
  - RV relaxation and compliance
  - The phase of the respiratory cycle, preload, and atrial fibrillation.

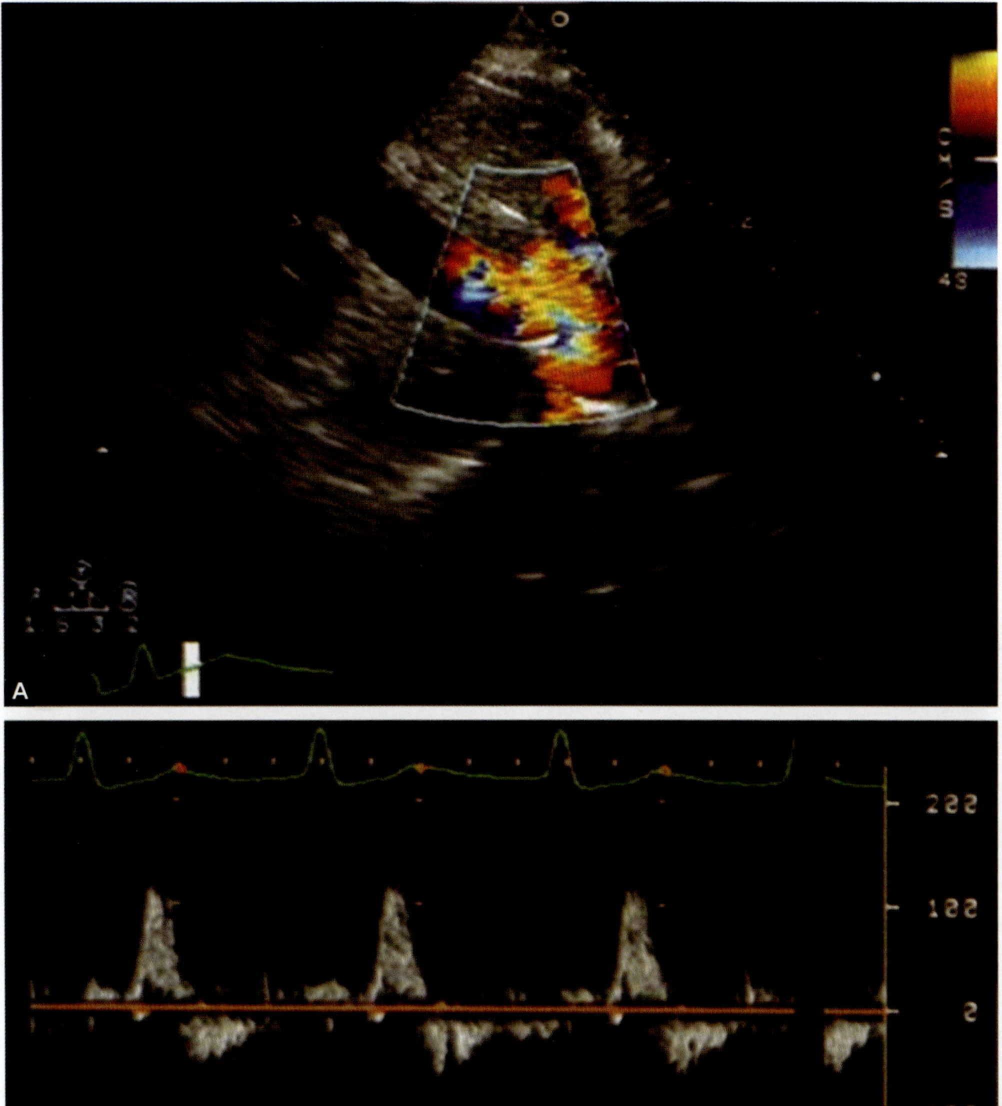

Figures 40A and B

Pulse wave Doppler in tricuspid regurgitation

MEASUREMENT OF THE VENA CONTRACTA

Tribouilloy et al. found a vena contracta width of 6.5 mm or more highly sensitive and specific in identifying severe TR. Yang et al. found a vena contracta width of > 7 mm to be a strong independent predictor of heart failure, TV surgery, and death. This group of investigators defined severe TR as jet area greater than 30 percent of right atrial area or an absolute jet area of >10 cm^2 or systolic flow reversal in a hepatic vein. A dense continuous wave Doppler TR spectral waveform suggests more significant TR as compared to a less dense envelope. This is because the density of the waveform depends on the number of reflectors, in this case the blood cells, present within the Doppler envelope. In severe TR the continuous wave Doppler waveform may change from its usual U or parabolic configuration to an asymmetric triangular shape. This is related to a marked increase in the right atrial pressure produced by the large regurgitant volume with consequent decrease in the pressure difference between the right ventricle and right atrium. An important point to remember is that mild TR detected by color Doppler is seen in many normal individuals and therefore, should not be construed as a pathologic finding. Because of the difficulty in assessing right atrial area accurately during a transesophageal study, determination of the maximum jet area is most often used in clinical practice for estimating TR severity. A jet area measuring 10 cm^2 or more indicates severe TR **(Fig. 41)**.

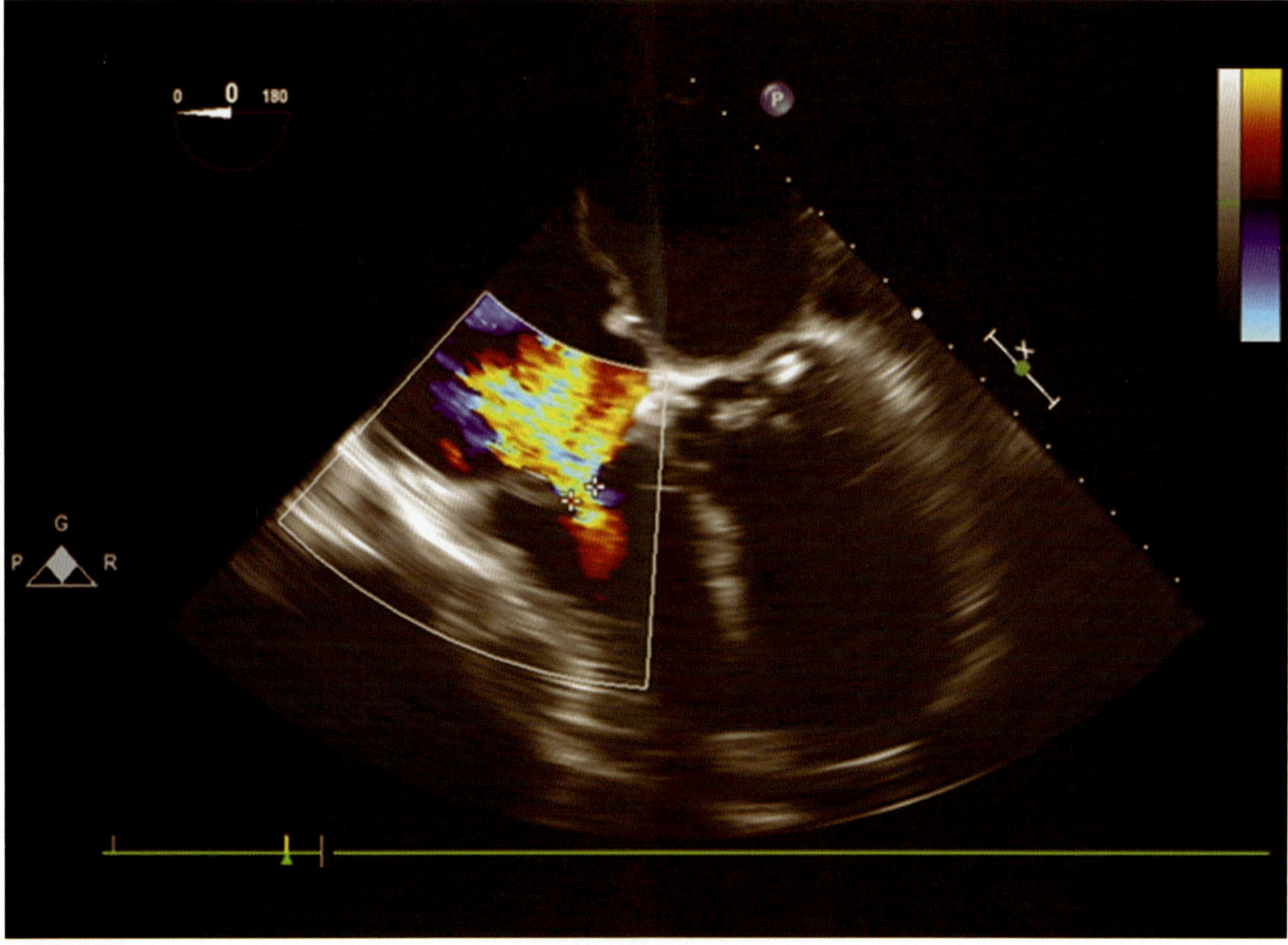

Figure 41

Measurement of vena contracta in severe tricuspid regurgitation

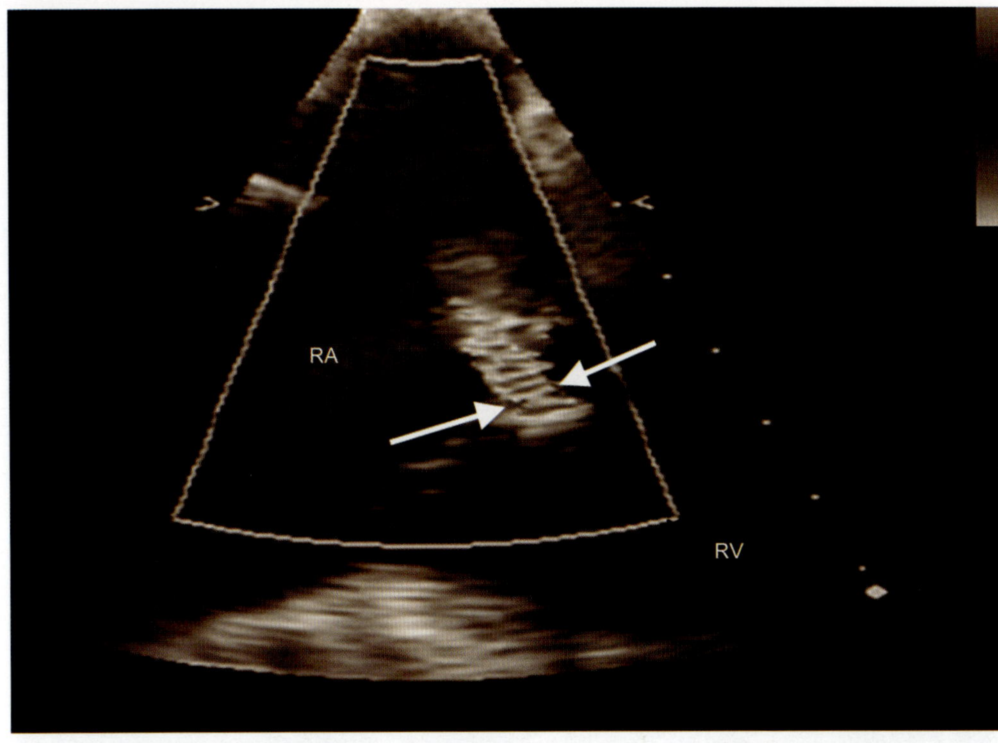

Figure 42

Twenty measurement of the vena contracta in a midesophageal 4 chamber view in a 40-year-old male

The narrowest width of the regurgitant jet that is immediately downstream to the flow convergence area—provides a more hemodynamically independent estimate of the TR severity **(Fig. 42)**. By TTE, this method has been shown to correlate well with the effective orifice area. A VC greater than 6.5 mm indicates severe tricuspid regurgitation on TEE.

MODERATE TRICUSPID REGURGITATION DURING MITRAL VALVE SURGERY

The pathogenesis of MV disease causing TR explains why patient survival would be expected to worsen as severity of TR worsens. Multiple factors such as ischemia, rheumatic heart disease or dilated cardiomyopathy lead to MV disease, which causes an increase in left atrial pressure. This leads to pulmonary hypertension and left atrial dilatation (which can lead to atrial fibrillation), which can cause tricuspid annulus dilatation. Pulmonary hypertension leads to RV dilatation and impaired function **(Fig. 43)**. The degree of TR is dependent on the degree of tricuspid annulus dilatation, RV dilatation and impaired function affecting afterload. Organic tricuspid valve disease from rheumatic heart disease can also cause TR. As TR worsens, this causes further right ventricular dilatation and reduced function, leading to worsened tricuspid annulus dilatation, leading to a worsening cycle of right heart failure.[59] Thus, patients who have progressed further along this pathway and exhibit more severe TR are more likely to have heart failure compared with patients with a lesser degree of TR **(Fig. 44)**.

This is also likely to explain why there was a significant difference in functional outcome TVR and non-TVR group. Both of these groups had TR ≥2+, with the

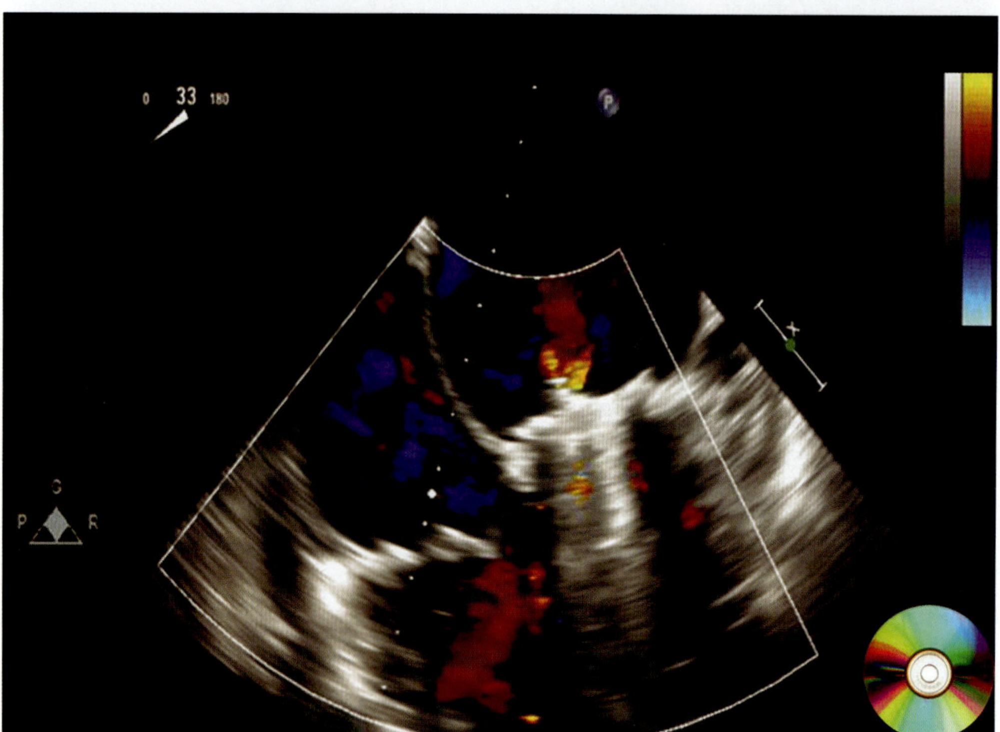

Figure 43 (VIDEO 31)

Tricuspid regurgitation with mitral stenosis

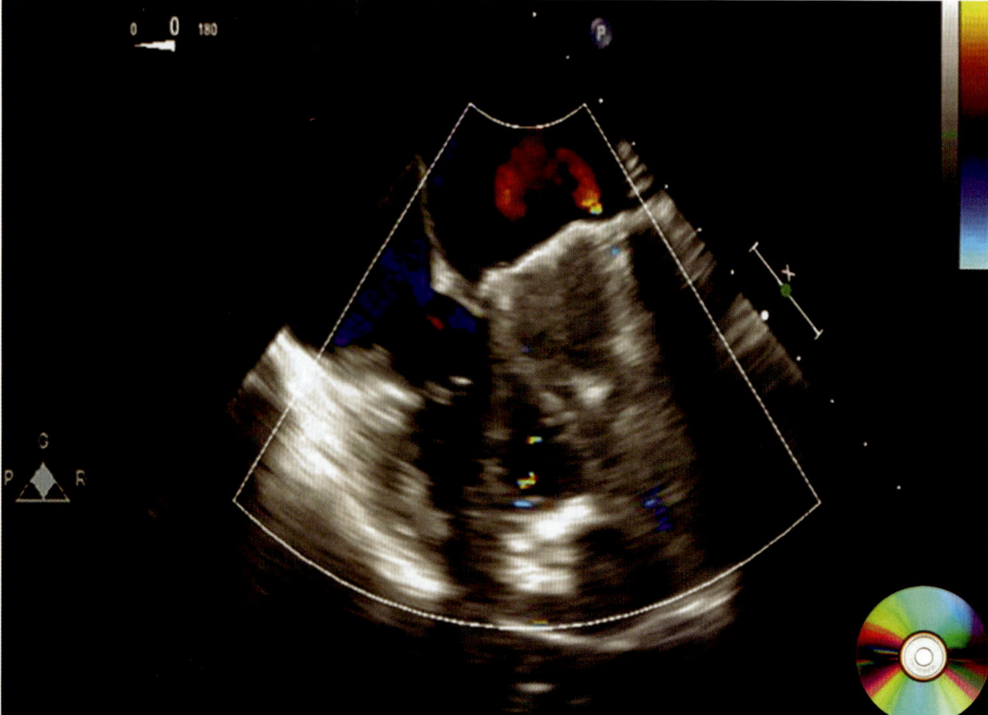

Figure 44 (VIDEO 32)

Mitral stenosis with TR

majority of patients in each group classed as a moderate level of TR; however, this means that significant annular dilatation, RV dilatation and dysfunction has already occurred, and this damage is likely to be irreversible.[60] A potential reason why the non-TVR group was found to have a significantly better functional outcome was that the higher levels of TR in this group allowed the RV to decompress compared with the TVR group.

ENDOCARDIAL LEAD INDUCED TRICUSPID REGURGITATION

A pacing lead impinges on the tricuspid valve leaflet and thus, prevents it from competent closure. Failure to diagnose this condition leads to progressive right heart failure—thus a high index of suspicion is needed as a preventive strategy in fixing the endocardial leads on the right ventricle.

The mechanism of endocardial lead—induced tricuspid regurgitation caused by a mechanical interference of the pacing lead with the tricuspid valve, may be characterized as (a) impingement (described in the majority of cases), (b) perforation, (c) entanglement or (d) adhesion as reported by some authors.[61]

A case discussed by Khoshbin et al.[62] in which a patient with pacemaker lead in which case, the endocardial lead had not only appeared to perforate the septal leaflet, but also appeared adherent to the chords and it was difficult to exclude entanglement of the lead with the chords. The authors concluded that identification of the lesion as one of the above alone was impossible.

The calcific attachments of the lead to the right atrium had a leverage effect on the valve making it difficult to sustain optimal positioning. Hence the ventricular lead was excised and replaced by an epicardial lead. These calcific adhesions may be responsible for the long-term mechanism which is known as impingement of the septal leaflet **(Fig. 45)**.

Associated Features of TR

If tricuspid regurgitation is present

- **Assess any coexistent tricuspid stenosis**
- **Assess any coexistent disease affecting the other valves (as patients undergoing tricuspid valve surgery may also require any other valvular abnormalities to be corrected at the same time)**
- **Assess the size of the RA, RV and IVC—these chambers are usually dilated if tricuspid regurgitation is severe**
- **Assess RV dimensions and function**
- **Calculate pulmonary artery systolic pressure to assess if there is pulmonary hypertension.**

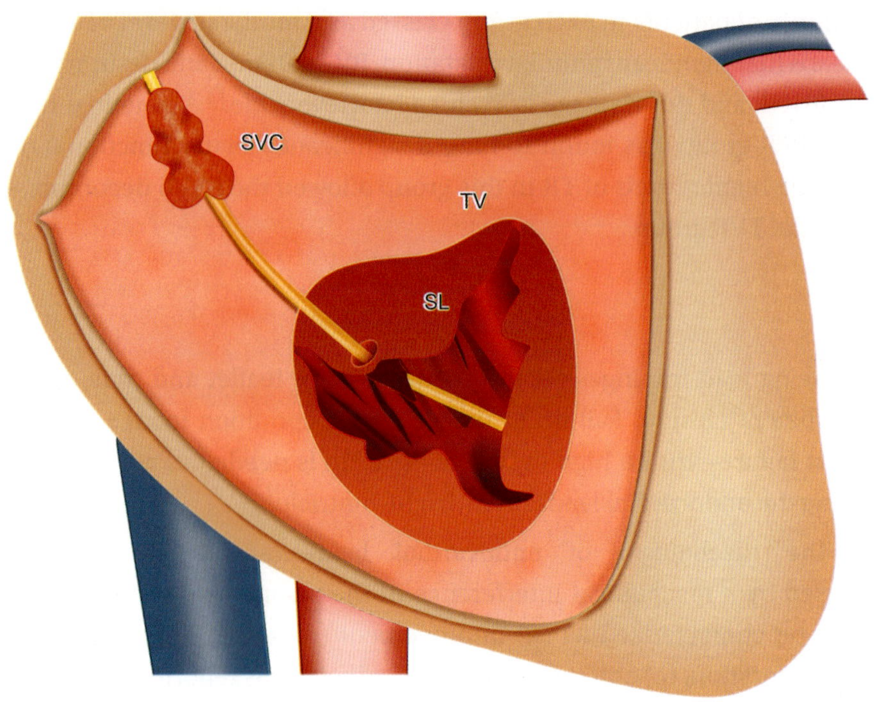

Figure 45

Transvenous pacing wire wedging the valve open as well as piercing through the septal leaflet of the tricuspid valve

TRICUSPID VALVE ANATOMY ON REAL TIME 3D ECHOCARDIOGRAPHY

The tricuspid valve has been less explored by 3DE than the mitral and aortic valves. However, considering that it is not possible to visualize all three tricuspid valve leaflets and their attachment in the annulus simultaneously in one cross-sectional view, using 2D echocardiography, 3D echocardiography developed our imaging interpretation, allowing valve and apparatus visualization from any perspective **(Fig. 46)**.

Using instantaneous full-volume echocardiography, we can assess the entire tricuspid valve and apparatus with one heart beat **(Fig. 47)** and analyze it in detail. This may improve our understanding of the pathophysiological mechanisms underlying tricuspid valve diseases. It was already described that the 3DE measurements of the tricuspid annulus are accurate compared with magnetic resonance imaging and may have an important implication in the surgical decision making processes. When comparing the tricuspid annulus with the mitral annulus using 3DE, it appears less nonplanar with a round or oval shape.[63]

Regarding functional tricuspid regurgitation, secondary to pulmonary hypertension, additional geometric changes were characterized by 3DE, showing enlargement of tricuspid tenting volume and dilatation of the annulus.[64]

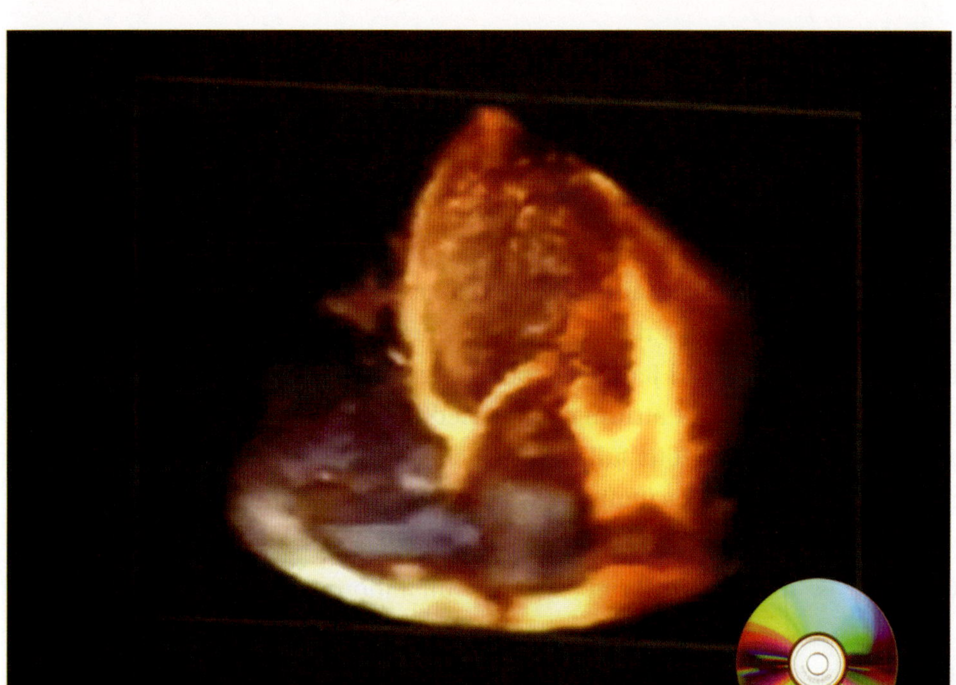

Figure 46 (VIDEO 33)

Three dimensional echocardiography of tricuspid regurgitation

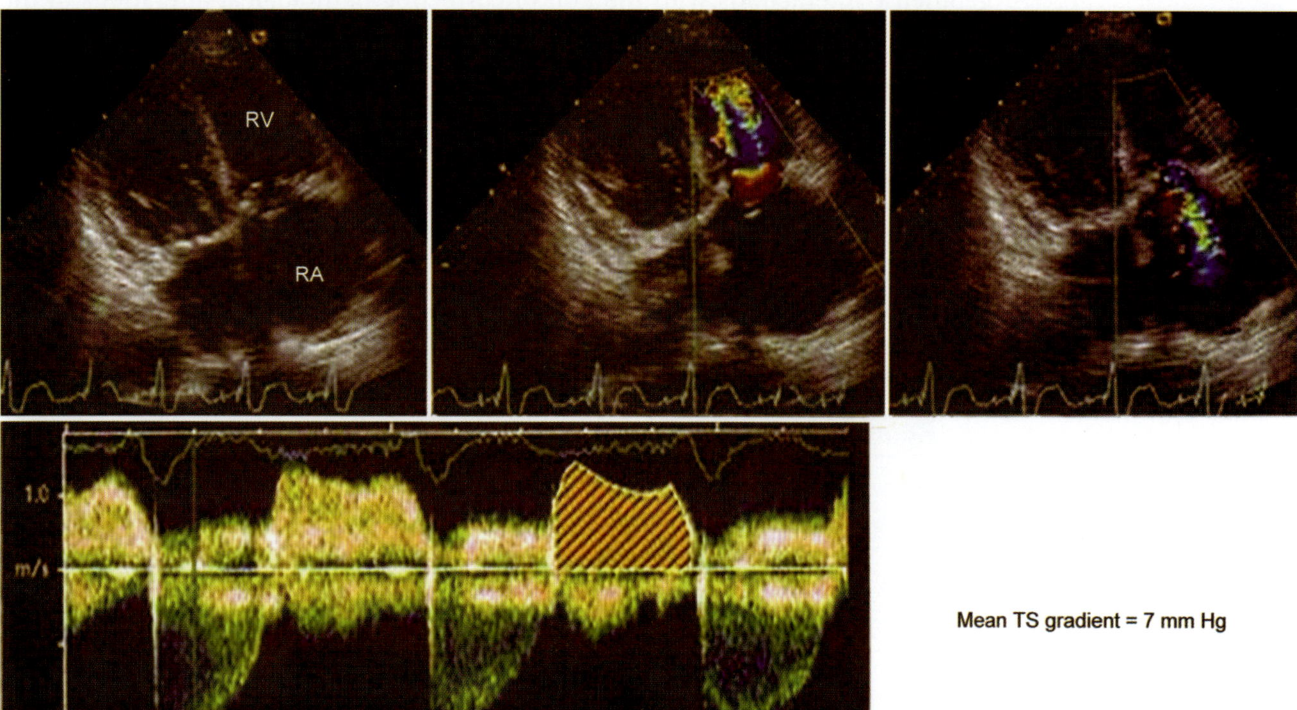

Figure 47

Rheumatic tricuspid regurgitation and stenosis

In addition, the concepts of 3DE color flow and instantaneous full-volume color Doppler echocardiography pertaining to mitral valve regurgitation might be also applied to tricuspid regurgitation assessment. The feasibility of obtaining the area of vena contracta from the tricuspid regurgitant jet has already been confirmed. It can be achieved by cropping the 3DE color Doppler data in a precise parallel level to the tricuspid valve orifice. However, a poor correlation is found between the area of the vena contracta obtained by 3DE and its width measured by 2DE. Similar to mitral regurgitation, this data supported the concept that the vena contracta of the regurgitant tricuspid jet has a complex geometry and, when obtained, the en face view from the right atrium can be used for estimating severity of tricuspid regurgitation.[65] Instantaneous full volume echocardiography allows an automatic calculation of 3D PISA, thus it might present these measurements in an easier and more accurate manner.

While it is understood that annular dilatation contributes to tricuspid regurgitation (TR), other factors are less clear **(Fig. 48)**. The geometry of the right ventricle (RV) and left ventricle (LV) may alter tricuspid annulus size and papillary muscle (PM) positions leading to TR. Alterations in ventricular geometry can lead to TR by altering both tricuspid annulus size and PM position. Understanding these geometric interactions with the aim of correcting pathological alterations of the tricuspid valve apparatus may lead to more robust tricuspid valve repairs.

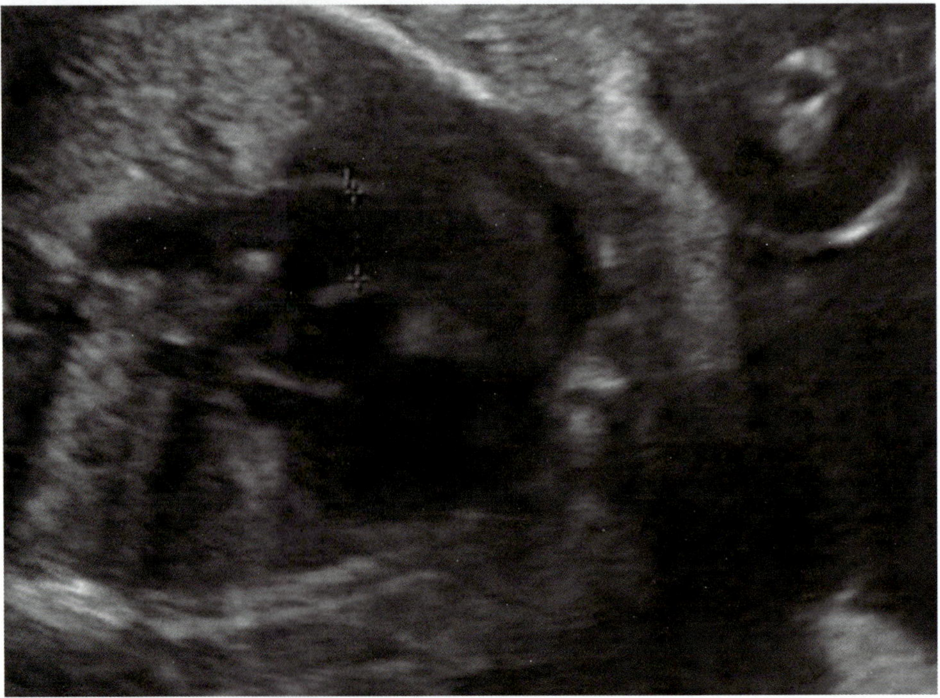

Figure 48

3D echo of tricuspid regurgitation

Spinner Em et al.[66] correlated the occurrence of tricuspid regurgitation on 3D echo with variables like pulmonary artery pressure, ventricular geometry, annular dilation and papillary muscles displacement. Using the GE vivid 7 ultrasound system, they used the end-diastolic area was used to classify ventricle geometry: GE echo PAC was used to measure annulus area and position of the PM tips. Patients with RV dilatation had significant ($P \leq 0.05$) displacement of all PMs apically and the septal PM and posterior PM away from the center of the RV toward the LV. Patients with LV dilatation had significant ($P \leq 0.05$) apical displacement of the anterior PM. Pulmonary arterial pressure ($r = 0.66$), annulus area ($r = 0.51$), apical displacement of the anterior PM ($r = 0.26$), posterior PM ($r = 0.49$), and septal PM ($r = 0.40$), lateral displacement of the septal PM ($r = 0.37$) and posterior PM ($r = 0.40$), and tenting area and height ($r = 0.54, 0.49$), were significantly ($P \leq 0.05$) correlated to the grade of TR, in their study **(Fig. 49)**.

One goal of 3D imaging is to provide a more accurate assessment of the vena contracta, PISA calculations and jet volumes. Live 3D TTE and TEE color Doppler measurements of VC area can be used for qualitative assessment of TR and its quantification. It is evident that technology is growing by leaps and bounds and that 3D developers are getting closer to their goal of providing more accurate quantitative information for the healthcare field **(Fig. 50)**.

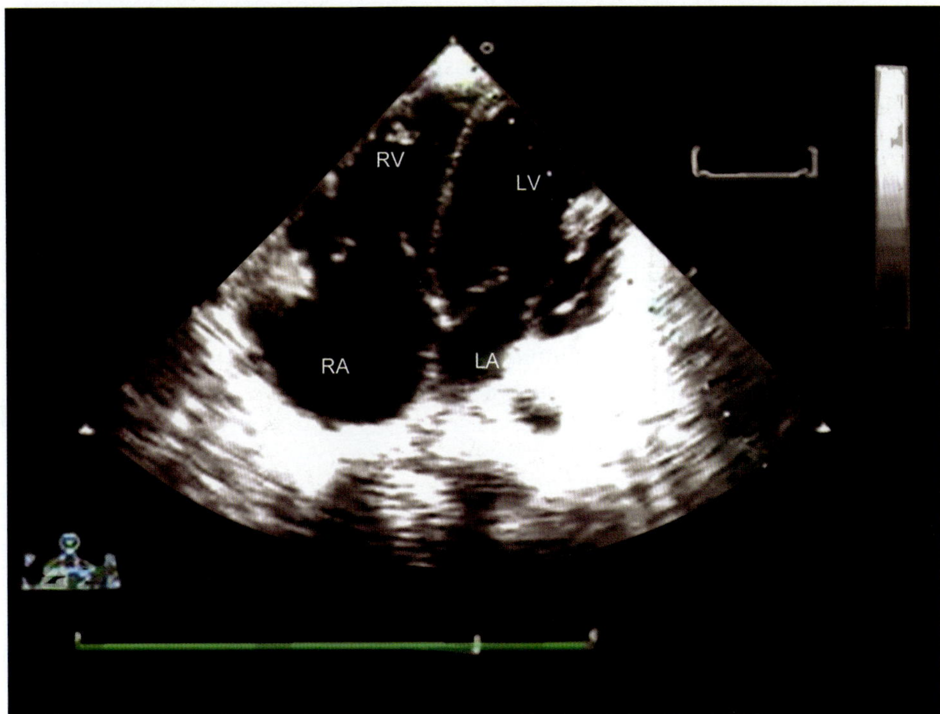

Figure 49

Three dimensional echocardiography of tricuspid regurgitation

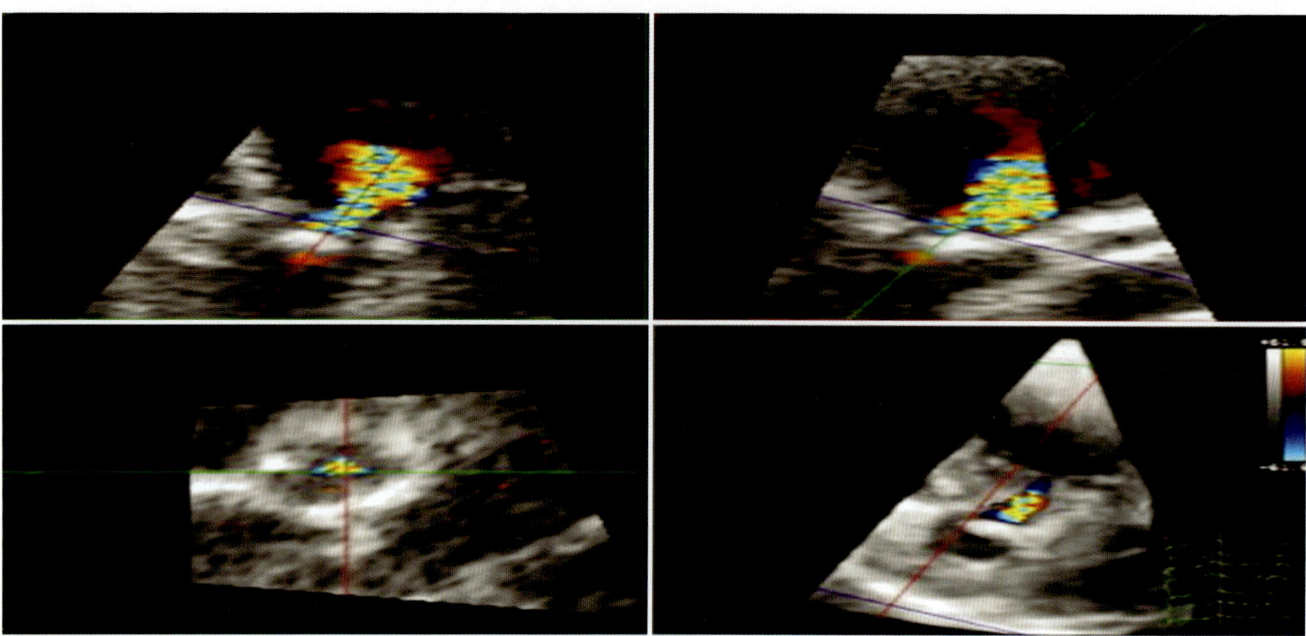

Figure 50

Three dimensional color Doppler echocardiography

TRAUMATIC TRICUSPID REGURGITATION ON 3D TEE

Tricuspid regurgitation (TR) secondary to blunt chest trauma is rare. 3D TEE provides a 'surgeon view' of the valve to aid surgical planning. While functional TR secondary to right ventricular dilation is most common cause of TR, valve injury from device-lead or catheter placement/removal is increasing in incidence. 2D TEE is unable to completely visualize the intracardiac course of a lead or catheter as it usually does not lie in a single imaging plane. 3D TEE has the ability to define 3D spatial relationship of the TV with nearby intracardiac devices in real time. This report illustrates the diagnostic capability of 3D TEE in providing incremental anatomic information of the TV and its relation to adjacent structures and/or devices for prevention and management of traumatic TR has been described by traumatic tricuspid regurgitation **(Figs 51A to F)**.

USEFULNESS OF LIVE 3D ECHOCARDIOGRAPHY IN TRICUSPID REGURGITATION

In a study done in 1993 consecutive patients using three dimensional transthoracic echocardiography measurements of vena contracta area to quantify the tricuspid regurgitation. Navin Nanda et al. by using multiple echocardiographic techniques

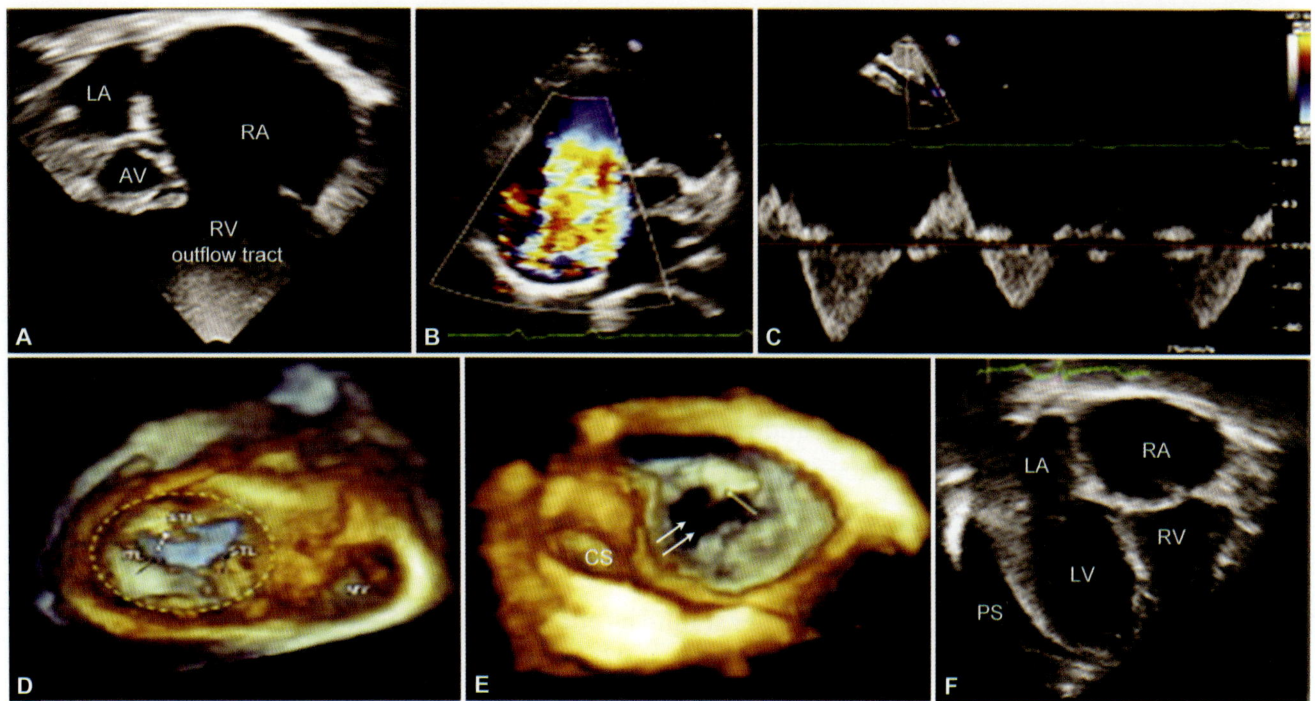

Figures 51A to F

Traumatic tricuspid regurgitation on 3D TEE

compared 2D and live 3D transthoracic echocardiography (TTE) to quantify the best tricuspid regurgitation parameter. The maximum area of vena contracta visible in systole was obtained by systematic cropping of the 3D TTE dataset in different planes by the authors. When more than one vena contracta were seen for a TR jet in a patient, the maximum vena contracta area of all was summed up. Assessment of this vena contracta by 3D TTE was compared with ratio of TR regurgitant jet area to right atrial area (RJA/RAA), RJA alone and vena contracta width on 2D TTE examination **(Table 7)**.[67] The authors concluded in their study of about 100 patients that live 3D TTE color Doppler measurements of vena contracta can be used for quantitative assessment of TR and offer incremental value for quantification particularly severe regurgitant lesions. The best echocardiographic quantification of TR by 2D TTE remains the vena contracta width. But in the case of tricuspid valve the geometry makes the vena contracta with vary and thus the vena contracta measured is not very accurate. Using an improved and comprehensive 3D TTE modality of visualizing the vena contracta width more accurately than 2D TTE especially in c/o eccentric jets. The authors found a new index of TR jet measurement and grading by using vena contracta width. The proposed criteria for vena contracta area assessment of TR is as:

Table 7: Grading of tricuspid according to vena contracta area

	Grade	*Vena contracta area*
TR grade	1	< 0.5 cm^2
TR grade	2	0.5–0.75 cm^2
TR grade	3	> 0.75 cm^2

The same authors reported on 3D TEE usefulness in measuring vena contracta width, potentially providing a more detailed and exact quantification of effective tricuspid regurgitation orifice size and shape.[68,69] 3D TEE can also define and diagnose size of the vegetation and any abscess formation and their site and extent of involvement and also postoperatively in determining prosthetic valve function and adequacy of repair by systemic enface cropping.

TRICUSPID REGURGITATION 3D COLOR FLOW DOPPLER

3D Color flow Doppler should be added to the multiple-beat acquisition in patients with tricuspid regurgitation and/or stenosis. Similar to the technique for acquiring noncolor Doppler multiple-beat imaging, obtaining a 3D color flow Doppler data set initially requires the identification of a region of interest in the orthogonal planes. The size of the region of interest should be limited to the tricuspid apparatus and color flow Doppler jet to optimize frame rate. In addition, although a high line density may be desirable, a lower line density will permit a larger sector to be displayed. Finally, the largest number of individually gated component subvolumes (4-6 beats) should always be attempted when electrocardiographic gating and reasonable acquisition times can be achieved.

Inferior vena cava: This venous structure runs in the retroperitoneal space, to the right of the vertebral body, and enters directly into the right atrium from the abdominal cavity. The hepatic vein is the last tributary to the inferior vena cava. Both venous structures may be important to image or Doppler for hemodynamic assessment of right atrial pressures, severity of tricuspid regurgitation and abnormal RV filling patterns.

REFERENCES

1. Sagie A, Schwammenthal E, Padial LR, Vazquez de Prada JA, Weyman AE, Sagie A, Schwammenthal E, Padial LR, Vazquez de Prada JA, et al. Plete tricuspid valve closure: Doppler color flow study of 109 patients. J Am Coll Cardiol. 1994;446-53.
2. Nucifora G, Badano LP, Allocca G, Gianfagna P, Proclemer A, Cinello M, et al. Severe tricuspid regurgitation due to entrapment of the anterior leaflet of the valve by a permanent pacemaker lead: role of real time three-dimensional echocardiography. Echocardiography. 2007;24:649-52.

3. Schnabel R, Khaw AV, von Bardeleben RS, Strasser C, Kramm T, Meyer J, et al. Assessment of the tricuspid valve morphology by transthoracic real-time-3D-echocardiography. Echocardiography. 2005;22:15-23.
4. Ahlgrim AA, Nanda NC, Berther E, Gill EA. Three-dimensional echocardiography: an alternative imaging choice for evaluation of tricuspid valve disorders. Cardiol Clin. 2007;25:305-9.
5. Pothineni KR, Duncan K, Yelamanchili P, Nanda NC, Patel V, Fan P, et al. Live/real-time three-dimensional transthoracic echocardiographic assessment of tricuspid valve pathology: incremental value over the two-dimensional technique. Echocardiography. 2007;24:541-52.
6. Parranon S, Abadir S, Acar P. New insight into the tricuspid valve in Ebstein anomaly using three-dimensional echocardiography. Heart. 2006;92:1627.
7. Anwar AM, Attia WM, Nosir YF, et al. Unusual bileaflet tricuspid valve by real time three-dimensional echocardiography. Echocardiography. 2008;25:534-6.
8. Reddy VK, Nanda S, Bandarupalli N, et al. Traumatic tricuspid papillary muscle and chordae rupture: emerging role of three-dimensional echocardiography. Echocardiography. 2008;25:653-7.
9. Lancellotti P, Moura L, Pierard LA, et al. European Association of Echocardiography. European Association of Echocardiography recommendations for the assessment of valvular regurgitation. Part 2: mitral and tricuspid regurgitation (native valve disease). Eur J Echocardiogr. 2010;11(4):307-32.
10. Velayudhan DE, Brown TM, Nanda NC, et al. Quantification of tricuspid regurgitation by live three-dimensional transthoracic echocardiographic measurements of vena contracta area. Echocardiography. 2006;23(9):793-800.
11. Zamorano J, Almería C, Alfonso F, et al. Transesophageal Doppler analysis of coronary sinus flow a new method to assess the severity of tricuspid regurgitation. Echocardiography. 1997;14(6 Pt 1):579-88.
12. Tribouilloy CM, Enriquez-Sarano M, Bailey KR, et al. Quantification of tricuspid regurgitation by measuring the width of the vena contracta with Doppler color flow imaging: a clinical study. J Am Coll Cardiol. 2000;36(2):472-8.
13. Yang WI, Shim CY, Kang MK, et al. Vena contracta width as a predictor of adverse outcomes in patients with severe isolated tricuspid regurgitation. J Am Soc Echocardiogr. 2011;24(9):1013-9.
14. Chopra HK, Nanda NC, Fan P, et al. Can two-dimensional echocardiography and Doppler color flow mapping identify the need for tricuspid valve repair? J Am Coll Cardiol. 1989;14(5):1266-74.
15. Blaustein AS, Ramanathan A: Tricuspid valve disease. Cardiol Clin. 1998;16(3):551-72.
16. Braunwald NS, Ross J Jr., Morrow AG. Conservative management of tricuspid regurgitation in patients undergoing mitral valve replacement. Circulation. 1967;35:I63-9.
17. Gürsoy et al. Long-term prognosis of mild functional tricuspid regurgitation after mitral valve replacement: an observational retrospective study. Anadolu Kardiyol Derg. 2013; 13(0): 000-000. doi:10.5152/akd.2013.239.
18. Roberts WC, Eways EA. Clinical and anatomic observations in patients having mitral valve replacement for pure mitral regurgitation and simultaneous tricuspid valve replacement. Am J Cardiol. 1991;68:1107-11.

19. Ubago JL, Figueroa A, Ochoteco A, Colman T, Duran RM, Duran CG. Analysis of the amount of tricuspid valve anular dilation required to produce functional tricuspid regurgitation. Am J Cardiol. 1983;52:155-8.

20. Sugimoto T, Okada M, Ozaki N, et al. Long-term evaluation of treatment for functional tricuspid regurgitation with regurgitant volume: characteristic differences based on primary cardiac lesion. J Thorac Cardiovasc Surg. 1999;117:463-71.

21. Fukuda S, Song JM, Gillinov AM, et al. Tricuspid valve tethering predicts residual tricuspid regurgitation after tricuspid annuloplasty. Circulation. 2005;111:975-9.

22. Antunes MJ, Barlow JB. Management of tricuspid valve regurgitation. Heart. 2007;93:271-6.

23. Hannoush H, Fawzy ME, Stefadouros M, Moursi M, Chaudhary MA, Dunn B. Regression of significant tricuspid regurgitation after mitral balloon valvotomy for severe mitral stenosis. Am Heart J. 2004;148:865-70.

24. Song H, Kang DH, Kim JH, et al. Percutaneous mitral valvuloplasty versus surgical treatment in mitral stenosis with severe tricuspid regurgitation. Circulation. 2007;116:I246-50.

25. Kim HK, Kim YJ, Kim KI, et al. Impact of the maze operation combined with left-sided valve surgery on the change in tricuspid regurgitation over time. Circulation. 2005;112:I14-9.

26. Henein MY, O'Sullivan CA, Li W, et al. Evidence for rheumatic valve disease in patients with severe tricuspid regurgitation long after mitral valve surgery: the role of 3D echo reconstruction. J Heart Valve Dis. 2003;12:566-72.

27. Simon R. Size and motion of the tricuspid annulus. Circulation. 1983;67:709.

28. Fukuda S, Saracino G, Matsumara Y, Daimon M, Tran H, Greenberg NL, Hozumi T, Yoshikawa J, Thomas JD, et al. Three-dimensional geometry of the tricuspid annulus in healthy subjects and in patients with functional tricuspid regurgitation: a real-time, 3-dimensional echocardiographic study. Circulation. 2006;114:I-492-I-498.

29. Singh JP, Evans JC, Levy D, Larson MG, Freed LA, Fuller DL, et al. Prevalence and clinical determinants of mitral, tricuspid, and aortic regurgitation (the Framingham Heart Study). Am J Cardiol. 1999;83:897-902.

30. Klein A, Burstow D, Tajik A, Zachariah P, Taliercio C, Taylor C, et al. Age-related prevalence of valvular regurgitation in normal subjects: a comprehensive color-flow examination in 118 volunteers. J Am Soc Echocardiogr. 1990;3:54-63.

31. Sukmawan R, Watanabe N, Ogasawara Y, Yamaura Y, Yamamoto K, Wada N, et al. Geometric changes of tricuspid valve tenting in tricuspid regurgitation secondary to pulmonary hypertension quantified by novel system with transthoracic real-time 3-dimensional echocardiography. J Am Soc Echocardiogr. 2007;20:470-6.

32. Kim HK, Kim YJ, Park JS, Kim KH, Kim KB, Ahn H, et al. Determinants of the severity of functional tricuspid regurgitation. Am J Cardiol. 2006;98:236-42.

33. Joon Bum Kim, Dong Gon Yoo, Gwan Sic Kim, et al. Mild-to-moderate functional tricuspid regurgitation in patients undergoing valve replacement for rheumatic mitral disease: the influence of tricuspid valve repair on clinical and echocardiographic outcomes. Heart. 2012;98:24-30.

34. Gonzalez-Vilchez F, Zarauza J, Vazquez de Prada JA, et al. Assessment of tricuspid regurgitation by Doppler color flow imaging: angiographic correlation. Int J Cardiol. 1994;44:275e83.

35. Bonow RO, Carabello BA, Chatterjee K, de Leon AC, Faxon DP, Freed MD, Gaasch WH, Lytle BW, Nishimura RA, O'Gara PT, O'Rourke RA, Otto CM, Sha PM, Shanewise JS. 2008 focused update incorporated into the ACC/AHA 2006 guidelines for the management of patients

with valvular heart disease: a report of the American College of Cardiology/American Heart Association Task Force on Practice Guidelines (Writing Committee to revise the 1998 guidelines for the management of patients with valvular heart disease). Endorsed by the Society of Cardiovascular Anesthesiologists, Society for Cardiovascular Angiography and Interventions, and Society of Thoracic Surgeons. J Am Coll Cardiol. 2008;52:e1–e142.

36. Vahanian A, Alfieri O, Andreooti F, Antunes M, Baro´ n- Esquivias G, Baumgartner H, Borger MA, Carrel TP, De Bonis M, Evangelista A, Falk V, Iung B, Lancellotti P, Pierard L, Price S, Schaefers H-J, Schuler G, Stepinska J, Swedberg K, Takkenberg J, Von Oppel UO, Windecker S, Zamorano JL, Zembala M. Guidelines on the Management of Valvular Heart Disease (Version 2012). Eur Heart J. 2012;33:2451-96.

37. Uretzky G, Puga FJ, Danielson GK, Hagler DJ, McGoon DC. Reoperation after correction of tetralogy of Fallot. Circulation. 1982;66(2):I202-8.

38. Mahle WT, Parks WJ, Fyfe DA, et al. Tricuspid regurgitation in patients with repaired Tetralogy of Fallot and its relation to right ventricular dilatation. Am J Cardiolo. 2003;92(5): 643-5.

39. Kobayashi J, Kawashima Y, Matsuda H, Nakano S, Miura T, Tokuan Y, et al. Prevalence and risk factors of tricuspid regurgitation after correction of tetralogy of Fallot. J Thorac Cardiovas Cardiolo. 1991;102(4):611-6.

40. Jong Won Ha et al. E' velocity is well preserved in patients with isolated CP even when there is no characteristic respiratory variation of E velocity. J Am Soc Echocardiogr 2002;15:1468-71.

41. Himelman RB, Lee E, Schiller NB. Septal bounce, vena cava plethora and pericardial adhesion: Informative two-dimensional echocardiophic signs in the diagnosis of pericardial constriction. J Am Soc Echocardiogr. 1988;1:333-40.

42. Goldstein JA. Cardiac tamponade, constructive pericarditis and restrictive cardiomyopathy. Curr Probl Cardiol. 2004;29(9):503-67.

43. Ommen SR, Nishimura RA, Appleton CP, Miller FA, Oh JK, Redfield MM, et al. Clinical utility of Doppler echocardiography and tissue Doppler imaging in the estimation of left ventricular filling pressures: A comparative simultaneous Doppler-catheterization study. Circulation. 2000;102:1788-94.

44. Nakamura T, Masai T, Yamauchi T, Higuchi T, Ito H, Toyoshima Y, et al. Successful surgical management for severe mitral regurgitation unmasked after pericardiectomy for chronic constrictive pericarditis. Ann Thorac Surg. 2008;86:1994-6.

45. Buckingham RE Jr, Furnary AP, Weaver MT, et al. Mitral insufficiency after pericardiectomy for constrictive pericarditis. Ann Thorac Surg. 1994;58:1171-4.

46. Terada Y, Mitsui T, Yamada S. Mitral regurgitation after pericardiectomy for constrictive pericarditis. Jpn J Thorac Cardiovasc Surg. 1999;47:27-30.

47. TEE of tricuspid and puolmonary valves – chapter 4 in Atlas of Transesophageal Echocardiography by Navin C. Nanda, Michael J Domanski. Lippincott Williams & Wilkins. 2007;2:191-2.

48. Fisher EA, Goldman ME. Simple, rapid method of quantification of tricuspid regurgitation by two-dimensional echocardiography. Am J Cardiol. 1989;63:1375-8.

49. Abi-Saleh B, Schoondyke JW, Abboud L, Downs CJ, Haddadin TZ, Iskandar SB. Tricuspid valve involvement in carcinoid disease. Echocardiography. 2007;24:439-42.

50. Attenhofer Jost CH, Connolly HM, Dearani JA, et al. Ebstein's anomaly. Circulation. 2007;115;277-85.

51. Quιrι JP, Tribouilloy C, Enriquez-Sarano M. Vena contracta width measurement: Theoretic basis and usefulness in the assessment of valvular regurgitation severity. Curr Cardiol Rep. 2003;5:110-5.

52. Shapira Y, Porter A, Wurzel M, et al. Evaluation of tricuspid regurgitation severity: Echocardiographic and clinical correlation. J Am Soc Echocardiogr. 1998;11:652-9.

53. Grossmann G, Stein M, Kochs M, Hϕher M, Koenig W, Hombach V, et al. Comparison of the proximal flow convergence method and the jet area method for the assessment of the severity of tricuspid regurgitation. Eur Heart J. 1998;19:652-9.

54. Yamachika S, Reid CL, Savani D, Meckel C, Paynter J, Knoll M, et al. Usefulness of color Doppler proximal isovelocity surface area method in quantitating valvular regurgitation. J Am Soc Echocardiogr. 1997;10:159-68.

55. Quiρones MA, Otto CM, Stoddard M, Waggoner A, Zoghbi WA; Doppler Quantification Task Force of the Nomenclature and Standards Committee of the American Society of Echocardiography. Recommendations for quantification of Doppler echocardiography: A report from the Doppler Quantification Task Force of the Nomenclature and Standards Committee of the American Society of Echocardiography. J Am Soc Echocardiogr. 2002; 15:167-84.

56. Nimura Y, Miyatake K, Okamoto M, Beppu S, Kinoshita N, Sakakibara H. Pulsed Doppler echocardiography in the assessment of tricuspid regurgitation. Ultrasound Med Biol. 1984;10(2):239-47.

57. Pennestrν F, Loperfido F, Salvatori MP, Mongiardo R, Ferrazza A, Guccione P, et al. Assessment of tricuspid regurgitation by pulsed Doppler ultrasonography of the hepatic veins. Am J Cardiol. 1984;54:363-8.

58. Nagueh SF, Kopelen HA, Zoghbi WA. Relation of mean right atrial pressure to echocardiographic and Doppler parameters of right atrial and right ventricular function. Circulation. 1996;93:1160-9.

59. Shiran A, Sagie A. Tricuspid regurgitation in mitral valve disease; incidence, prognostic implications, mechanisms and management. J Am Coll Cardiol. 2009;53:401-8.

60. Rogers JH, Bolling SF. The tricuspid valve: current perspective and evolving management of tricuspid regurgitation. Circulation. 2009;119: 2718-25.

61. Lin G, Nishimura RA, Connolly HM, et al. Severe symptomatic tricuspid valve regurgitation due to permanent pacemaker or implantable cardioverter-defibrillator leads. J Am Coll Cardiol. 2005;45:1672-5.

62. Espeed Khoshbin, Abdelrahman Abdelbar, Stuart Allen, et al. The mechanism of endocardial lead-induced tricuspid regurgitation BMJ Case Rep 2013. doi:10.1136/bcr-2012-008191

63. Heaven DJ, Henein MY, Sutton R. Pacemaker lead related tricuspid stenosis: a report of two cases. Heart. 2000;83:351-2.

64. Krishanan A, Moulick A, Sinha P, Kuehl K, Kanter J, Slack M, Kaltman J, Mereader M, Moak JP. Severe tricuspid valve stenosis secondary to pacemaker leads presenting as ascites and liver dysfunction: a complex problem requiring a multidisciplinary therapeutic approach. J Interv Card Electrophysiol. 2009;24:71-75.

65. Hussain T, Knight WB, Mcleod KA. Lead-induced tricuspid stenosis successful management by ballon angioplasty. Pacing Clin Electrophysiol. 2009;32:140-2.

66. Spinner EM, Lerakis S, Higginson J, Pernetz M, Howell S, Veledar E, et al. Correlates of tricuspid regurgitation as determined by 3D echocardiography: pulmonary arterial pressure, ventricle geometry, annular dilatation, and papillary muscle displacement. Circ Cardiovasc Imaging. 2012;5(1):43-50.

67. Patel V, Hsiung MC, Nanda NC, Miller AP, Fang L, Yelamanchili P, Mehmood F, Gupta M, Duncan K, Singh A, Rajdev S, Fan P, Naftel DC, McGiffin DC, Pacifico AD, et al. Echocardiography. 2006;23(6):513-8.

68. Galloway AC, Colvin SB, Baumann FG, et al. A comparison of mitral valve reconstruction with mitral valve replacement: Intermediate-term results. Ann Thorac Surg. 1989;47:655-2.

69. Hellemans IM, Pieper EG, Ravelli AC, et al. Prediction of surgical strategy in mitral valve regurgitation based on echocardiography. Interuniversity Cardiology Institute of The Netherlands. Am J Cardiol. 1997;79:334-8.

5 Tricuspid Stenosis

Poonam Malhotra Kapoor, Arindam Choudhury, Manju Mani

ETIOLOGY OF TRICUSPID STENOSIS

Tricuspid stenosis (TS) is currently the least common of the valvular stenosis lesions given the low incidence of rheumatic heart disease. In India, rheumatic heart disease is the most common cause of tricuspid stenosis. Less likely causes include congenital malformation, carcinoid syndrome, and an obstructing mass. Most commonly, TS is accompanied by regurgitation so that the higher flows through the valve further increase the transvalvular gradient and contribute to a greater elevation of right atrial pressures.

In the west regions where rheumatic heart disease is still prevalent, as in India TS is rarely an isolated disorder; more often, it is accompanied by MS or TR. Other causes of TS include carcinoid syndrome (always combined with TR which is commonly predominant), rare congenital malformations. **Figure 1** shows carcinoid disease valvular or pacemaker endocarditis and pacemaker-induced adhesions, lupus valvulitis, and mechanical obstruction by benign or malignant tumors.

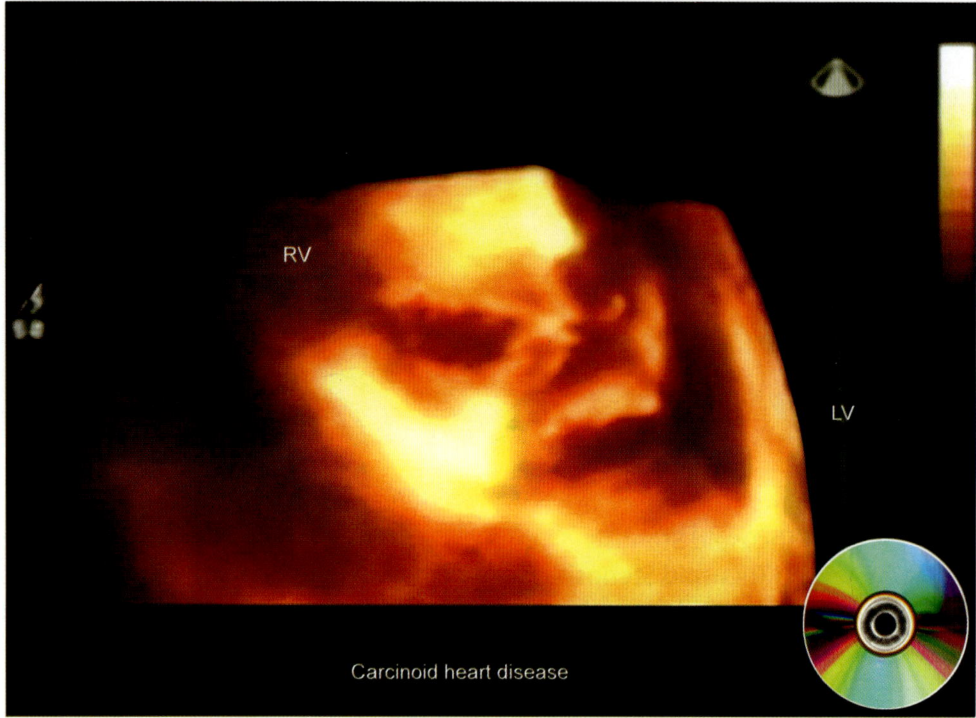

Figure 1 (VIDEO 1)

Tricuspid stenosis on 3D TEE with thickened TV cusps

Transesophageal echocardiography (TEE) shows thickening and restricted mobility of the TV leaflets with a flat diastolic E-F slope on the M-mode and an absent A wave. The RA is enlarged and can be markedly delated when the stenosis is severe. 3D TEE provides reliable information of TS as it views the three leaflets enface simultaneously with thickening and calcification seen at one go.

RHEUMATIC IN TRICUSPID STENOSIS

Involvement of the TV is almost always in association with rheumatic mitral and aortic involvement, and seldom occurs as an isolated finding. Rheumatic tricuspid stenosis occurs in 10 to 15 percent of patients with rheumatic heart disease. Hemodynamically significant tricuspid stenosis is rare. Functionally significant tricuspid regurgitation is present in at least half the cases.

- **Most commonly, TS is accompanied by regurgitation so that the higher flows through the valve further increase the transvalvular gradient and contribute to a greater elevation of right atrial pressures.**

CARCINOID IN TRICUSPID STENOSIS

Carcinoid is the second most common etiology of tricuspid stenosis and is invariably associated with regurgitation, as discussed earlier. The carcinoid plaques are present on both the atrial and the ventricular surfaces of the valve. The thickened and rigid leaflets appear fixed in the open position **(Figs 2 and 3)**. Similar findings are seen with drug-related tricuspid stenosis.

Tricuspid Stenosis

- Most commonly of rheumatic etiology, other causes are congenital, endocarditis, carcinoid heart disease, endomyocardial fibrosis.
- *2D-examination:* Doming and thickening of leaflets, restricted leaflet motion and commissural fusion.
- *Doppler:* Peak velocities (E waves >1.5 m/sec).

EOSINOPHILIC IN TRICUSPID STENOSIS

Eosinophilic myocarditis (both tropical and nontropical or Loeffler's syndrome) usually presents as a combined lesion with tricuspid stenosis and regurgitation.

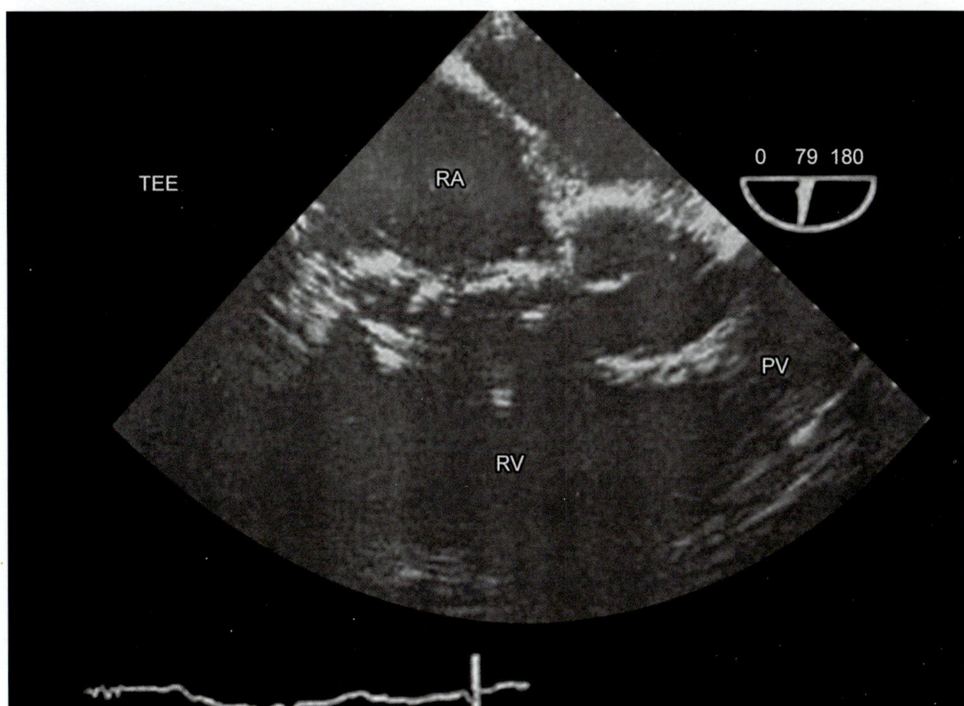

Figure 2

The ME RV inflow-outflow view showing both TV and PV

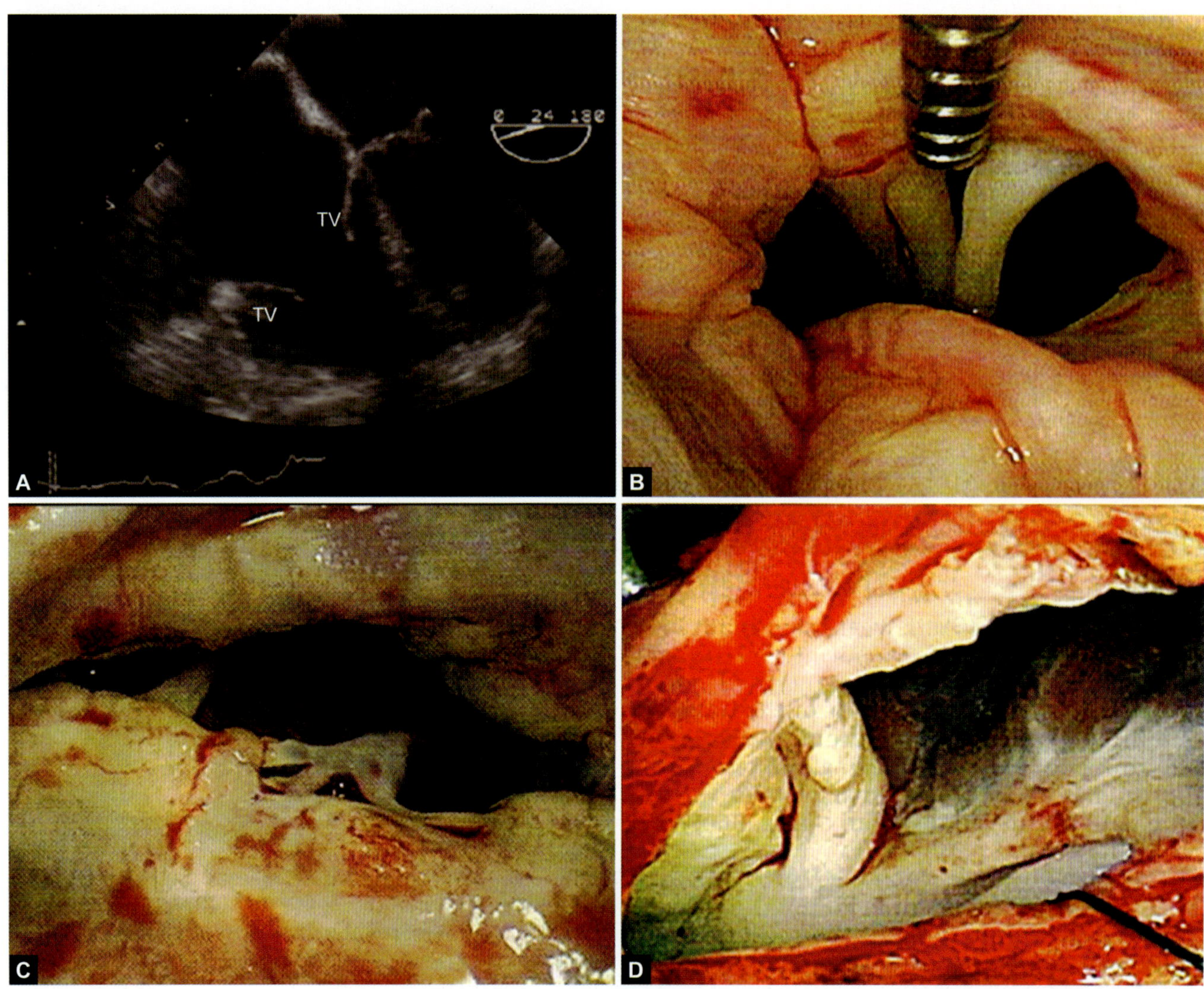

Figures 3A to D

Carcinoid DS involves right-sided valves more than left-sided valves. (A) Fixed, thickened and retracted leaflets (B to D) cut open surgical sections of tricuspid valve showing the 'frozen appearance' in carcinoid disease

There is involvement of the chordae in addition to the valve leaflets. Similar findings are seen with significant eosinophilia from other causes such as parasite infestation, leukemia, or conditions of hypersensitivity. Approximately 40 to 60 percent of patients with hypereosinophilic syndrome develop cardiac involvement and the condition is then referred to as Loeffler's syndrome. Loeffler in 1936 described two patients with heart failure and eosinophilia who at autopsy showed endomyocardial fibrosis. Toxins secreted by eosinophils have been implicated in the damage to cardiac myocytes with subsequent development of fibrosis and thrombus formation. Both ventricular apices may show marked thickening and thrombus formation together with diffuse thickening of the TV and/or mitral valve. The aortic valve is rarely affected and pulmonary valve involvement was recently reported by our group for the first time, to our knowledge. The lesions of this syndrome regress partially or completely with a tyrosine kinase inhibitor or corticosteroids.

LIVE 3D ECHOCARDIOGRAPHY IN CARCINOID DISEASE

Unlike 2D TTE which may show thickened anterior and septal leaflets of the tricuspid valve with restricted motion, but it is unable to show the posterior leaflet of TV or the right anterior PV leaflet or any area suggestive of carcinoid deposits.

Live 3D TTE, however shows all three leaflets of TV simultaneously enface alongwith restricted motion as has been described in an adult patient of metastatic carcinoid disease of the heart by Bhavin Dumaswala et al. from University of Alabama, Birmingham. 3D TTE by these authors helped to determine accurately the extent of carcinoid involvement of all three leaflets of the tricuspid valve, thus better determining the need for valve replacement. Live 3D TEE also accurately quantifies the TR of carcinoid by measuring the vena contract width and the elevated RA volumes and also the diminished RA systolic function thus telling us about the detailed cardiac chamber involvement and also the extent of hepatic metastases. 3D echocardiography thus provides information over and above echo in carcinoid disease of the heart.

METABOLIC AND OTHERS ABNORMALITIES IN TRICUSPID STENOSIS

Metabolic abnormalities such as Fabry's disease, Whipple's disease, and methysergide toxicity can cause endocardial fibrosis and are among the rarer etiologies of tricuspid stenosis. A right atrial mass such as a large tumor, thrombus, TV vegetations, or thrombus in transit from the venous bed can cause RV inflow stenosis and may simulate tricuspid stenosis. Gradients with these conditions, however, are rarely very high.

PACEMAKER LEAD-INDUCED SEVERE TRICUSPID VALVE STENOSIS

Severe tricuspid valve stenosis due to pacemaker leads is uncommon. Tricuspid valve stenosis secondary to transvenous leads are reported to be treated with surgical replacement, surgical valvuloplasty or percutaneous balloon valvuloplasty. Cardiac CT can provide supportive evidence of the anatomic mechanism of valve dysfunction and planning of treatment strategy.

INFECTIVE ENDOCARDITIS IN PROSTHETIC TRICUSPID VALVE

Unlike infective endocarditis involving native valves, prosthetic valve infections are not uncommonly associated with stenosis of the valve orifice. In a review of 22 necropsy patients with endocarditis involving left-sided mechanical prosthetic cardiac valves, Arnett and Roberts, found six cases with evidence of valvular stenosis. Nunez and associates, reviewed a series of 20 patients with infective endocarditis involving left-sided bioprosthetic valves and found (in the group of II patients who did not respond to medical treatment) evidence of leaflet thickening or vegetation formation by echocardiography, as well as large transprosthetic gradients by cardiac catheterization. Pathologic findings included severe stenosis of the valves and extensive thrombotic vegetation formation. These authors suggested that bioprosthetic valves may be more prone to obstruction during infective endocarditis and that this complication may render medical therapy ineffective. The first documented case of valve obstruction in association with tricuspid prosthetic valve endocarditis. Although two-dimensional echocardiography revealed the presence and growth of vegetations during serial evaluation, the magnitude of the obstruction induced by the vegetations was determined by Doppler examination. In fact, the continuous wave Doppler tracing was indistinguishable from that seen in native tricuspid or mitral stenosis.

OTHER MISCELLANEOUS ETIOLOGY OF TRICUSPID VALVE

Right ventricular (RV) fibroelastoma may be seen as vegetation on one of the valve leaflets as shown in **Figure 4**.

Tricuspid stenosis can result from tricuspid atresia or from abnormalities of the tricuspid valve leaflets. Tricuspid atresia is a well-recognized entity, and results from agenesis of the tricuspid valve. In contrast, stenosis originating with the tricuspid valve leaflets most often occurs as part of a syndrome involving multiple valvular abnormalities; isolated tricuspid stenosis is rare. A 17-year-old patient who had been cyanotic at birth, who's ECG had a left anterior fascicular block, and who had an ostium secundum atrial septal defect was reported with isolated tricuspid valvular stenosis. Schlesinger et al. reported a 50-year-old subject with normal axis of the ECG, and tricuspid stenosis with no atrial septal defect. Similarly, Oeconomos et al. reported a 19-year-old case with right atrial enlargement with a normal axis on ECG, and tricuspid stenosis without atrial septal defect. Congenital tricuspid valve stenosis with abnormal chordal insertions and an ostium secundum atrial septal defect has been reported in literature. This resulted in tricuspid stenosis with no insufficiency, and right to left shunting at the atrial level. Her ECG showed a left anterior fascicular block and no associated right atrial enlargement. Ostium

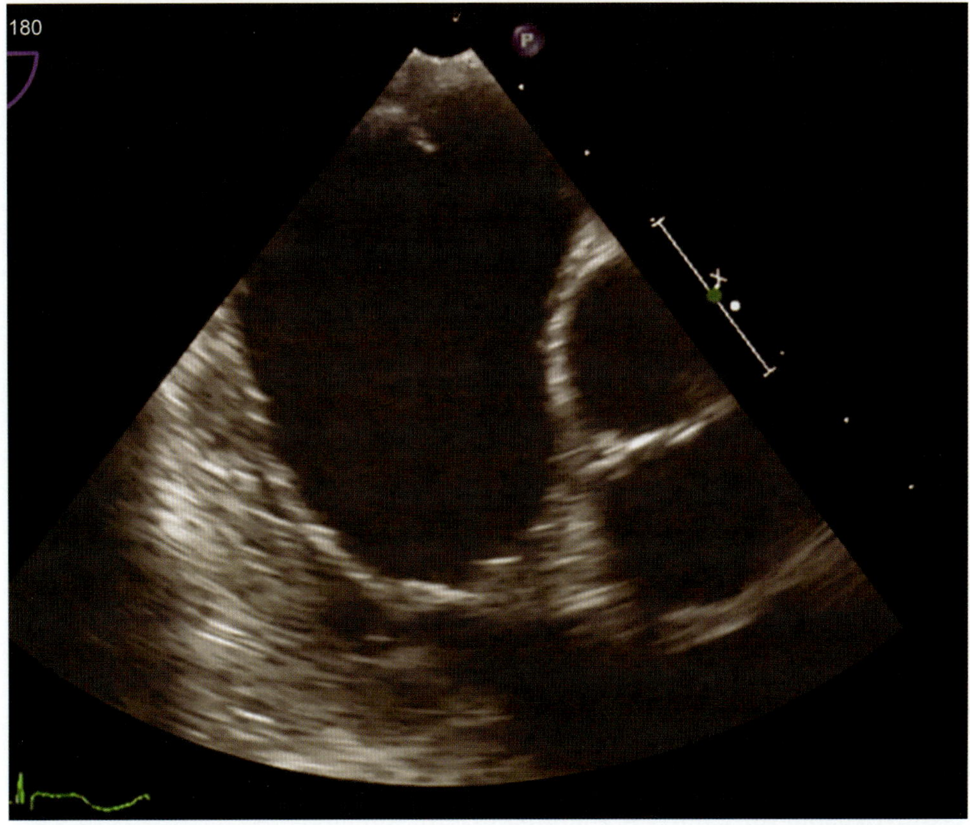

Figure 4
Right ventricular (RV) fibroelastoma seen as a vegetation on TV leaflet

secundum defects are occasionally associated with electrocardiographic complete or incomplete right bundle branch block, but not with left axis deviation.

The left anterior fascicular block most likely is part of the clinical syndrome and, unusually, is associated with the secundum atrial septal defect. The lack of marked right atrial enlargement, both by ECG and by echocardiogram, is likely due to decompression of the increased right atrial pressure into the left atrium.

PATHOPHYSIOLOGY OF TRICUSPID VALVE

Tricuspid stenosis results from alterations in the structure of the tricuspid valve that precipitate inadequate excursion of the valve leaflets. The most common etiology is rheumatic fever, and tricuspid valve involvement occurs universally with mitral and aortic valve involvement. With rheumatic tricuspid stenosis, the valve leaflets become thickened and sclerotic as the chordae tendineae become shortened. The restricted valve opening hampers blood flow into the right ventricle and, subsequently, to the pulmonary vasculature. Right atrial enlargement is observed as a consequence. The obstructed venous return results in hepatic enlargement, decreased pulmonary blood flow, and peripheral edema. Other rare causes of tricuspid stenosis include carcinoid syndrome, endocarditis, endomyocardial fibrosis, systemic lupus erythematosus, and congenital tricuspid atresia. Also cause an increase in RA size and resistance of flow through the pulmonary vasculature.

In the rare instances of congenital tricuspid stenosis, the valve leaflets may manifest various forms of deformity, which can include deformed leaflets, deformed chordae, and displacement of the entire valve apparatus. Other cardiac anomalies are usually present.

Views of Transesophageal Echocardiography

As with all valve lesions, the initial evaluation starts with an anatomical assessment of the valve by 2D echocardiography using multiple windows such as ME four chamber, RV inflow-outflow and modified bicaval view. Echo assessment of tricuspid stenosis.

2D and M-mode

Use 2D and M-mode echo to assess the structure of the valve:

- Is the tricuspid valve normal, rheumatic or myxomatous?
- Is there evidence of Ebstein's anomaly?
- Are the valve leaflets (anterior, posterior, septal) normal? Is there thickening, and does this affect the tips or the body of the leaflet(s)?
- Is there leaflet calcification, and is this focal (anterior, posterior, septal) or diffuse?
- Is leaflet mobility normal or reduced? How much is it reduced?
- Is there any doming or prolapse of the leaflets?
- Is there any evidence of papillary muscle rupture?
- Are there any tricuspid valve vegetations or abscesses?
- Is the tricuspid annulus normal, dilated or calcified?

The normal tricuspid annulus in adults has a diameter of 28 ± 5 mm in the modified apical four-chamber view. Significant dilatation is defined by a diastolic annular diameter >35 mm (or, when indexed for body surface area, >21 mm/m^2).

- **The most common etiology is rheumatic fever, and tricuspid valve involvement occurs universally with mitral and aortic valve involvement.**

Color Doppler

Use color Doppler to look for any coexistent tricuspid regurgitation. The color jet can also help in obtaining correct alignment of the probe for continuous wave (CW) and pulsed-wave (PW) Doppler recordings.

Continuous Wave and Pulsed Wave Doppler

Use Doppler to record forward flow through the tricuspid valve from a modified ME four-chamber view. Ignore traces obtained from ectopic beats (and the beat following an ectopic), and if the patient is in AF, average the measurements taken from several beats. From the trace, measure the mean tricuspid valve gradient (trace the velocity time integral (VTI) of the tricuspid inflow) **(Fig. 5)**.

SEQUELAE OF TRICUSPID STENOSIS

The sequelae of significant tricuspid stenosis are clinically readily apparent (peripheral edema and limitations in functional class). While clinical evaluation is essential in the management of tricuspid stenosis, 2D and Doppler examination help document the valvular hemodynamics. Indirect parameters of significant tricuspid stenosis include enlarged right atrial size and plethoric vena cava and hepatic veins, with preservation of RV size and function. However, these signs

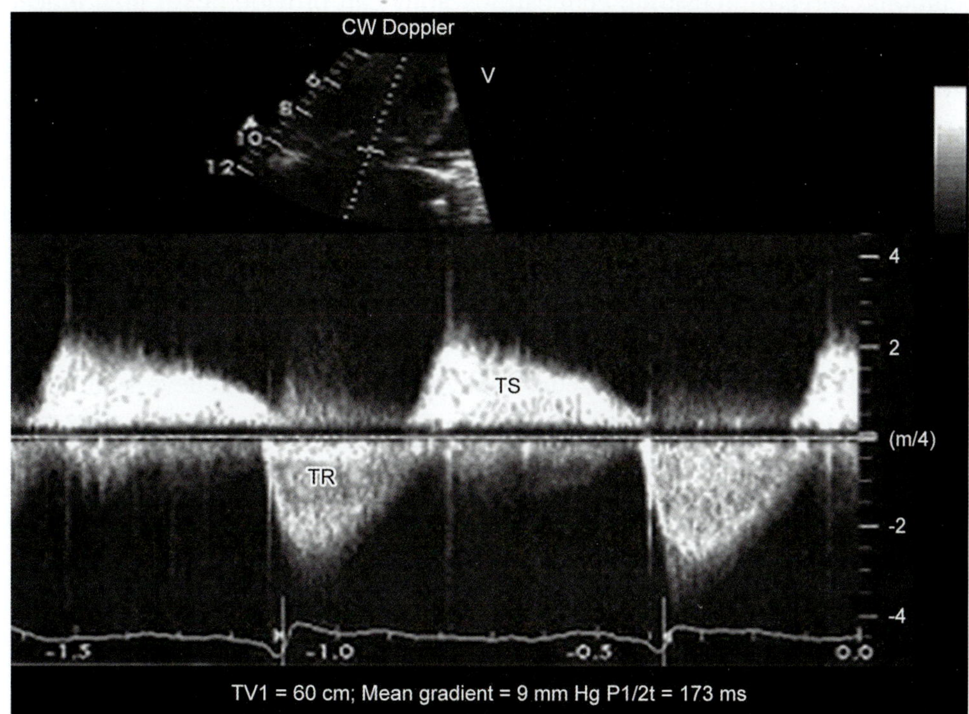

Figure 5

Continuous wave Doppler (CWD) showing the TV1 and mean gradient across TV are not specific for tricuspid stenosis. Imaging of the stenotic valve—essential in evaluating its morphology is etiology—is poorly predictive of its severity. Doming of the anterior leaflet and/or significant restriction of valvular motion is a prerequisite to the presence of a hemodynamically significant lesion. Thickening and restriction of the posterior leaflet can be seen with milder lesions. Direct planimetry of the tricuspid valve area, unlike for the mitral valve, is more difficult to accomplish. This is due to suboptimal cross-sectional alignment of the imaging plane consequent to the position and orientation of the TV.

ANATOMIC PRESENTATION OF TRICUSPID STENOSIS

As the etiology is mostly rheumatic the leaflets appear thickened and with restricted motion secondary to commissural fusion, leading to a relatively fixed orifice. Diastolic doming of the leaflets is typical of rheumatic involvement. Due to the increased gradient across the valve, the right atrium is enlarged. The severe cases that are still in sinus rhythm, there may be prominent reversal of flow in the inferior vena cava during atrial systole.

One looks for valve thickening and/or calcification, restricted mobility with diastolic doming, reduced leaflet separation at peak opening, and right atrial enlargement. In carcinoid syndrome, one sees severe immobility of the leaflets, described as a 'frozen' appearance **(Figs 6A to H)**. Echocardiography also allows for the detection of valve obstruction by atrial tumors, metastatic lesions, or giant vegetations. Three-dimensional echocardiography can provide better anatomical detail of the relation of the three leaflets to each other and assessment of the orifice area. Using color flow Doppler one can appreciate narrowing of the diastolic inflow jet, higher velocities that produce mosaic color dispersion, and associated valve regurgitation. The RA size is invariably enlarged.

HOW TO GRADE TRICUSPID STENOSIS?

From a clinical standpoint, the importance of an accurate assessment of TS is to be able to recognize patients with hemodynamically significant stenosis in whom a surgical- or catheter-based procedure may be necessary to relieve symptoms of right-sided failure. In the presence of anatomic evidence by 2D echo of TS, the findings listed in **Table 1** are consistent with significant stenosis with or without regurgitation.

The hallmark of a stenotic valve is an increase in transvalvular velocity recorded by CWD. Peak inflow velocity through a normal tricuspid valve rarely exceeds 0.7 m/s. Tricuspid inflow is normally accentuated during inspiration; consequently, with TS, it is common to record peak velocities ~1.0 m/s that may approach 2 m/s during inspiration. The transvalvular gradients (peak and mean) should be obtained

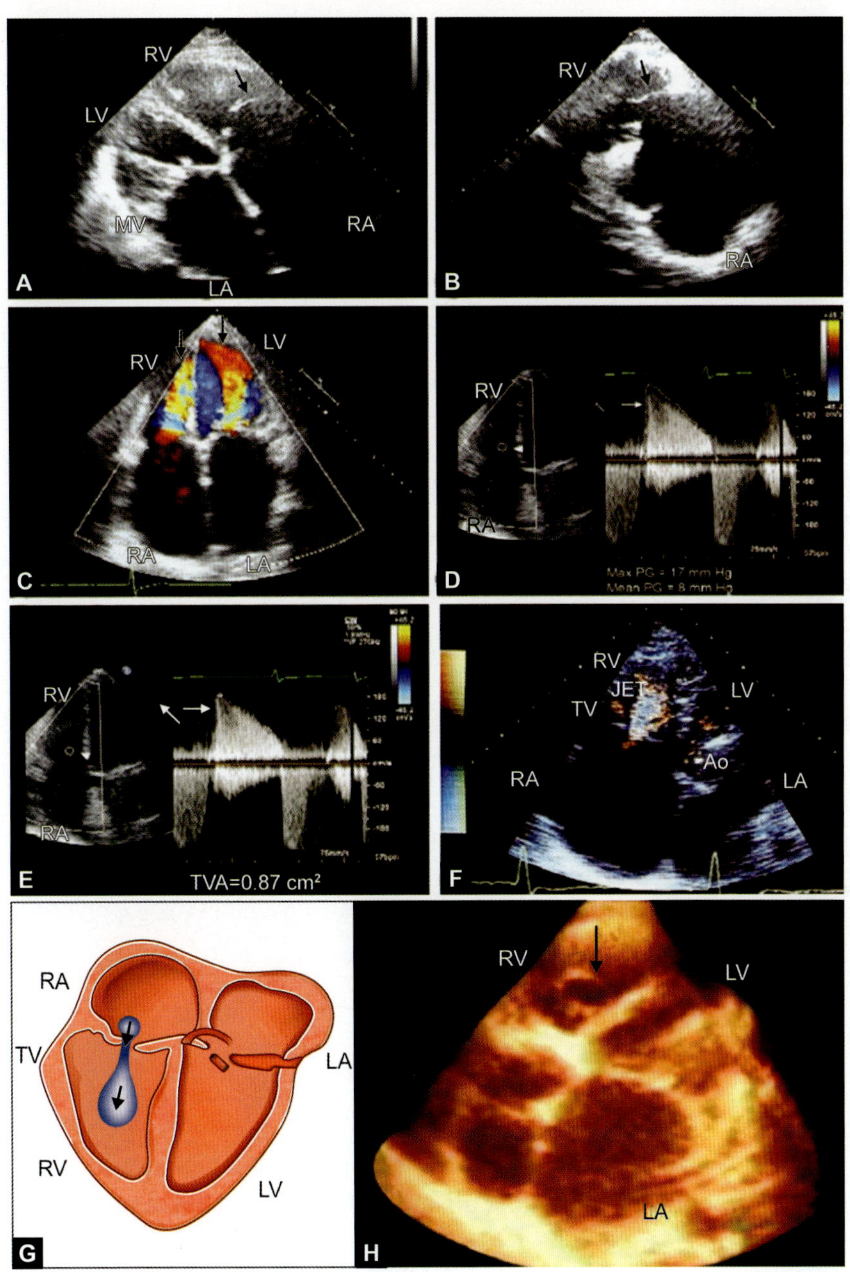

Figures 6A to H

Tricuspid valve stenosis in a 65-year-old female with rheumatic heart disease. (A to G) Two-dimensional transthoracic echocardiography. (A and B) Apical four-chamber (A) and modified right ventricular two-chamber (B) views. Arrow points to diastolic doming of the tricuspid valve (TV) consistent with stenosis. Mitral valve (MV) is also thickened and stenotic; (C) Shows turbulent stenotic jets originating from TV (left arrow) and MV (right arrow). Also, note the eccentric tricuspid regurgitation (TR) jet (D and E) Arrow in (D) shows the Doppler velocity waveform obtained by continuous wave Doppler interrogation of the TV with maximum and mean diastolic pressure gradients high at 17 and 8 mm Hg, respectively. In (E) TV area (TVA) calculated using the pressure half-time method is 0.87 cm^2 consistent with severe stenosis. Arrowheads in (D) and (E) point to the Doppler cursor line; (F and G) Apical four-chamber view in a 50-year-old woman who had aortic and mitral valve replacement shows mosaic signals of tricuspid stenosis (TS) in the right ventricle during diastole originating from the tricuspid valve (TV). These signals are very narrow at the origin, implying severe stenosis, and widen considerably farther in the right ventricle (RV) because of a large diastolic pressure gradient between the right atrium (RA) and the RV. (G) is a schematic; (H) Live/real time three-dimensional transthoracic echocardiography. Rheumatic tricuspid valve stenosis/tricuspid regurgitation. Arrow points to the tricuspid orifice in a patient with tricuspid valve stenosis. The orifice area measured 2.02 cm^2 in diastole. *Abbreviations:* Ao, aorta; LA, left atrium; LV, left ventricle; RA, right atrium; RV, right ventricle

Table 1: Tricuspid stenosis echocardiography findings	
TTE findings	• Leaflet thickness, extent of commissural fusion and area planimetry can be readily obtained in rheumatic disease. • 3D TTE provides new opportunities for improving the quantitative assessment of valve disease severity (tricuspid valve stenosis and regurgitation, isolated or associated) • RT3D-TTE allowed a detailed assessment of TV leaflets (thickness, mobility, and calcification) as well as measurement of TV area in our patients with TV stenosis.
TEE findings	• Confirmed the preoperative diagnosis of mild tricuspid stenosis • Leaflet and chordal thickening
2D findings	• Thickening of leaflet with restricted motion, • Commissural fusion and doming of leaflets in diastole. • Decreases size of the tricuspid valve orifice
3D findings	• Commissural width • Planimetry of valve area
Doppler findings	• Increases pressure gradient • $T_{1/2}$ valve area • Peak velocities nearly twice normal, velocities >1.5 m/s

Table 2: Tricuspid stenosis: Grading scales				
	Normal	*Mild*	*Moderate*	*Severe*
Valve area (cm^2)	7–9			<2
Mean gradient (mm Hg)	<2	2–3	3–6	>7
Peak gradient (mm Hg)	<4			>25
Peak velocity (m/s)	<1	1–1.5	1.5–2.5	>2.5
Continuous wave Doppler signal		Steep deceleration		Delayed deceleration, dense signal

from 2 different views. Importantly, the gradients are very dependent on flow—thus significant TR may be associated with a high gradient even in the absence of a stenotic orifice. In the absence of significant TR, a mean gradient of greater than 7 mm Hg indicates severe TS, and a gradient of 2 to 6 mm Hg indicates moderate TS. Calculation of the valve area with the pressure half time method has been described using a constant of 190 (TVA = 190/PHT) rather the 220 used for the MV. An area of 1 cm^2 or less is severe **(Table 2)**.

As a general rule, the mean pressure gradient derived using the $4v_2$ equation is lower in tricuspid than in MS, usually ranging between 2 and 10 mm Hg, and averaging around 5 mm Hg. Higher gradients may be seen with combined stenosis and regurgitation.

The primary consequence of TS is elevation of right atrial pressure and development of right-sided congestion. Because of the frequent presence of TR, the transvalvular gradient is clinically more relevant for assessment of severity and decision-making than the actual stenotic valve area. In addition, because anatomical valve orifice area is difficult to measure (not withstanding future developments in 3D), and TR is so frequently present, the typical CWD methods for valve method (T½) has been applied in a manner analogous to MS. Some authors have used the same constant of 220, while others have proposed a constant of 190 with valve area determined as: (190/T½). Although validation studies with TS are less than those with MS, valve area by the (T½) method may be less accurate than in MS. This is probably due to differences in atrioventricular compliance between the right and left side, and the influence of right ventricular relaxation, respiration, and TR on the pressure half-time. However, as a general rule, a longer (T½) implies a greater TS severity with values -190 frequently associated with significant (or critical) stenosis.

In theory, the continuity equation should provide a robust method for determining the effective valve area as SV divided by the tricuspid inflow VTI as recorded with CWD. The main limitation of the method is obtaining an accurate measurement of the inflow volume passing through the tricuspid valve. In the absence of significant TR, one can use the SV obtained from either the left or right ventricular outflow; a valve area of -1 cm^2 is considered indicative of severe TS. However, as severity of TR increases, valve area is progressively underestimated by this method. Nevertheless, a value -1 cm^2, although it is not accounting for the additional regurgitant volume, may still be indicative of a significant hemodynamic burden induced by the combined lesion **(Table 3)**.

Patients may present with fatigue, peripheral edema or symptoms relating to an underlying cause (e.g. flushing in carcinoid syndrome) or coexistent condition (e.g. mitral stenosis). Physical signs include a prominent 'a' wave in the JVP, a tricuspid opening snap and a diastolic murmur at the left sternal edge.

Table 3: Findings indicative of hemodynamically significant tricuspid stenosis	
Specific findings	
• Mean pressure gradient	≥ 5 mm Hg
• Inflow time-velocity	> 60 cm
• $T_{1/2}$	≥ 190 ms
• Valve area by continuity equation[a]	≤ 1 cm^2
Supportive findings	
• Enlarged right atrium ≥ moderates	
• Dilated inferior vena cava	

[a]Wave in the JVP

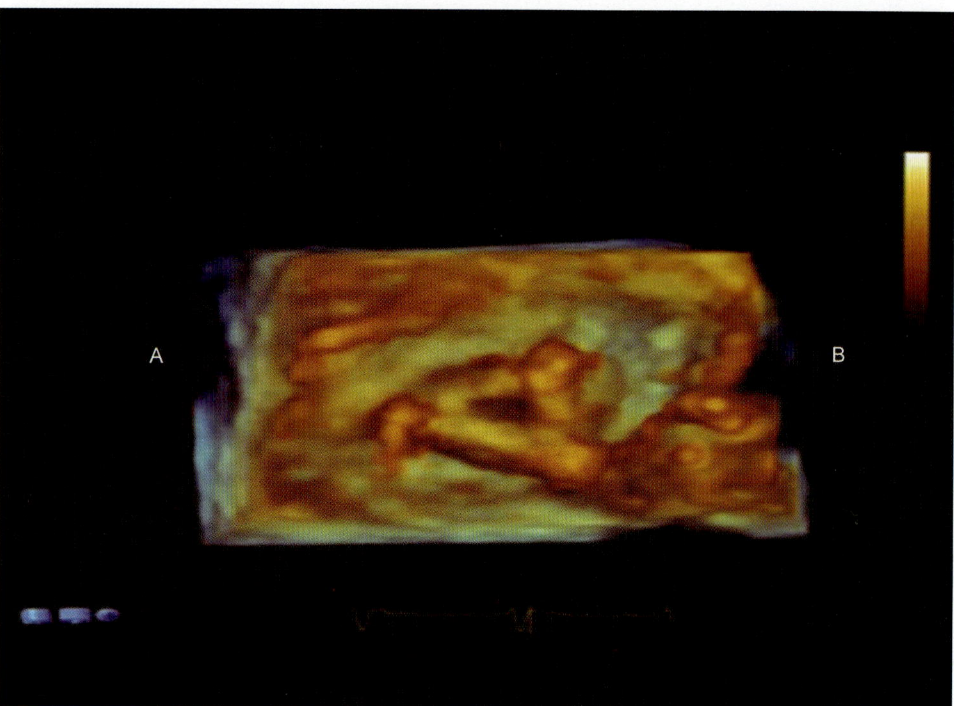

Figure 7

3D echocardiography showing severely calcified and stenotic bioprosthetic tricuspid valve, ventricular view. (A) Interventricular septum; (B) Right ventricular free wall

APPROACHES TO THREE-DIMENSIONAL IMAGING OF THE TRICUSPID VALVE STENOSIS

In tricuspid valve stenosis, the same approach as mitral stenosis can be used keeping in mind that thee hemodynamic assessment of the tricuspid valve varies with respiration. The mean gradient is the clinically used index to assess tricuspid stenosis severity.

PERCUTANEOUS TRANSCATHETER VALVE-IN-VALVE IMPLANTATION IN STENOSED TRICUSPID VALVE BIOPROSTHESIS

It has been reported by Van garsse et al, in a patient with a previous MVR now coming for a percutaneous tricuspid valve replacement in which the cannulae for CPB were percutaneously placed via the right femoral vessels under LA and a pacemaker wire was placed in the LV via the left femoral artery.

Transesophageal echocardiography viewing of the TV is partial it being obstructed by the scatter of the mechanical mitral valve which was already *in situ* in this patients with good LV function so an intracardiac echocardiographic probe was inserted in the left femoral view into the RA for preoperative imaging **(Fig. 7)**.

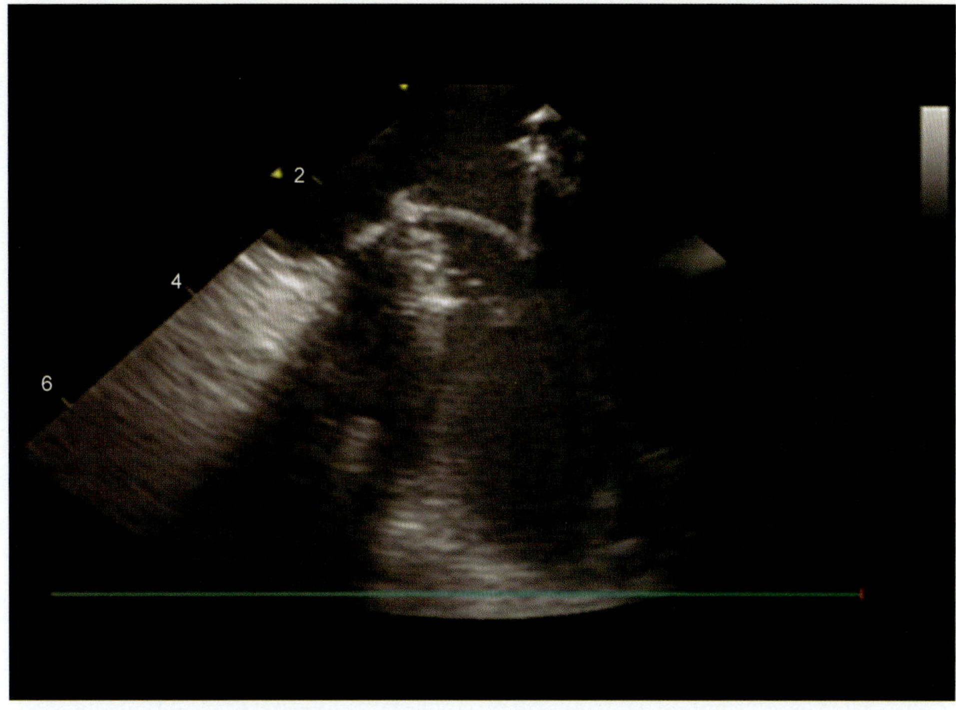

Figure 8
Intracardiac echocardiography showing adequate position and function of the tricuspid transcatheter bioprosthesis

The authors described the first human percutaneous transcatheter tricuspid valve-in-valve implantation. Although valve positioning was fluoroscopy-guided, intracardiac echocardiography provides reliable monitoring when transesophageal echocardiographic was inadequate.

Parallel position of the tricuspid valve to the caval veins can hamper the balloon to cross the heavily calcified tricuspid bioprosthesis. This case report Percutaneous valve-in-valve implantation in degenerated bioprostheses in tricuspid valve position is a feasible treatment option in selected cases **(Fig. 8)**.

SUMMARY

General Comments of Tricuspid Valve Stenosis

- Because the TV has the greatest cross-sectional area, flow velocities across the valve are lowest (<0.7 m/s).
- Significant TS is suggested when peak flow velocity exceeds 1.5 m/s.
- Many conditions that cause TS also result in significant TR.
- Measurement of peak gradients with spectral Doppler is heavily dependent on loading conditions, the compliance of the RA and RV, and the correct alignment of the ultrasound beam with the direction of antegrade blood flow.

- TV leaflets affected by carcinoid disease are often fixed and retracted whereas those involved in rheumatic disease demonstrated characteristic commissural fusion and doming during diastole.

BIBLIOGRAPHY

1. Acikel M, Erol MK, Yekeler I, Ozyazicioglu A. A case of free-floating ball thrombus in right atrium with tricuspid stenosis. Int J Cardiol. 2004;94(2-3):329-30 [Medline].
2. Ames DE, Asherson RA, Coltart JD, Vassilikos V, Jones JK, Hughes GR. Systemic lupus erythematosus complicated by tricuspid stenosis and regurgitation: successful treatment by valve transplantation. Ann Rheum Dis. 1992;51:120-2.
3. Arnett EN, Roberts WC. Prosthetic valve endocarditis. Clinicopathologic analysis of 22 necropsy patients with comparison of observations in 74 necropsy patients with 12 active infective endocarditis involving natural left-sided cardiac valves. Am J Cardiol. 1976;38:281-92
4. Chrissos DN, Stougiannos PN, Mytas DZ, Katsaros AA, Andrikopoulos GK, Kallikazaros IE. Multiple cardiac metastases from a malignant melanoma. Eur J Echocardiogr. 2008;9:391-2.
5. Coelho E. Physiopathologic study (clinical and experimental) of the tricuspid valve. Amer J Cardiol. 1959;3:517.
6. Cohen ML, Spray T, Gutierrez F, Barzilai B, Bauwens D. Congenital tricuspid valve stenosis with atrial septal defect and left anterior fascicular block. Clin Cardiol. 1990;13:497-9.
7. Dervanian P, Mace L, Bucari S, Folliguet TA, Grinda JM, Neveux JY. Valved conduit bypass for extensively calcified tricuspid valve stenosis. Ann Thorac Surg. 1995;60:450-2.
8. DutRoziEz P. Du Retrecissement de La Tricuspide Gaz Hop Paris. 1868;41:310.
9. Hatle L, Angelsen B, Tromsdal A. Noninvasive assessment of atrioventricular pressure half-time by Doppler ultrasound. Circulation. 1979;60:1096-1104.
10. Heaven DJ, Henein MY, Sutton R. Pacemaker lead related tricuspid stenosis: a report of two cases. Heart. 2000;83:351-2.
11. Hussain T, Knight WB, Mcleod KA. Lead-induced tricuspid stenosis successful management by ballon angioplasty. Pacing Clin Electrophysiol. 2009;32:140-2.
12. Krishanan A, Moulick A, Sinha P, Kuehl K, Kanter J, Slack M, Kaltman J, Mereader M, Moak JP. Severe tricuspid valve stenosis secondary to pacemaker leads presenting as ascites and liver dysfunction: a complex problem requiring a multidisciplinary therapeutic approach. J Interv Card Electrophysiol. 2009;24:71-5.
13. Kuralay E, Cingoz F, Gunay C, Demirkilic U, Tatar H. Huge right atrial myxoma causing fixed tricuspid stenosis with constitutional symptoms. J Card Surg. 2003;18:550-3.
14. Mehta V, Sengupta PP, Banerjee A, Arora R, Datt V. Congenital tricuspid stenosis and membranous right ventricular outflow tract obstruction in an adult. Ann Card Anaesth. 2003;6:152-5.
15. Nishida H, Grooters RK, Coster D, Soltanzadeh H, Thieman KC. Metastatic right atrial tumor in colon cancer with superior vena cava syndrome and tricuspid obstruction. Heart Vessels. 1991;6:125-7.
16. Nunez L, De Ia Llana R, Aguado MG, Iglesias A, Larrea JL, Celemin D. Bioprosthetic valve endocarditis. Indicators for surgical intervention. Ann Thorac Surg. 1983;35:262-70.

17. Old WD, Paulsen W, Lewis SA, Nixon JV. Pacemaker lead-induced tricuspid stenosis: diagnosis by Doppler echocardiography. Am Heart J. 1989;117:1165-7.
18. Ootaki Y, Yamaguchi M, Yoshimura N, Tsukuda K. Congenital heart disease with hyper-eosinophilic syndrome. Pediatr Cardiol. 2003;24:608-10.
19. Pearlman AS. Role of echocardiography in the diagnosis and evaluation of severity of mitral and tricuspid stenosis. Circulation. 1991;84(3 Suppl):1193-7.
20. Pothineni KR, Duncan K, Yelamanchili P, Nanda NC, Patel V, Fan P, et al. Live/real time three-dimensional transthoracic echocardiographic assessment of tricuspid valve pathology: incremental value over the two-dimensional technique. Echocardiography. 2007;24:541-52.
21. Saito T, Horimi H, Hasegawa T, Kamoshida T. Isolated tricuspid valve stenosis caused by infective endocarditis in an adult: report of a case. Surg Today. 1993;23:1081-4.
22. Salazar E, Levine HD. Rheumatic tricuspid regurgitation. Amer J Med. 1962;33:111.
23. Taira K, Suzuki A, Fujino A, Watanabe T, Ogyu A, Ashikawa K. Tricuspid valve stenosis related to subvalvular adhesion of pacemaker lead: a case report. J Cardiol. 2006;47:301-6.
24. Thatipelli MR, Uber PA, Mehra MR. Isolated tricuspid stenosis and heart failure: a focus on carcinoid heart disease. Congest Heart Fail. 2003;9:294-6.
25. Uribe-Etxebarria N, Voces R, Rodriguez MA, Llorente A, Perez P, Aramendi JI. Reversible tricuspid valve stenosis due to a metastatic dissemination of a noncardiac sarcoma. Ann Thorac Surg. 2005;80:e1-2.
26. Waller BF. Morphological aspects of valvular heart disease: Part I. Curr Probl Cardiol. Oct 1984;9(7):1-66 [Medline].
27. Waller BF. Morphological aspects of valvular heart disease: Part II. Curr Probl Cardiol. Nov. 1984;9(8):1-74 [Medline].
28. Yousof AM, Shafei MZ, Endrys G, Khan N, Simo M, Cherian G. Tricuspid stenosis and regurgitation in rheumatic heart disease: a prospective cardiac catheterization study in 525 patients. Am Heart J. 1985;110(1 Pt 1):60-4.

II

TRANSESOPHAGEAL ECHOCARDIOGRAPHY OF PULMONARY VALVE

muralidhar kanchi
section editor

6 Pulmonary Stenosis

Poonam Malhotra Kapoor, Sarvesh Pal Singh

- Anatomy of Pulmonary Valve
- Valve Anatomy
- What is Pulmonary Stenosis? Pathophysiology of Pulmonary Stenosis
- Physiology of Pulmonary Stenosis
- Infundibular Pulmonary Stenosis
- Pulmonary Artery and Vein Stenosis
- Why is Pulmonary Stenosis a Concern?
- Color Wave and Pulse Wave Doppler and Pressure Gradients Across the Pulmonary Stenosis
- Pressure Gradient Across the Pulmonary Stenosis
- Severity Definitions of Pulmonary Stenosis

INTRODUCTION

Echocardiography plays a major role in the assessment and management of pulmonary valve stenosis.[1] It is useful in detecting the site of the stenosis, quantifying severity, determining the cause of the stenosis, and is essential in determining an appropriate management strategy.[2] Ancillary findings with pulmonary stenosis such as right ventricular hypertrophy may also be detected and assessed. Although the majority of pulmonary stenosis is valvular, narrowing of the right ventricular outflow tract (RVOT) below the valve from concurrent right ventricular hypertrophy may occur as may narrowing of the pulmonary artery sinotubular junction above the valve.

ANATOMY OF PULMONARY VALVE

- Pulmonary valvular apparatus consists of the 3 cusps, associated sinuses of valsalva and a sinotubular junction similar to aortic valve.
- The 3 cusps are named the anterior, the left and right.
- Valve area is approximately 2 cm/m^2.

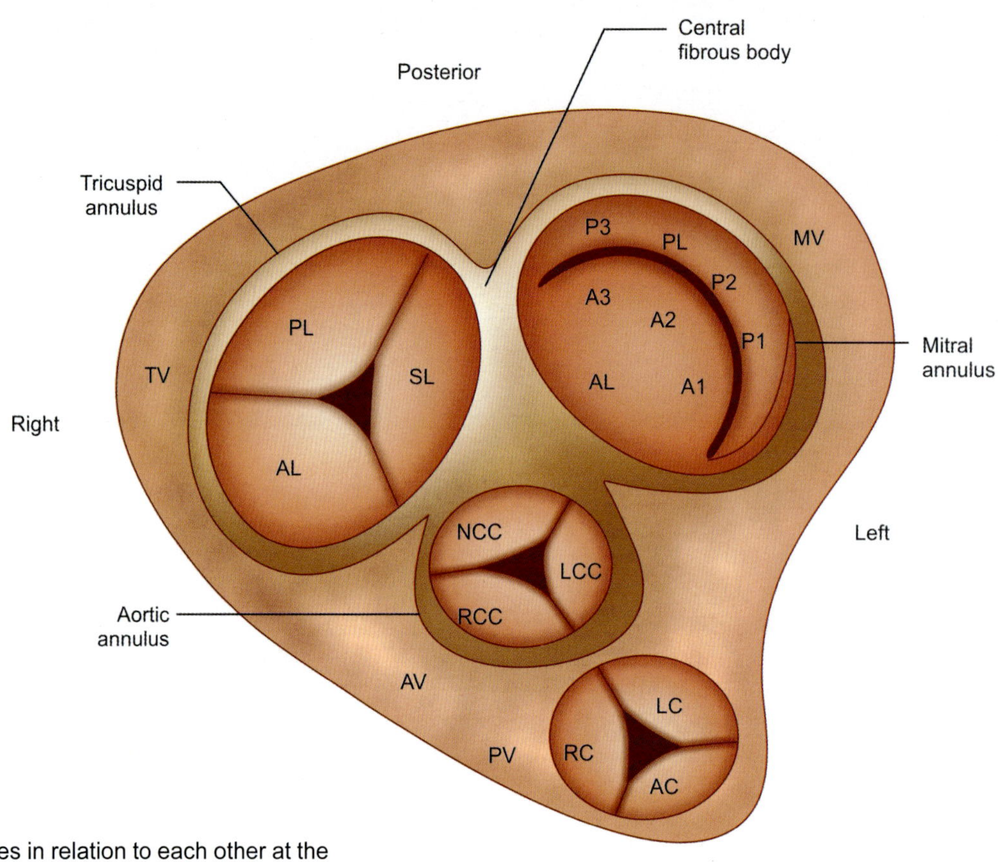

Figure 1

The relationship of the 4 valves in relation to each other at the base of the heart

- PA: Slightly dilated forming sinus.
- Normally AV and PV lie at 90· planes to each other. Imaging the AV in ME SAX (PV long axis view—**Fig. 1**) as in ME RVOT, AV in LAX (PV is a very anterior structure).

VALVE ANATOMY

Evaluation of anatomy is important in defining where the stenosis is maximal, as discussed above. Valve morphology is often evident especially the thin mobile leaflets seen with the dome-shaped valve. Dysplastic leaflets move little and are rarely associated with the post-stenotic dilatation common in dome-shaped leaflets. However, the size of the pulmonary annulus should be measured in order to define the optimal balloon size for successful dilatation of the valve.[3]

WHAT IS PULMONARY STENOSIS? PATHOPHYSIOLOGY OF PULMONARY STENOSIS

Pulmonary stenosis is a condition characterized by obstruction to blood flow from the right ventricle to the pulmonary artery. This obstruction is caused by narrowing

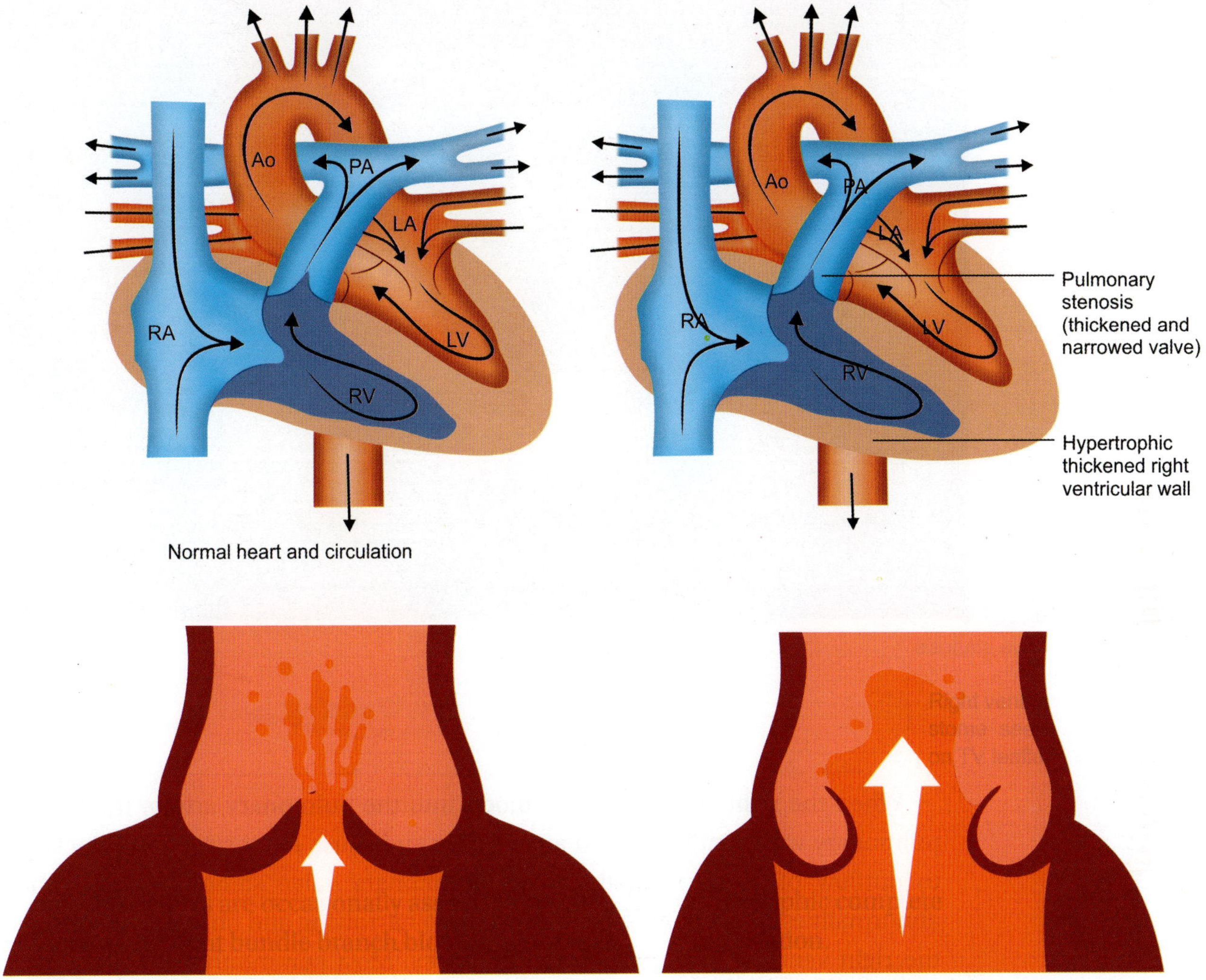

Pulmonary stenosis (thickened and narrowed valve)

Hypertrophic thickened right ventricular wall

Normal heart and circulation

Pulmonary stenosis

Healthy pulmonary valve

Figure 2

Normal pulmonary valve consists of three thin and pliable valve leaflets

or stenosis at one or more of several points from the right ventricle to the pulmonary artery. It includes obstruction from thickened muscle below the pulmonary valve, narrowing of the valve itself, or narrowing of the pulmonary artery above the valve. The most common form of pulmonary stenosis is obstruction at the valve itself, referred to as pulmonary valvular stenosis. The normal pulmonary valve consists of three thin and pliable valve leaflets **(Fig. 2)**.

- **Calcification of the valve is relatively rare so the valve appearance does not play a huge role in decisions for balloon valvuloplasty**

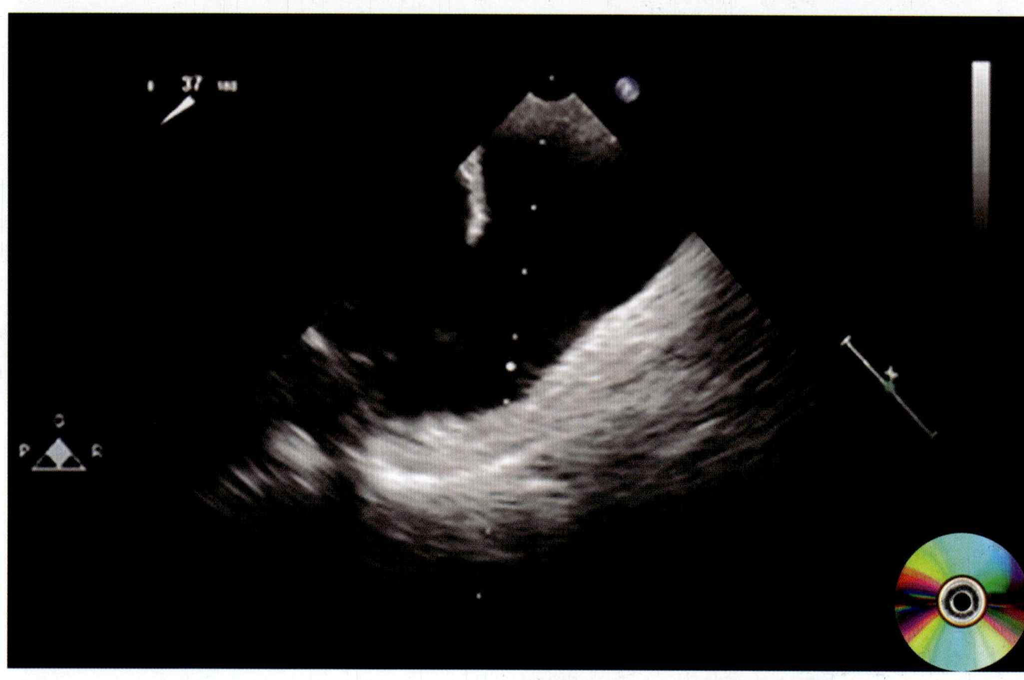

Figure 3 (VIDEO 1)

TEE of pulmonary valve stenosis

When the right ventricle ejects blood into the pulmonary artery, the normal pulmonary valve leaflets spread apart easily and cause no obstruction (blockage) to outflow of blood from the heart. Pulmonary valve stenosis occurs when abnormalities of the pulmonary valve lead to narrowing and obstruction between the right ventricle and the pulmonary artery. Most commonly with pulmonary valvar stenosis, the pulmonary valve leaflets are thickened and fused together along their separation lines (commissures). The increased right ventricular muscle, known as hypertrophy, is rarely a problem in itself, but instead is an indication that significant valve obstruction exists **(Fig. 3)**.

PHYSIOLOGY OF PULMONARY STENOSIS

When the pulmonary valve is severely obstructed, especially in newborns with critical degrees of pulmonary stenosis, the right ventricle cannot eject sufficient volume of blood flow into the pulmonary artery **(Figs 4A and B)**. In these instances, blue blood bypasses the right ventricle flowing from the right atrium to left atrium, through the foramen ovale, a communication or "hole" between these two chambers that is normally present in newborns. Newborns with critical pulmonary stenosis therefore will have cyanosis (blue discoloration of the lips and nail beds) due to lower oxygen levels in their blood.

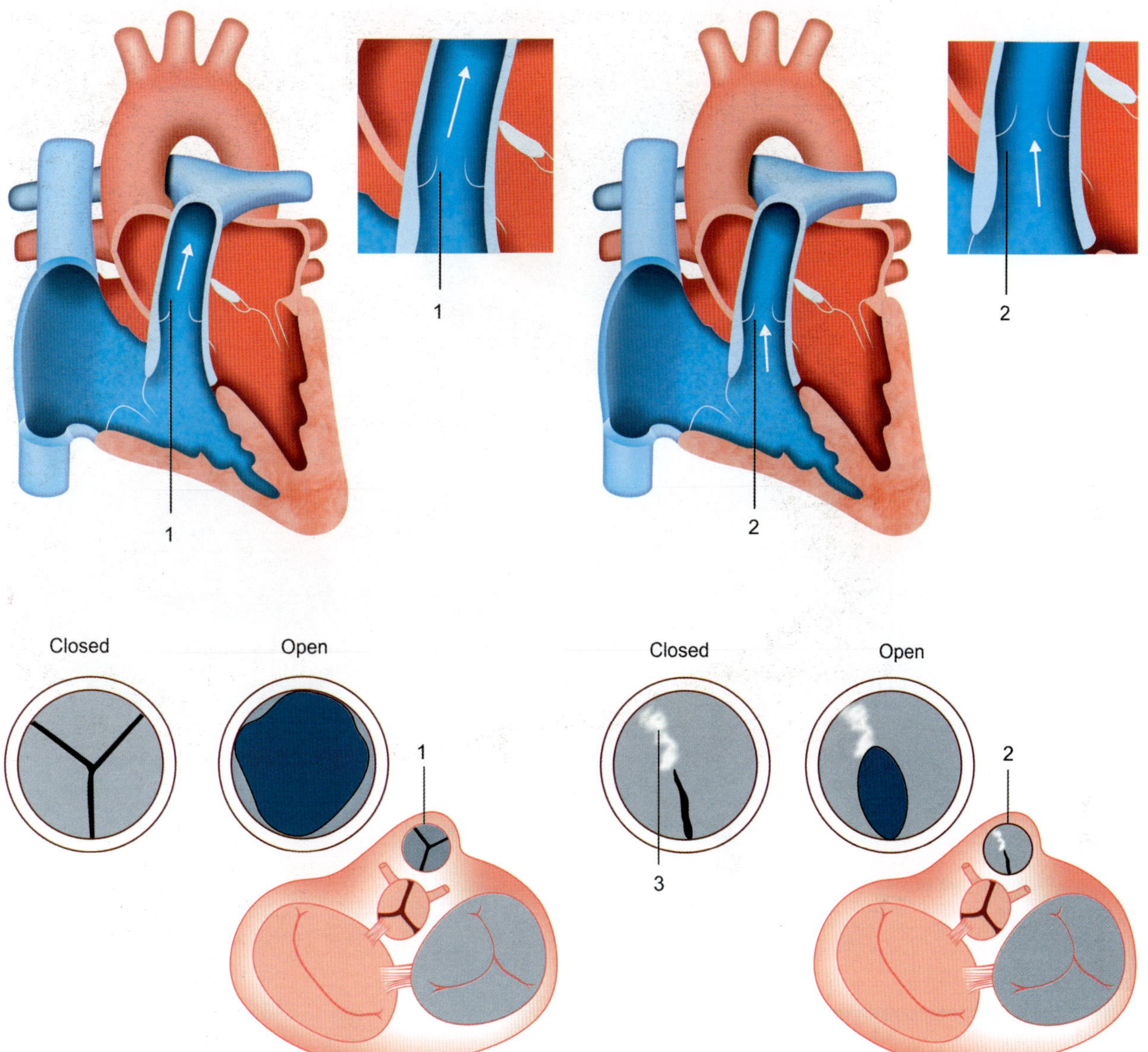

1. Normal heart in systole (during ventricular ejection) showing pulmonic valve opening completely.
2. Pulmonic stenosis with thickened and fused valve leaflets preventing full opening during systole.
3. Fusion of a commissure in a malformed, bicuspid pulmonic valve.

Figure 4A

Pulmonary valve in systole

There are four different types of pulmonary stenosis:

1. *Valvular pulmonary stenosis:* The valve leaflets are thickened and/or narrowed.
2. *Supravalvar pulmonary stenosis:* The pulmonary artery just above the pulmonary valve is narrowed.

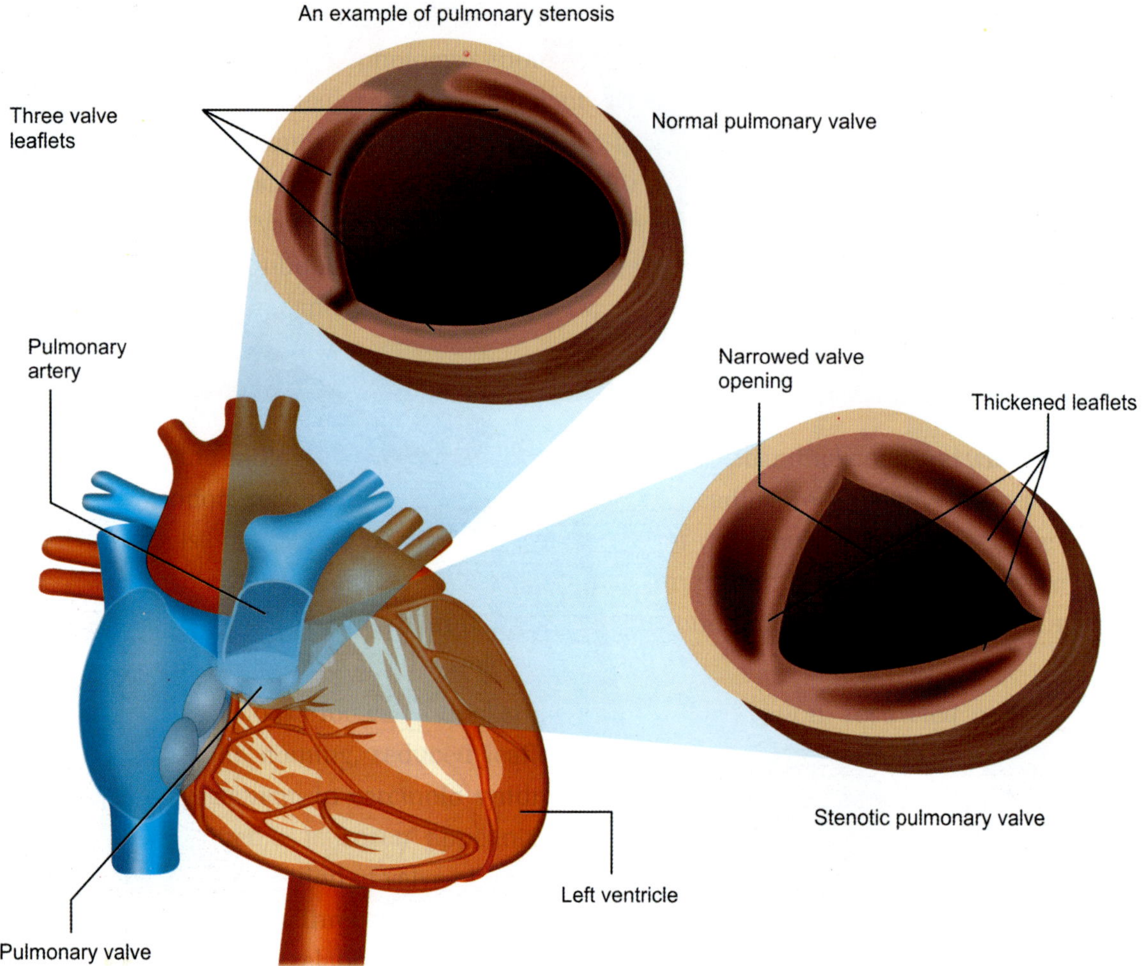

Figure 4B

An example of pulmonary stenosis in diastole

3. *Subvalvar (infundibular) pulmonary stenosis:* The muscle under the valve area is thickened, narrowing the outflow tract from the right ventricle.
4. *Branch peripheral pulmonic stenosis:* The right or left pulmonary artery is narrowed, or both may be narrowed.

Branch Peripheral Pulmonic Stenosis

Transient pulmonary branch stenosis (PBS) in preterm and term neonates is well recognized. In preterm infants, closure of a patent ductus arteriosus (PDA) seems to be an important factor in the development of PBS but in only one of the studies reported in literature was the natural history reported. The presence of a heart murmur a few days or weeks after closure of a PDA in a preterm infant is often thought to be due to reopening of the ductus arteriosus, but the relation between a murmur and PDA is poor, and in term infants it has been shown to be more often associated with PBS than with PDA.

Causes and Clinical Presentation

Congenital pulmonary stenosis occurs due to improper development of the pulmonary valve in the first 8 weeks of fetal growth. It can be caused by a number of factors, though most of the time this heart defect occurs sporadically (by chance), with no clear reason evident for its development. Pulmonary stenosis usually does not cause symptoms in infants or small children. As the child gets older, abnormal signs and symptoms may appear, including:

- Fatigue
- A heart murmur (an extra heart sound when a doctor listens with a stethoscope)
- Chest pain
- Fainting
- Heavy or rapid breathing
- Shortness of breath
- Rapid heart rate
- Swelling in the feet, ankles, face, eyelids, and/or abdomen
- Fewer wet diapers or trips to the bathroom.

Some congenital heart defects may have a genetic link, either occurring due to a defect in a gene, a chromosome abnormality, or environmental exposure, causing heart problems to occur more often in certain families. The normal pulmonary valve is trileaflet. The congenitally stenotic valve may be trileaflet, bicuspid, unicuspid, or dysplastic.[4]

Rheumatic pulmonary stenosis is rare even when the valve is affected by the rheumatic process.[5] Carcinoid disease is the most common cause of acquired pulmonary valve disease (combined stenosis and regurgitation with usually predominant regurgitation) and this may be sufficiently severe to require prosthetic replacement. Various tumors may compress the RV outflow tract leading to functional pulmonary stenosis. These tumors may arise from within the heart or associated vasculature or be external to the heart and compress from without.[6,7]

- **Pulmonary stenosis is almost always congenital in origin**
- **Acquired stenosis of the pulmonary valve is very uncommon**

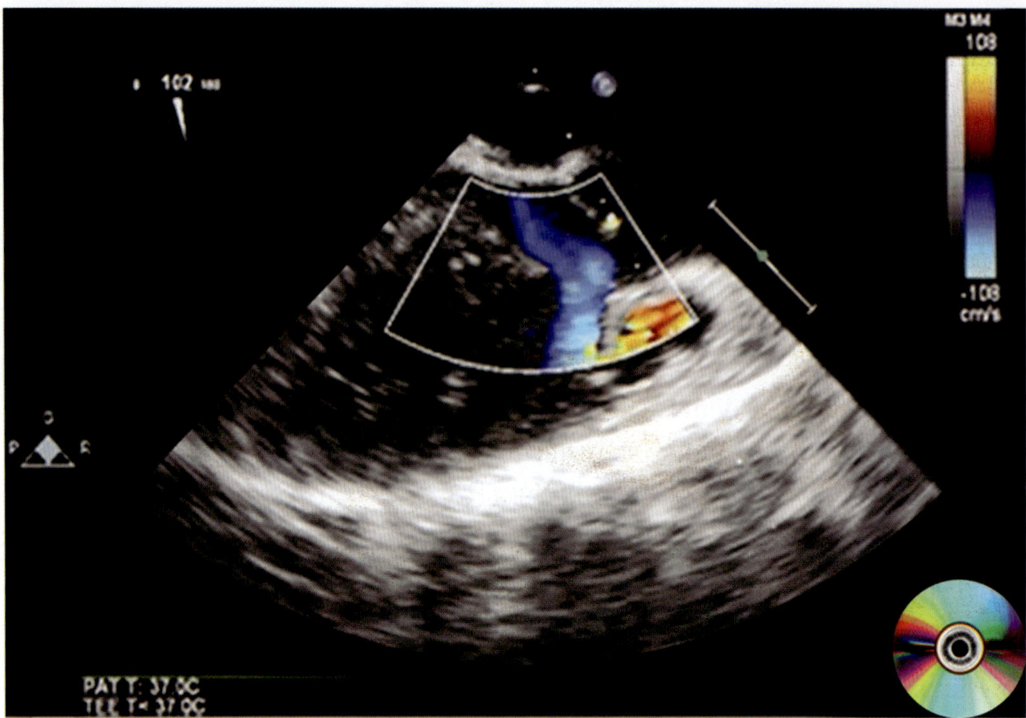

Figure 5 (VIDEO 2)

Tetralogy of Fallot in pulmonary stenosis

Pulmonary valve stenosis may also occur as part of more complex congenital lesions such as tetralogy of Fallot **(Fig. 5)**, complete atrioventricular canal, double outlet RV, and univentricular heart. Peripheral pulmonary artery stenosis may co-exist with valvular pulmonary stenosis such as in Noonan's syndrome and Williams's syndrome as shown later.

INFUNDIBULAR PULMONARY STENOSIS

Stenosis below (proximal to) the pulmonary valve may result from a number of causes, both congenital and acquired. Congenital ventricular septal defect (VSD) may also be associated with RV outflow tract obstruction secondary to development of obstructive midcavitary or infundibular muscle bundles (double chamber RV) **(Fig. 6)** or in rare cases as a result of the jet lesion produced by the VSD in this area. Severe right ventricular hypertrophy of any cause but in some cases caused by valvular pulmonary stenosis itself may be responsible for narrowing of the infundibular area below the pulmonary valve. Iatrogenic causes include prior surgery or intervention on this area. Other causes include hypertrophic or infiltrative processes such as hypertrophic obstructive cardiomyopathy or glycogen storage disorders and compression from a tumor or vascular structure.

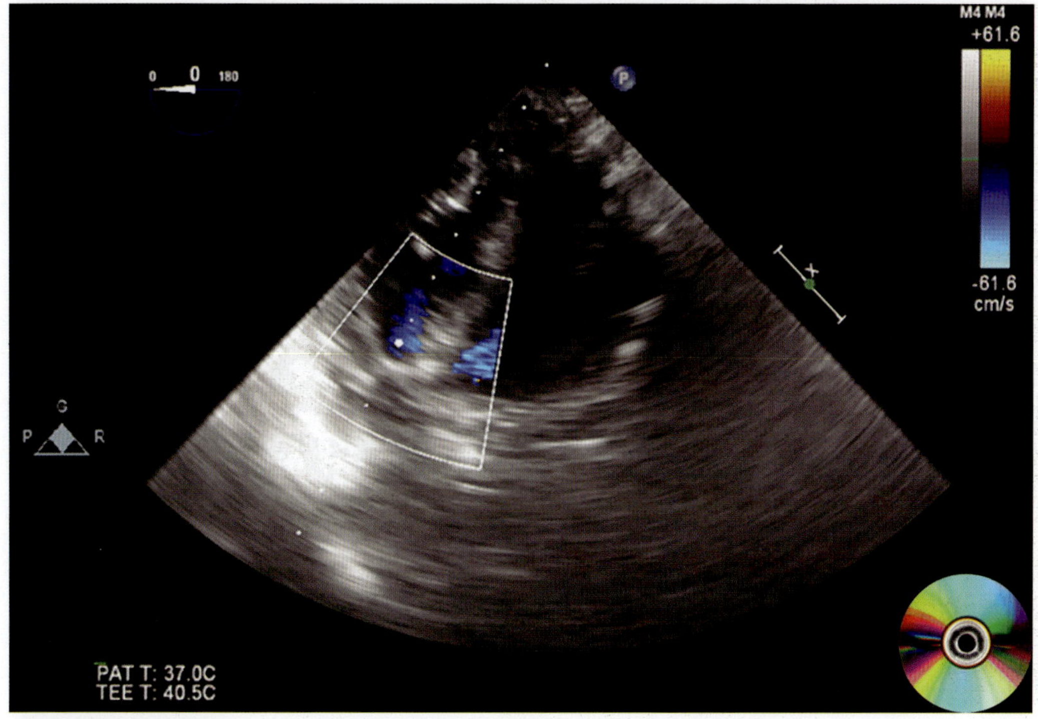

Figure 6 (VIDEO 3)

Double chamber right ventricular in pulmonary stenosis

PULMONARY ARTERY AND VEIN STENOSIS

Stenosis of the pulmonary artery above the valve (distal to the valve) may occur in the main pulmonary trunk at the bifurcation, or more distally in the branch vessels or in the pulmonary vein. In rare instances, a membrane just above the valve may cause stenosis. Pulmonary artery stenosis may occur as an isolated finding without other malformations.

WHY IS PULMONARY STENOSIS A CONCERN?

Mild pulmonary stenosis may not cause any symptoms. Problems can occur when pulmonary stenosis is moderate to severe, including the following:

- The right ventricle has to work harder to try to move blood through the tight pulmonary valve. Eventually, the right ventricle is no longer able to handle the extra workload, and it fails to pump forward efficiently. Pressure builds up in the right atrium, and then in the veins bringing blood back to the right side of the heart. Fluid retention and swelling may occur.
- There is a higher than average chance of developing an infection in the valves of the heart known as bacterial endocarditis.

COLOR WAVE AND PULSE WAVE DOPPLER AND PRESSURE GRADIENTS ACROSS THE PULMONARY STENOSIS

Use color wave (CW) Doppler to obtain a trace of forward flow through the pulmonary valve. Obtain traces from the right ventricular outflow view and the AV short axis view **(Fig. 7)**.

The CW Doppler trace will give peak transpulmonary velocity (V_{max}), which relates to peak transpulmonary pressure gradient (ΔP_{max}) via the simplified Bernoulli equation:

$$\Delta P_{max} = 4 \times V^2_{max}$$

If peak velocity in the RVOT is >1.0 m/s, use the full Bernoulli equation for greater accuracy:

$$\Delta P_{max} = 4 \times (V^2_2 - V^2_1)$$

Where V_2 is the peak transpulmonary velocity, assessed by CW Doppler and V_1 is the peak RVOT velocity, assessed by PW Doppler.

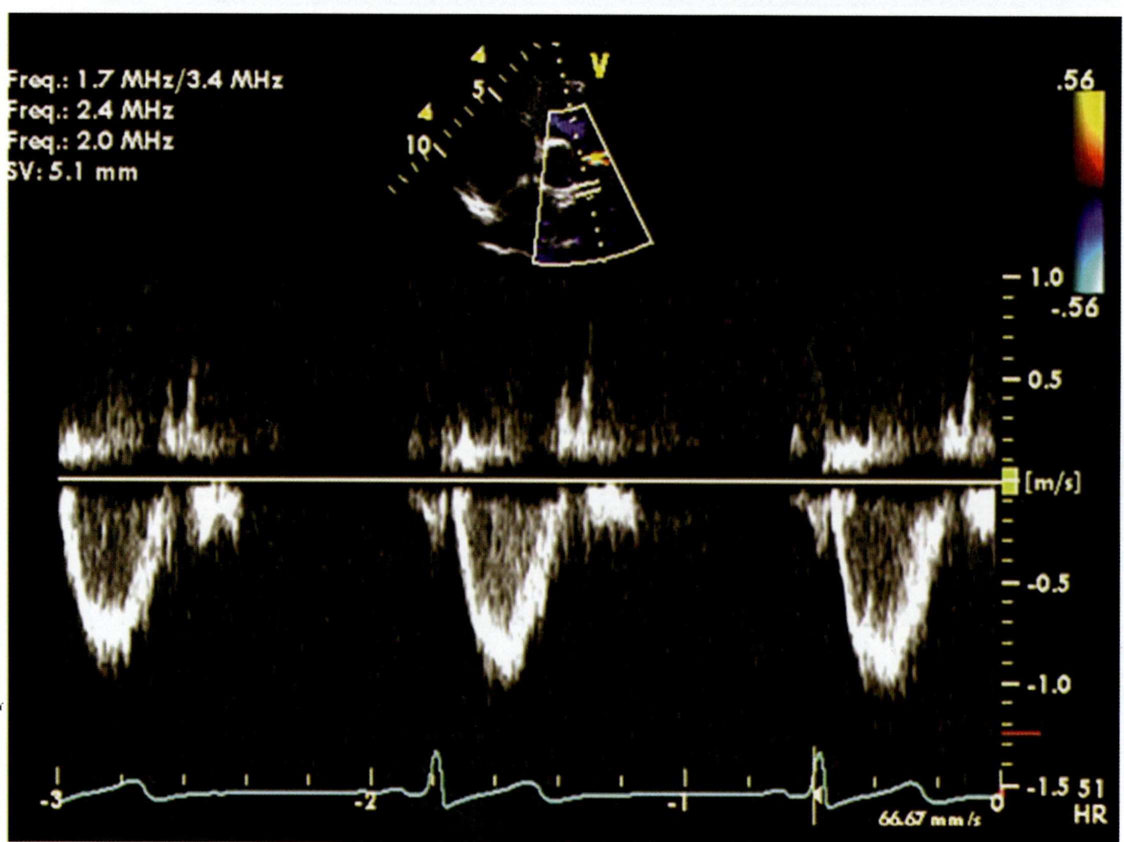

Figure 7

Patient with CWD in RVH and PS combined pulmonary valve stenosis and regurgitation

The mean transpulmonary pressure gradient (ΔP_{mean}) can be obtained by tracing the Dopple envelope, from which the echo machine can calculate a mean value by averaging the instantaneous gradients throughout the trace.

In complain of suspicion of infundibular or supravalvular stenosis stenosis, use PW Doppler to assess blood flow at different levels above and below the valve to detect where the main flow acceleration occurs. If color Doppler reveals pulmonary regurgitation, record a trace using CW Doppler to assess the density of the regurgitant signal (more dense = more severe) and also the angle of the downward (deceleration) slope (steeper slope = more severe) **(Figs 8 to 15)**.

Pulmonary vein stenosis in a child with VSD

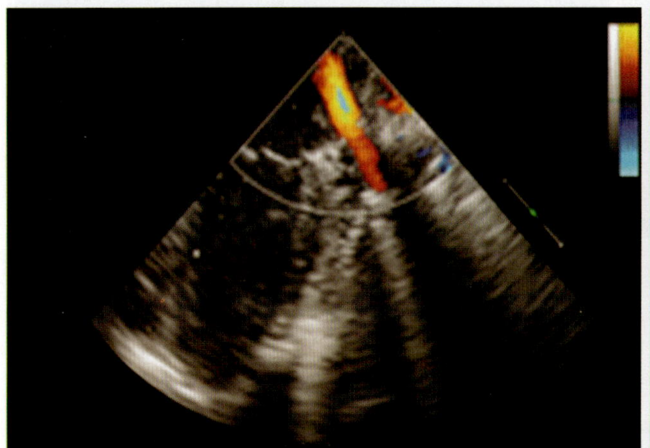

Figure 8

Color Doppler in midesophageal modified bicommissural view showing a discrete membrane obstructing the opening of left superior pulmonary vein (LSPV)

Figure 9

Color Doppler in midesophageal modified bicommissural view showing no obstruction to blood flow from the left superior pulmonary vein after resection of the membrane

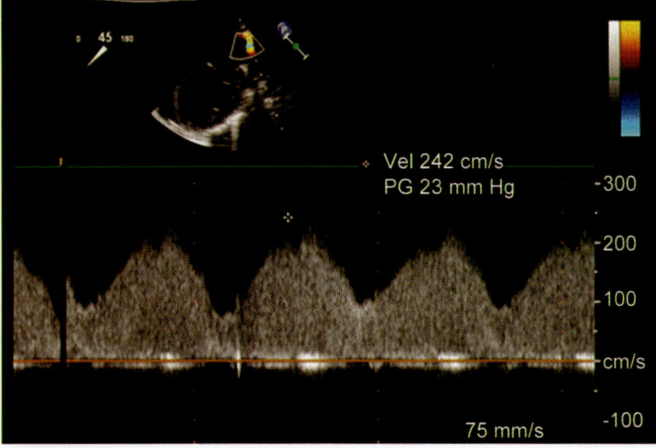

Figure 10

Continuous-wave Doppler showing a gradient of 23 mm Hg across the obstructing membrane

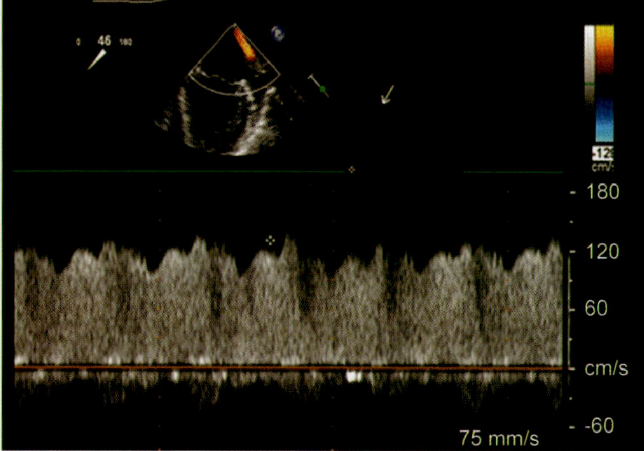

Figure 11

Continuous-wave Doppler showing a gradient of 7 mm Hg across left superior pulmonary vein after intracardiac repair

Pulmonic Valve Views (Figs 12A to D)

ME RV inflow-outflow (45–60°)
Right cusp: Near aortic valve
Anterior cusp: Laterally
Measure annulus (21 ± 3 mm)

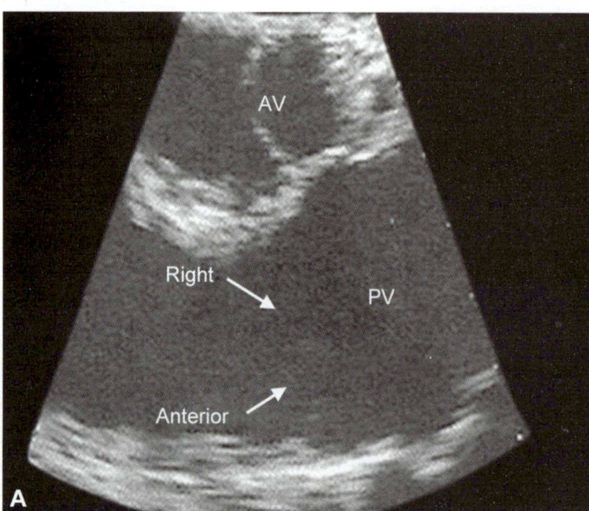

ME Ascending aorta SAX (0°)
Useful Doppler alignment for PA flow
Diameter main PA: 20 ± 5 mm

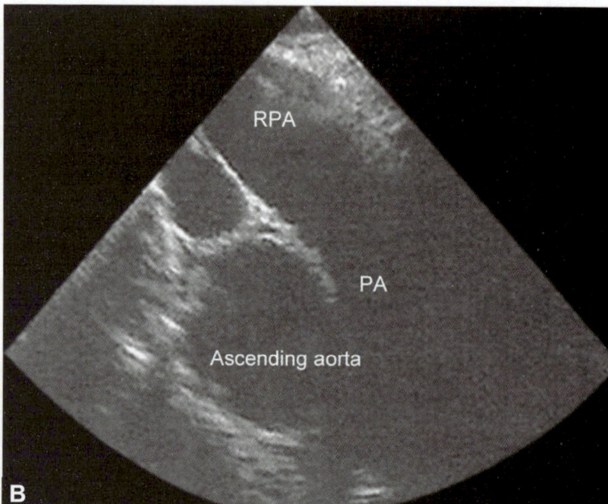

UE aortic arch SAX (60–90°)
Measure annulus
Doppler alignment for flow

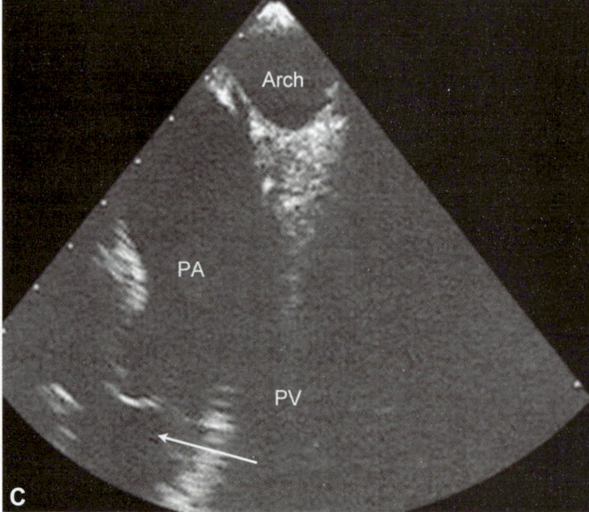

TG RV (modified 30–60°)
Useful Doppler alignment
Normal peak velocity 0.5–1.0 m/s

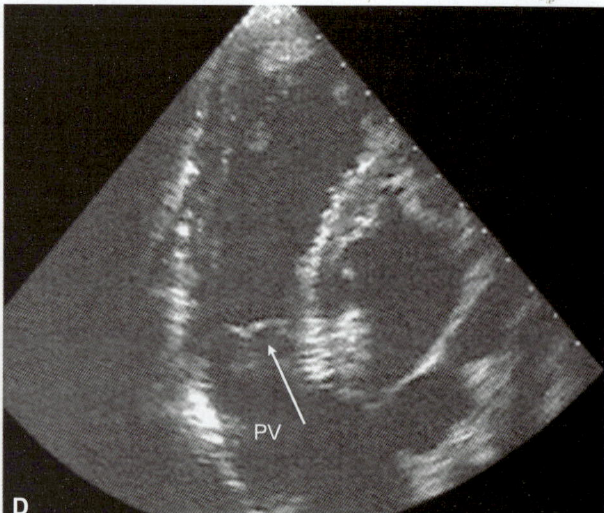

Figures 12A to D

Pulmonic valve views

TEE Views to assess Pulmonary Valve (Fig. 14)

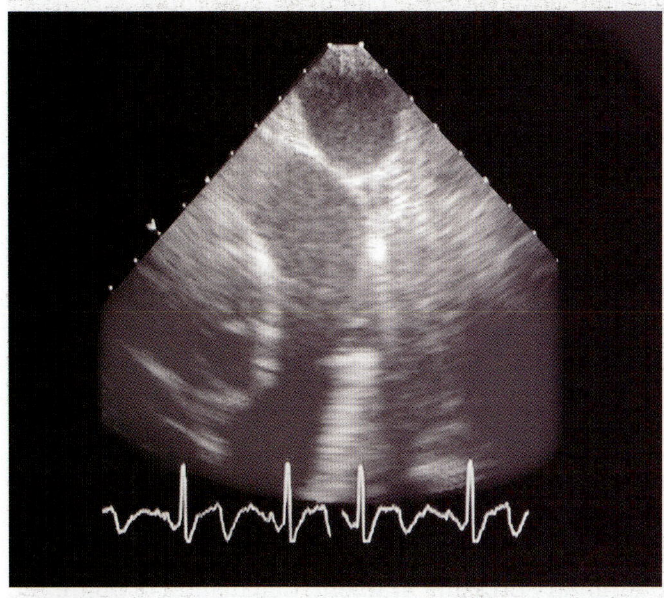

Figure 13

TEE views to assess pulmonary valve pulmonic valve and RVOT 70-110

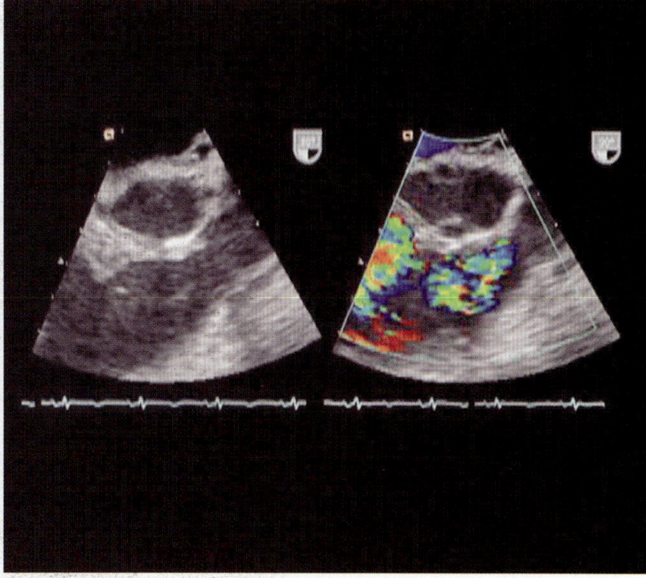

Figure 14

Tricuspid inflow and pulmonic regurgitation in diastole

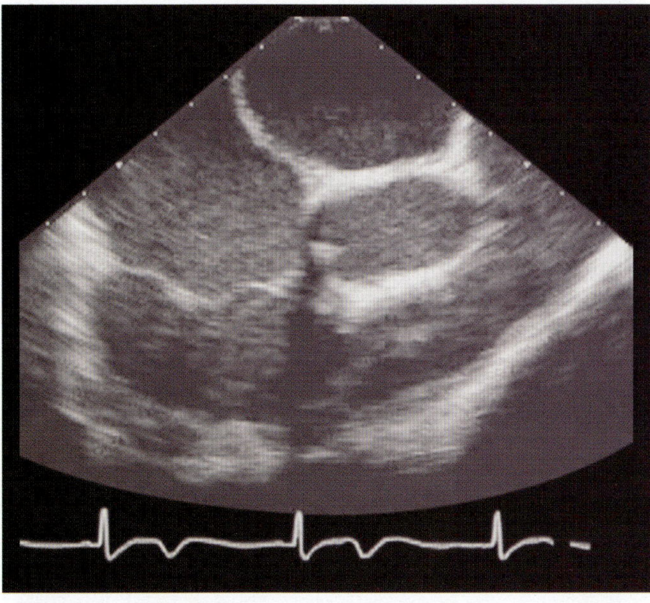

Figure 15

Pulmonary valve in RT sided inflow outflow view

Associated Features

Pulmonary stenosis is often associated with other congenital heart disorders, and so look carefully for any other structural heart defects (e. g. Tetralogy of Fallot). In addition:

- Assess any coexistent pulmonary regurgitation.
- Assess any coexistent tricuspid valve disease (carcinoid syndrome can affect both tricuspid and pulmonary valves.
- Assess RV dimensions and function. Obstruction to RV outflow by the pulmonary valve raises RV pressure, leading to RV hypertrophy and subsequently dilatation and impaired function.
- Assess pulmonary artery dimensions (pulmonary artery dilatation is a common finding in pulmonary stenosis).

Severity of Pulmonary Stenosis

Severity of pulmonary stenosis can be quantified by P_{max} **(Table 1)**.

How to Grade Pulmonary Stenosis?

Pulmonic stenosis severity quantitative assessment of pulmonary stenosis severity is based mainly on the transpulmonary pressure gradient. Calculation of pulmonic valve area by planimetry is not possible since the required image plane is in general not available. Continuity equation or proximal isovelocity surface area method, although feasible in principle, has not been validated in pulmonary stenosis and is rarely performed **(Fig. 16)**.

PRESSURE GRADIENT ACROSS THE PULMONARY STENOSIS

The estimation of the systolic pressure gradient is derived from the transpulmonary velocity flow curve using the simplified Bernoulli equation $P = 4v^2$. This estimation is reliable, as shown by the good correlation with invasive measurement using cardiac catheterization.[8] Continuous-wave Doppler is used to assess the severity

Table 1: Gradient of pulmonary stenosis

	Trivial	*Mild*	*Moderate*	*Severe*
Peak gradient	Less than 25 mm Hg	Between 25 and 49 mm Hg	Between 50 and 79 mm Hg	More than 80 mm Hg

Sample report

- **The pulmonary valve cusps are thin but the commissures are partially fused with 'doming' of the valve during systole. The transpulmonary peak velocity is 4.8 m/s (peak gradient 92 mm Hg, mean gradient 56 mm Hg). There is mild pulmonary regurgitation. The tricuspid, mitral and aortic valves are normal. There is moderate RV hypertrophy with good systolic function. The main pulmonary artery is mildly dilated. The findings are consistent with severe pulmonary stenosis.**

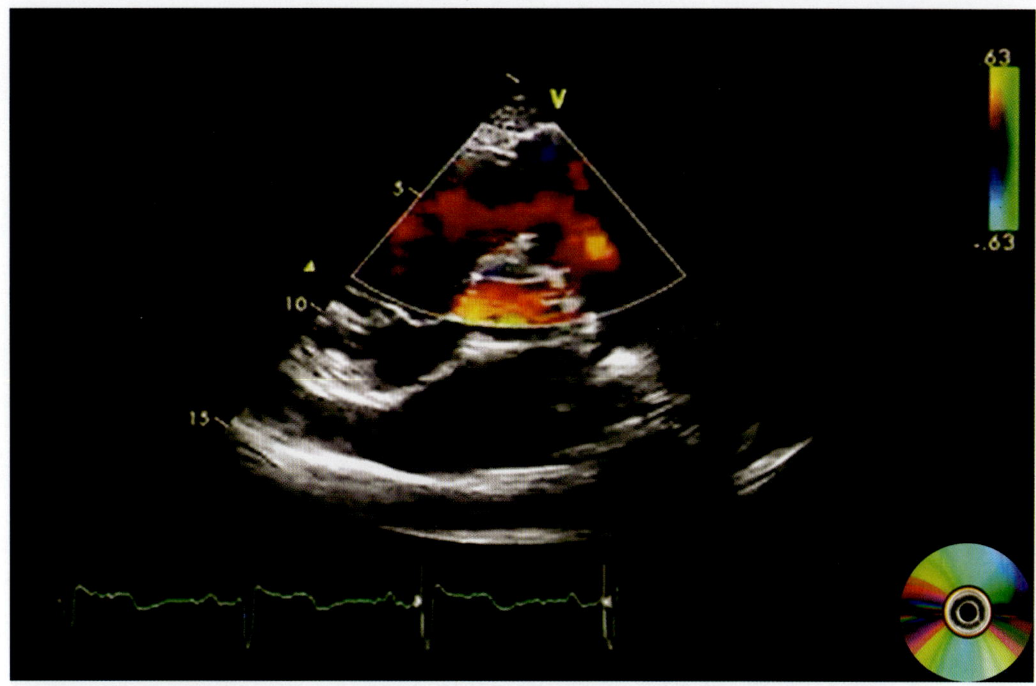

Figure 16 (VIDEO 4)
Pulmonary insufficiency

when even mild stenosis is present. It is important to line up the Doppler sample volume parallel to the flow with the aid of color flow mapping where appropriate. In adults, this is usually most readily performed from a aortic short-axis view but in children and in some adults the highest gradients may be found from UE AVSAX. A modified bicaval chamber view may also be used where the transducer is angled clockwise to bring in the RV outflow tract. Ideally, the highest velocity in multiple views should be used for the determination.[9,10]

In most instances of valvular pulmonary stenosis, the modified Bernoulli equation works well and there is no need to account for the proximal velocity as this is usually, 1 m/s. There are exceptions to this, however. In the setting of subvalvular or infundibular stenosis and pulmonary stenosis as part of a congenital syndrome or as a result of RV hypertrophy, the presence of two stenosis in series may make it impossible to ascertain precisely the individual contribution of each. In addition, such stenosis in series may cause significant PR resulting in a higher Doppler gradient compared with the net pressure drop across both stenosis.[11] Pulsed-wave Doppler may be useful to detect the sites of varying levels of obstruction in the outflow tract and in lesser degrees of obstruction may allow a full evaluation of it. Muscular infundibular obstruction is frequently characterized by a late peaking systolic jet that appears 'dagger-shaped,' reflecting the dynamic nature of the obstruction; this pattern can be useful is separating dynamic muscular obstruction from fixed valvular obstruction, where the peak velocity is generated early in systole.

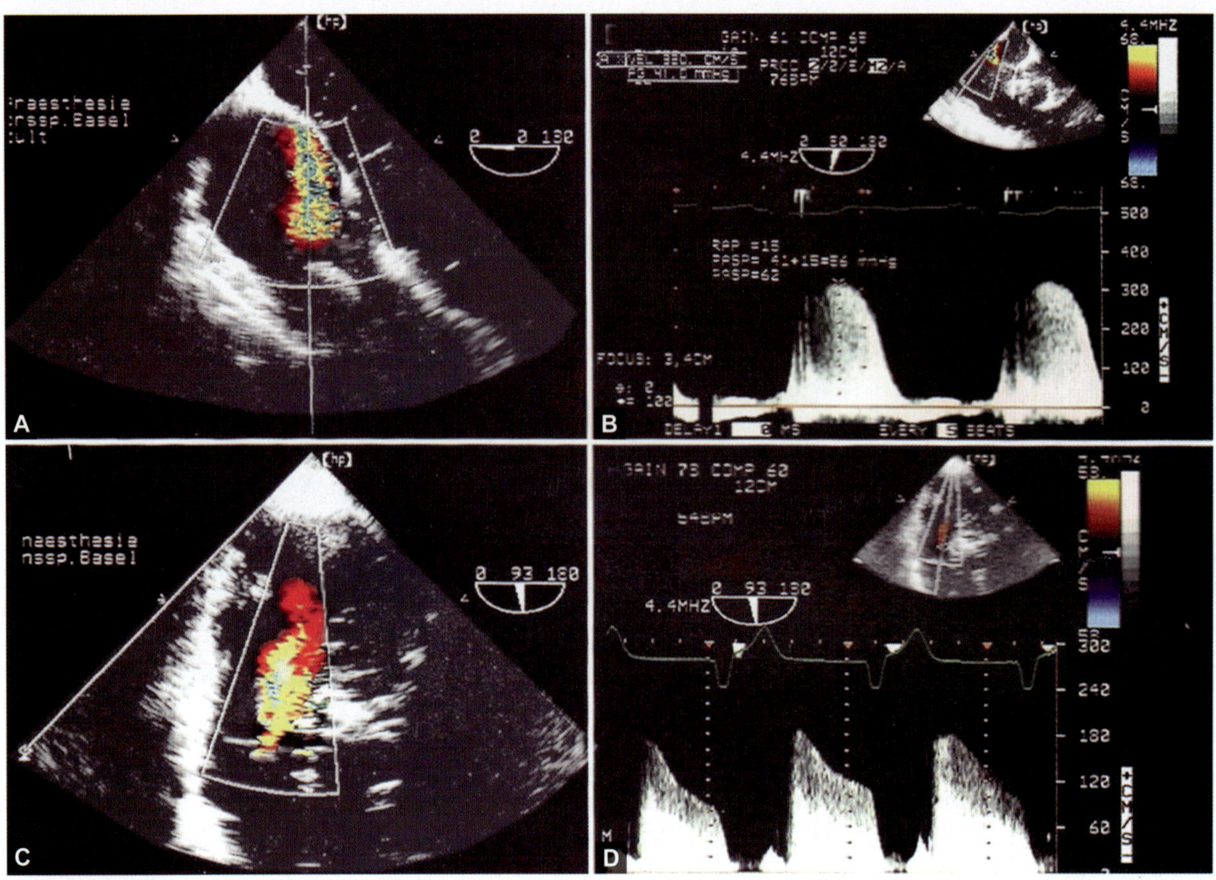

Figures 17A to D

Measurement of the pulmonary pressures on TEE in multiple views

Staging of Pulmonary Stenosis

The severity of pulmonary valve obstruction may be categorized (staged) as follows, based on peak-to-peak catheter-measured pulmonary valvar gradient. This severity classification is useful in categorizing patients for natural history studies and in formulating treatment algorithms.

In certain situations, TEE may allow a more accurate assessment of the pulmonary valve and RVOT than transthoracic echo. The pulmonary valve may be identified from a mid-esophageal window at varying transducer positions from 50 to 90, anterior to the aortic valve. The RVOT is often well seen in this view. It is in general impossible to line up CW to accurately ascertain maximal flow velocity. Other windows in which the pulmonary outflow tract may be interrogated include the deep transgastric view in which by appropriate torquing of the transducer, the RV inflow and outflow may be appreciated in a single image. This view can

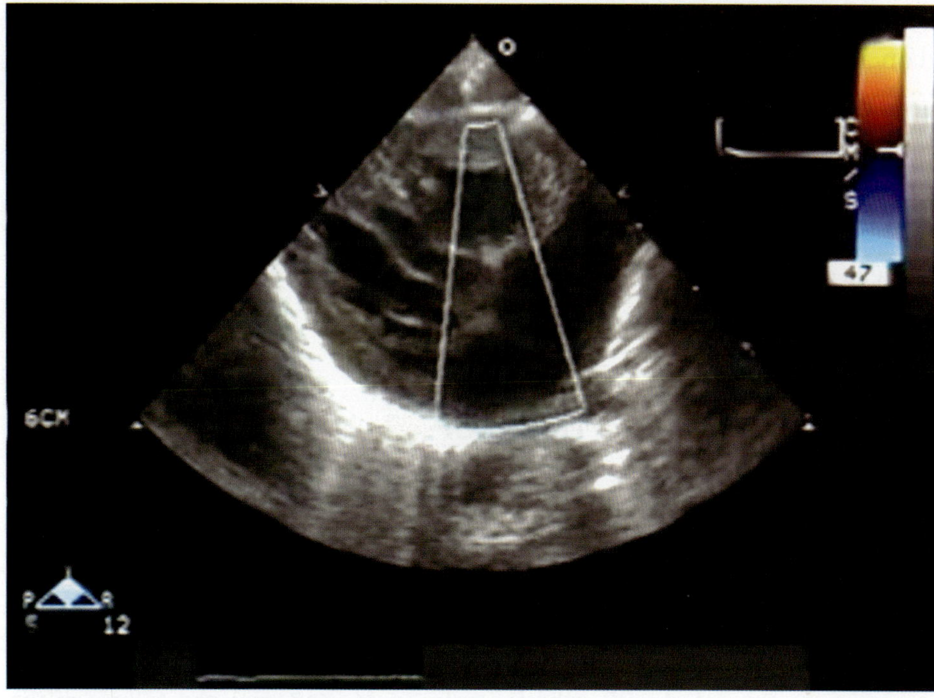

Figure 18
Pulmonary valve stenosis

allow accurate alignment of the Doppler beam with the area of subvalvar/valvular stenosis through the RV outflow tract **(Figs 17A to D)**.

In pulmonary valve stenosis, the pressure gradient across the valve is used to ascertain severity of the lesion more so than in left-sided valve conditions due in part to the difficulty in obtaining an accurate assessment of pulmonary valve area. The following definitions of severity have been defined in the 2006 American College of Cardiology/American Heart Association (ACC/AHA) guidelines on the management of valvular heart disease **(Fig. 18)**.

SEVERITY DEFINITIONS OF PULMONARY STENOSIS

Severe stenosis: A peak jet velocity 4 m/s (peak gradient 64 mm Hg)

Moderate stenosis: Peak jet velocity of 3–4 m/s (peak gradient 36–64 mm Hg)

Mild stenosis: Peak jet velocity is: 3 m/s (peak gradient less than 36 mm Hg).

- **Muscular infundibular obstruction is frequently characterized by a late peaking systolic jet that appears 'dagger-shaped', reflecting the dynamic nature of the obstruction.**
- **In pulmonary valve stenosis, the pressure gradient across the valve is used to ascertain severity of the lesion more so than in left-sided valve conditions due in part to the difficulty in obtaining an accurate assessment of pulmonary valve area.**

In determining the need for intervention, no specific Doppler gradients have been agreed on.

Severity of pulmonary stenosis using Doppler gradients has been based on catheterization data with demonstration of reasonable correlation between instantaneous peak Doppler gradients and peak-to-peak gradients obtained by catheterization. Typically though, Doppler peak gradients tend to be higher than peak-to-peak catheterization gradients. Doppler mean gradient has been shown in one study to correlate better with peak-to-peak atheterization gradient but is not commonly used.[12]

Other Indices of Severity: The RVSP

A useful index of severity is to determine the RV systolic pressure in patients with pulmonary stenosis from the tricuspid regurgitant velocity and the addition of an estimate of right atrial pressure. The pulmonary artery systolic pressure should be RV systolic pressure—pulmonary valve pressure gradient. In settings where there are multiple stenosis in the RV outflow tract or in the more peripheral pulmonary tree (sometimes associated with valvular pulmonary stenosis), the failure of the measured pulmonary valve gradient to account for much of the RV systolic pressure may be a clue for the presence of alternative stenosis.

Associated Lesions

Pulmonic stenosis especially when severe may be associated with right ventricular hypertrophy, eventually right ventricular enlargement, and right atrial enlargement. Given the unusual shape of the RV and its proximity to the chest wall, accurate estimation of RV hypertrophy and enlargement may be difficult. The parasternal long-axis and subcostal long-axis views are often best in assessing RV hypertrophy on transthoracic ECHO and the UE aortic SAX view the TG RV outflow view on TEE. The normal thickness of the RV is ~2 to 3 mm but given the difficulties in estimating thickness, a thickness of ~5 mm is usually considered abnormal. RV enlargement is typically assessed in the deep transgastric view.[13-15] As described above, pulmonary stenosis may form part of other syndromes or may be associated with other congenital lesions. Dilatation of the pulmonary artery beyond the valve is common and is due to weakness in the arterial wall in a manner analogous to bicuspid aortic valve and is not necessarily commensurate with the degree of obstruction. Detection of other lesions such as infundibular stenosis, VSD, or tetralogy of Fallot is all important in the assessment of these patients **(Fig. 19)**.

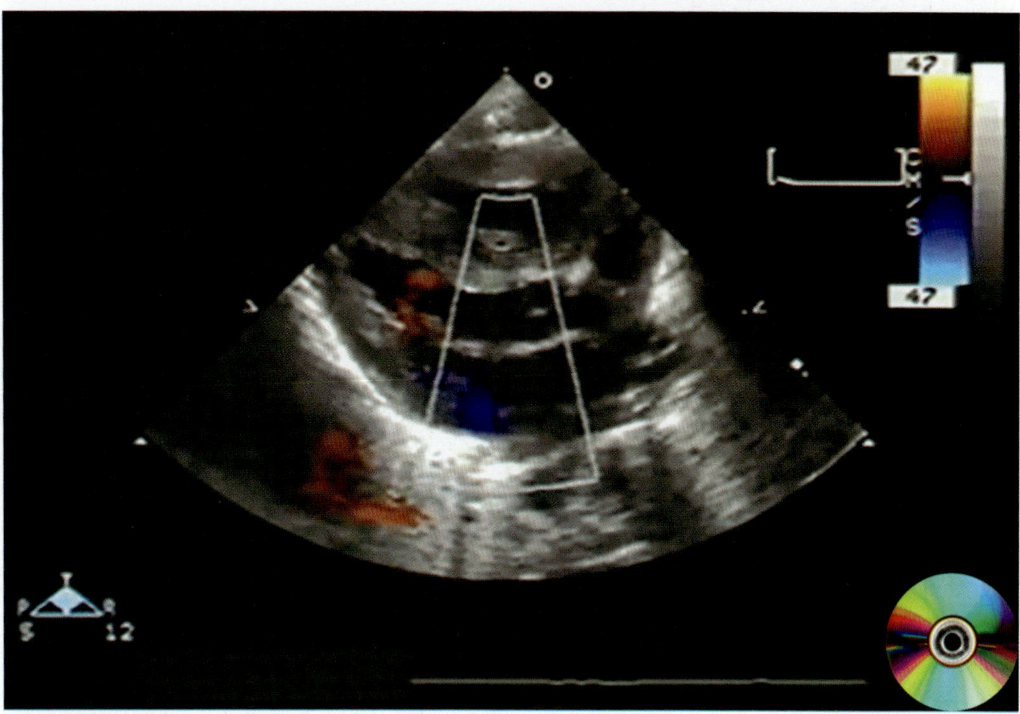

Figure 19 (VIDEO 5)

Associated lesions in pulmonary stenosis

Pulmonary Stenosis: TEE for TOF with Absent Pulmonary Valve

Tetralogy of Fallot (TOF) with absent pulmonary valve is a rare congenital anomaly characterized by features of tetralogy of Fallot with either rudimentary ridges or the complete absence of pulmonic valve tissue. Congenital absence of the pulmonary valve with an intact ventricular septum occurs, but this is much less common. The absence of mature pulmonary valve tissue leads to severe pulmonary regurgitation, which is often associated with massive dilatation of the pulmonary arteries and which is characteristic of this syndrome **(Fig. 20)**.

An interesting feature of this anomaly is that the ductus arteriosus is frequently absent. However, when the pulmonary valve is absent and the ventricular septum is intact, a normal ductus arteriosus is also generally present.

Pulmonary Stenosis with Arterial Septal Defect (ASD)

When pulmonary stenosis (PS) and atrial septal defect (ASD) occur together, the interatrial shunt could be patent foramen ovale, ostium secundum ASD, or ASDs of the ostium primum or sinus venous variety. Obstruction to the right ventricle (RV) outflow is usually caused by stenosis of the pulmonic valve (PV) and less commonly of the pulmorary artery (PA) and its branches. When a true ASD is present, coexisting PS is almost always valvular. In PV stenosis with intact ventricular septum, the coexisting right to left shunt (RTLS) is usually via a patent foramen ovale (PFO) rather than a true ASD **(Fig. 21)**.

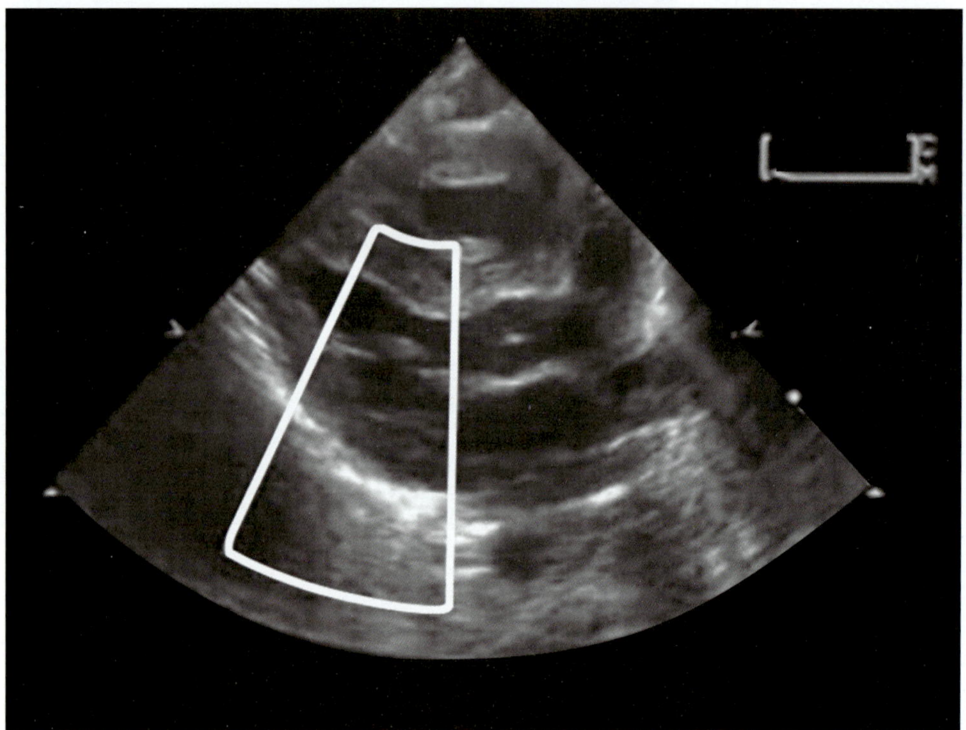

Figure 20

TEE view showing RVH and PS in TOF with absent PV

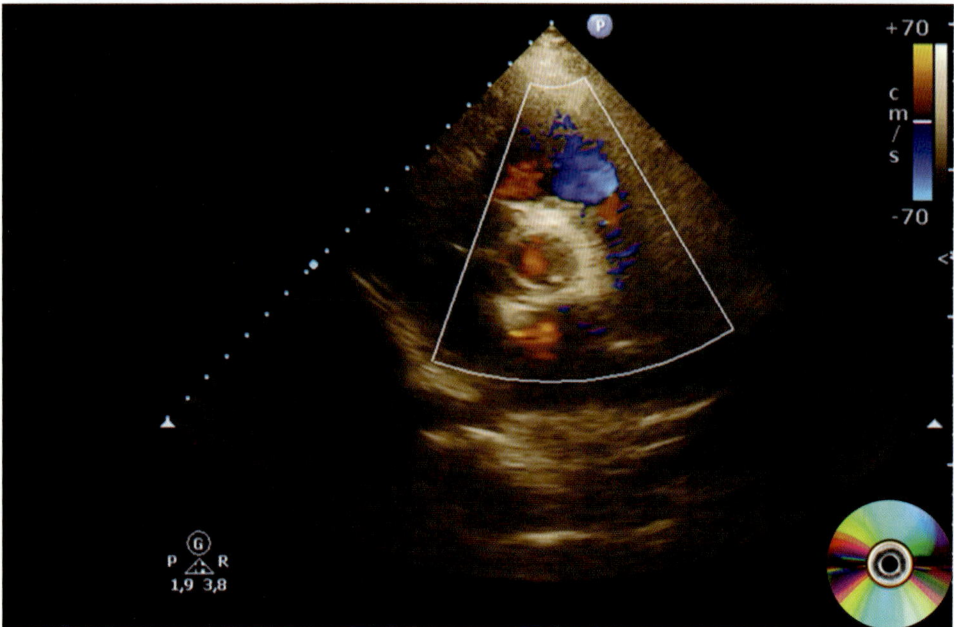

Figure 21 (VIDEO 6)

Arterial septal defect in pulmonary stenosis

PS: Does it only have Detrimental Effect on RV Mechanics after TOF Repair?

There was no doubt that PS must be completely removed during total repair of TOF. During the last 2 decades, while it was revealed that PR has been related to the most severe adverse outcomes at late follow-up, residual branch pulmonary artery stenosis has been recognized to have an adverse effect on RV deterioration caused by PR based on a report showing that transient balloon occlusion of the unilateral branch pulmonary artery increased PR. However, when we attempt the various modified techniques of RVOT enlargement in order to limit PR, we are faced with the distress that it is not possible to eliminate both PS and PR using an ideal technique. Even, a technique that gets rid of all PS and PR is referred to the 'Holy Grail'. However, some authors have in literature in an animal study that, PR combined with PS was associated with enhanced RV myocardial contractility and decreased RV diastolic compliance in marked contrast to the data in an isolated PR model. Additionally, in the clinical experience, patients with PS in addition to PR (PS + PR) have been able to tolerate chronic PR better than those with isolated PR.

Color/Doppler in TOF Patients

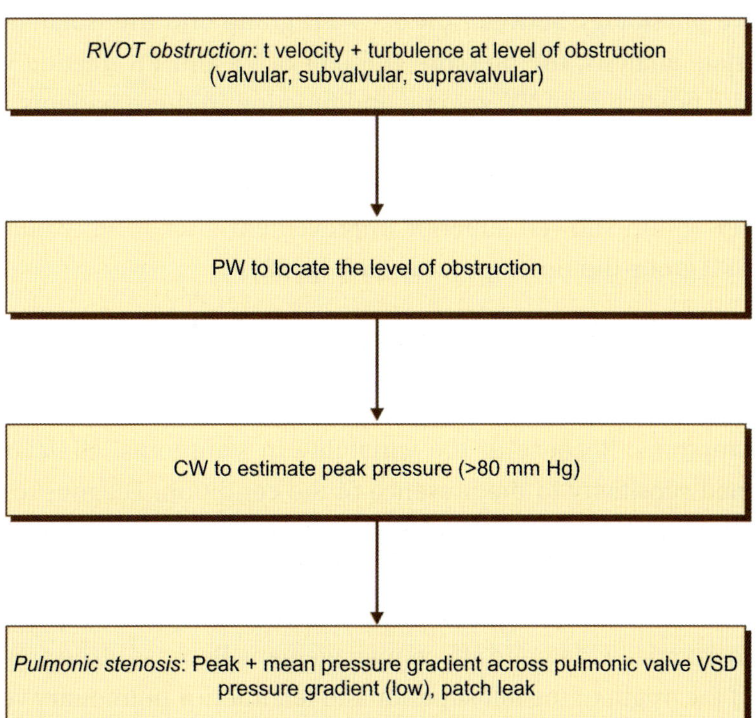

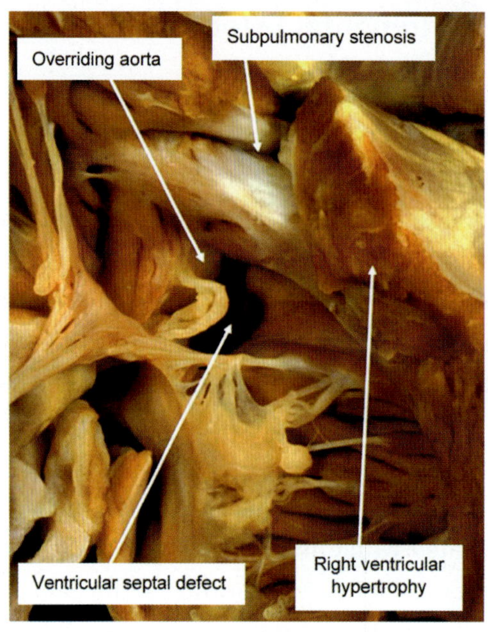

Figure 22

A surgical view of TOF showing its 4 components

The pressure gradient of PS in the PS + PR group was closely correlated with a smaller PR fraction and smaller RV volume indexes even though there was no difference in the PR fraction, the transannular patch ratio, or the frequency of restrictive physiology between the PS + PR group and the isolated PR group. In multivariate analysis, the pressure gradient of PS and PR fraction were revealed as definite predictors of RV volume and function in these patients. Furthermore, a recent report on percutaneous pulmonary valve implantation (PPVI) in patients with PS and/or PR revealed that both ventricular responses to exercise in the PS and/or PR group showed superior improvement after PPVI, while those in the isolated PR group did not improve at all **(Fig. 22)**.

In Treating PV, Stenosis with Stenting TEE is Essential

The more severe the stenosis and the greater number of stenosed veins result in more symptoms. Because of the variability in symptoms, clinicians must have heightened sensitivity to the presence of the condition. Diagnostic tests of value include magnetic resonance angiography and computed tomography. Although echocardiography has been used, it does not usually provide adequate assessment. Progression of stenosis is unpredictable and may be rapid. The specific anatomy of the stenosis varies widely and affects management. Because of the presence of antral fusion of the origin of the left superior and left inferior pulmonary vein, a stenosis involving 1 or the other can impinge and affect outcome. In this setting, bifurcation techniques familiar to interventional cardiology are very helpful **(Fig. 23)**.

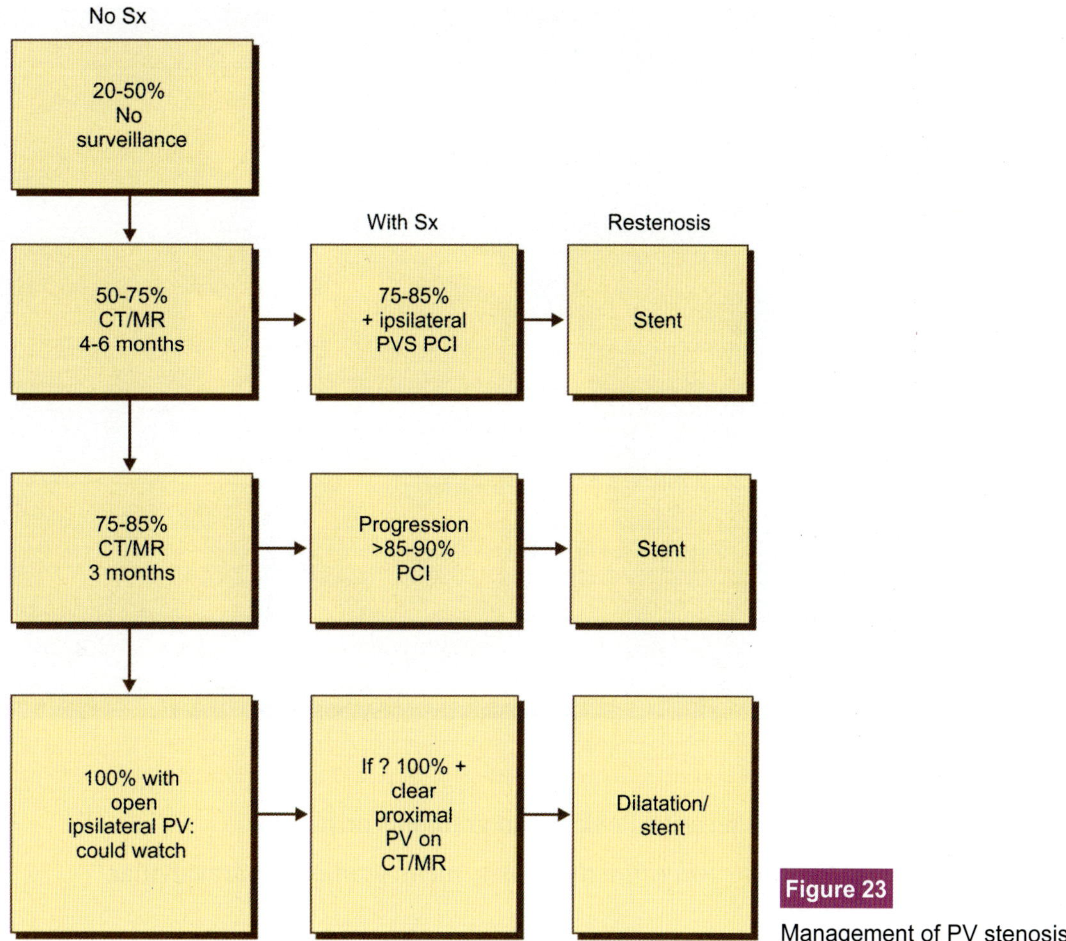

Figure 23
Management of PV stenosis

Controversy currently exists about the optimal treatment approach. The use of balloons and larger stents (approximately 10 mm) results in more optimal results than just balloon angioplasty alone; however, even with stent implantation, recurrent restenosis may occur in 30 to 50% of patients. Follow-up of these patients typically involves computed tomography imaging to document restenosis. If significant restenosis is identified, it should be treated promptly because of the potential for progression to total occlusion **(Fig. 24)**.

What to Tell the Surgeon?

Pre-CPB

- *Valve morphology:* Prosthetic failure post-stenotic PA dilatation > 20 mm annulus size 21 ± 3 mm **(Fig. 26)**

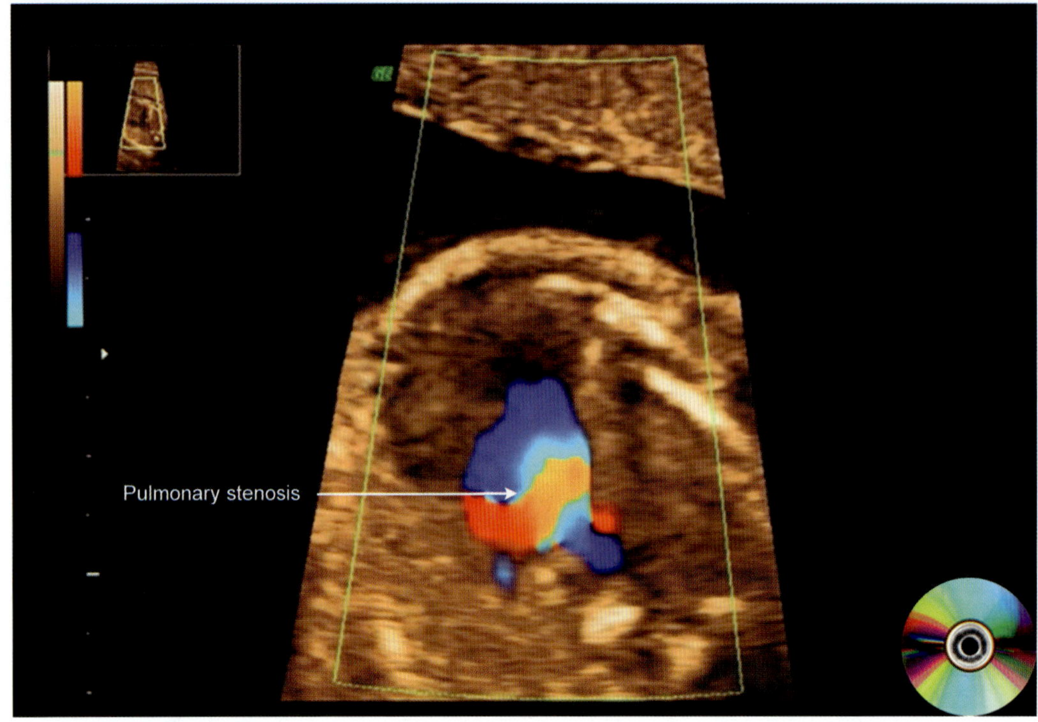

Figure 24 (VIDEO 7)

Fetal echocardiography in pulmonary stenosis

- *Stenosis severity:* Peak, mean gradients post-CPB
- *Prosthetic valve function:* Peak, mean gradients, paravalvular.

Perioperative CPB

- *Uncorrected:* VSD, RVOT level of obstruction, override aorta, RVH
- *Corrected:* VSD leak, pulmonic valve (PS/PI severity), RVOT obstruction
- RV size and function, aneurysmal RVOT if PI
- *Associated findings:* AI, LV function post CPB
- Residual VSD patch leak
- Pulmonic valve function (prosthetic)
- RV size and contractility
- Residual RVOT obstruction
- TR severity.

Postoperative (Figs 25A and B)

- Residual PR
- Post-PV stent ablation any PR.

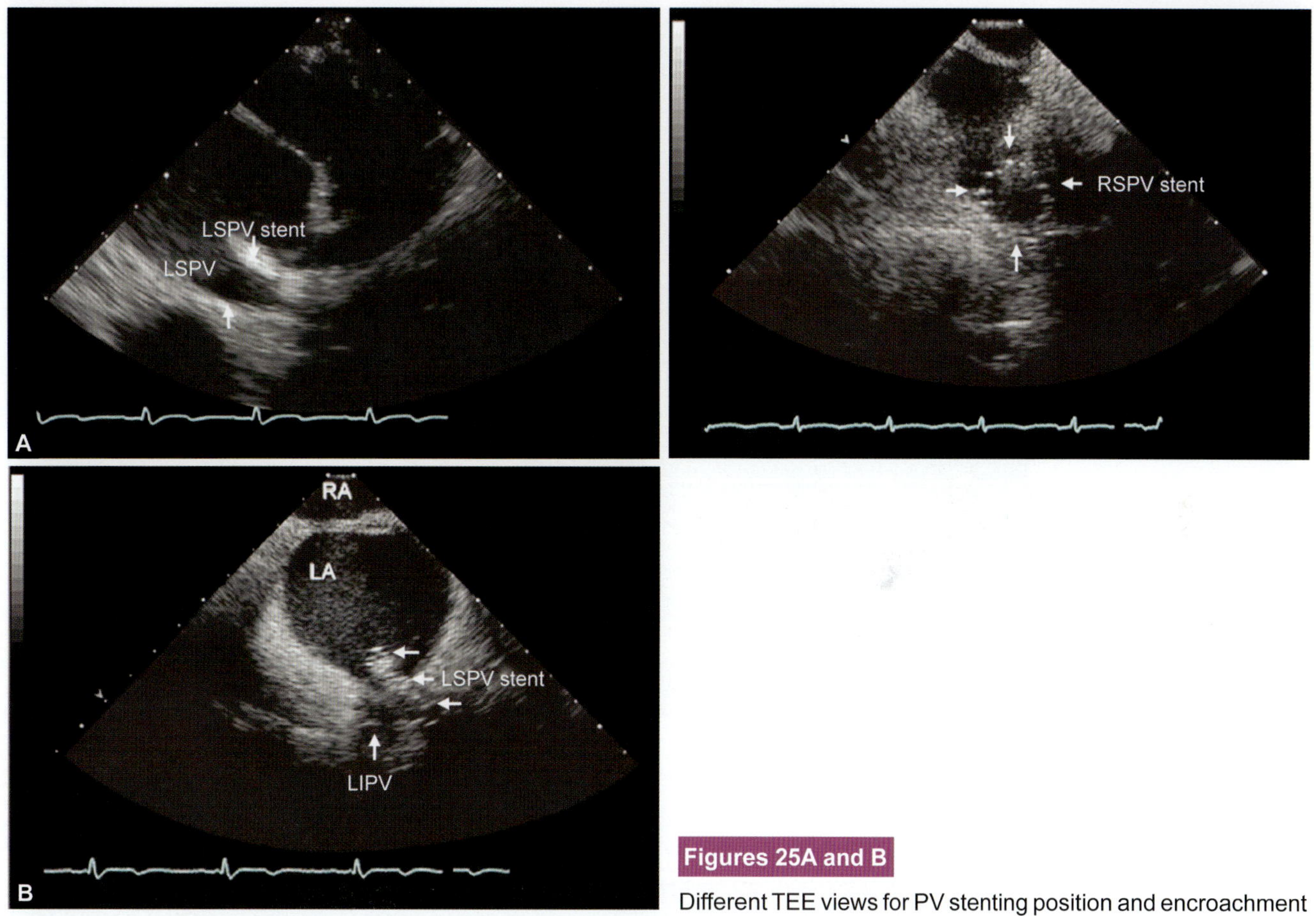

Figures 25A and B

Different TEE views for PV stenting position and encroachment

Etiology of Stenosis

- Normal valve area 2 cm^2/m^2
- *Valvular:* Rheumatic, carcinoid, prosthetic congenital
- Infundibular (RV).

2D Findings (Fig. 26)

- *Valve:* Thickened, calcified, immobile, systolic doming RVOT narrow in infundibular PS
- RVH (pressure overload), RV dilated
- Poststenotic PA dilatation (> 20 mm).

Doppler Findings (Fig. 27)

Color: Turbulent systolic flow at level of obstruction, also PI PW to locate level of obstruction

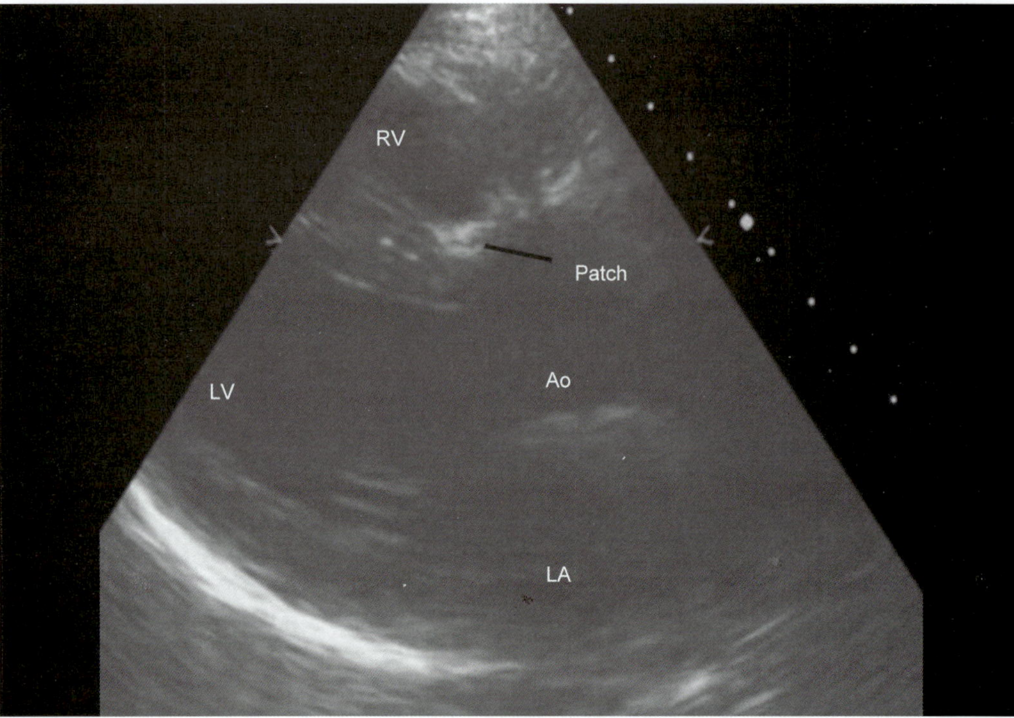

Figure 26

Gradient

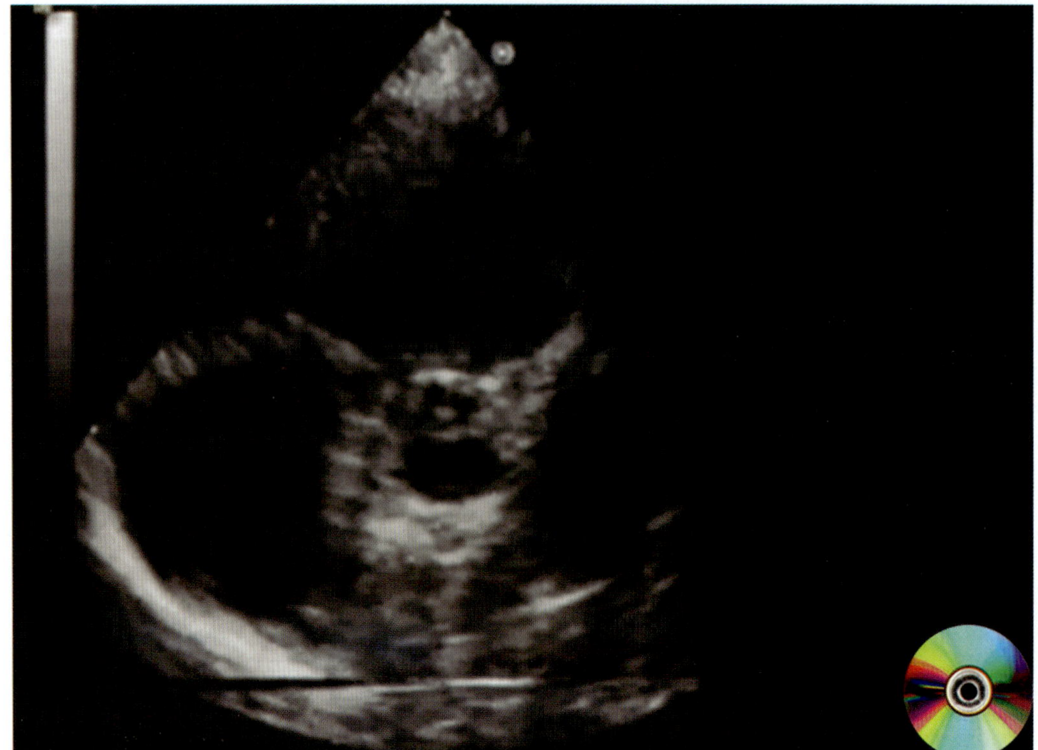

Figure 27 (VIDEO 8)

Severe pulmonary stenosis with color Doppler

Stenosis severity (severe)

- Peak velocity > 3.5 m/s
- Peak gradient > 80 mm Hg
- Continuity equation for valve area ≤ 0.5 cm^2).

Pulmonary Stenosis and Double Outlet Right Ventricle

In double outlet right ventricle (DORV), something goes wrong during the formation of the heart in the womb, and both great arteries are attached to the right ventricle. No arteries, or only a part of the aorta, are attached to the left ventricle. Children born with this congenital heart defect always have another heart defect called a ventricular septal defect (VSD). This is a hole in the septum, the wall that divides the right and left ventricle. The VSD is actually helpful—it allows the child to live. Without the VSD, blood that traveled to the lungs and back to the left side of the heart would have no place to go, since the aorta is not attached to the left ventricle, and no oxygenated blood would reach the body. The VSD allows oxygenated blood flowing into the left side of the heart to cross over to the right ventricle, and be pumped out to the body through the aorta. However, because it is a mix of the de-oxygenated blood in the right ventricle and the oxygenated blood from the left ventricle, the blood is not as high in oxygen as it should be, and this causes problems.

In some cases, because more blood than normal is flowing into the right ventricle, this heart defect means that too much blood is pumped to the lungs. Over time this uncontrolled flow can damage the lungs and heart, and heart failure can result.

In some cases, children with double outlet right ventricle also have pulmonary stenosis, a problem with the valve that leads out of the heart to the pulmonary artery. There may also be irregularities with the mitral valve, which separates the left atrium and left ventricle **(Fig. 28)**.

General Advice for the Future

Everyone who has pulmonary stenosis is at risk of getting infective endocarditis, both before and after surgery or treatment. Infective endocarditis is a rare condition where the inner lining of the heart, most commonly one of the heart valves, becomes infected. Infective endocarditis is a serious condition which can be life-threatening if it is not treated quickly. Get pulmonary atenosis treated early to prevent dvp of IE.

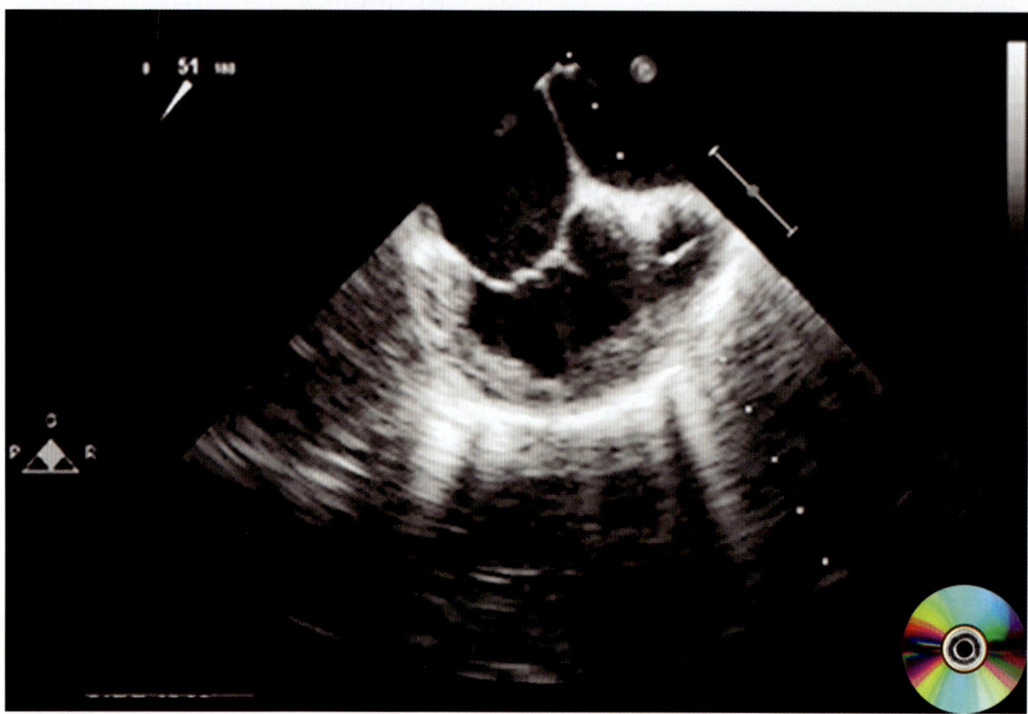

Figure 28 (VIDEO 9)

Double outlet right ventricle (DORV) with pulmonary stenosis

REFERENCES

1. Weyman AE, Hurwitz RA, Girod DA, Dillon JC, Feigenbaum H, Green D. Cross-sectional echocardiographic visualization of the stenotic pulmonary valve. Circulation. 1977;56:769-74.
2. Weyman AE, Dillon JC, Feigenbaum H, Chang S. Echocardiographic differentiation of infundibular from valvular pulmonary stenosis. Am J Cardiol. 1975;36:21-6.
3. Chen CR, Cheng TO, Huang T, Zhou YL, Chen JY, Huang YG, et al. Percutaneous balloon valvuloplasty for pulmonic stenosis in adolescents and adults. N Engl J Med. 1996;335:21-5.
4. Waller BF, Howard J, Fess S. Pathology of pulmonic valve stenosis and pure regurgitation. Clin Cardiol. 1995;18:45-50.
5. Bandin MA, Vargas-Barron J, Keirns C, Romero-Cardenas A, Villegas M, Buendia A. Echocardiographic diagnosis of rheumatic cardiopathy affecting all four cardiac valves. Am Heart J. 1990;120:1004-7.
6. Fox R, Panidis IP, Kotler MN, Mintz GS, Ross J. Detection by Doppler echocardiography of acquired pulmonic stenosis due to extrinsic tumor compression. Am J Cardiol. 1984;53:1475-6.
7. Van Camp G, De Mey J, Daenen W, Budts W, Schoors D. Pulmonary stenosis caused by extrinsic compression of an aortic pseudoaneurysm of a composite aortic graft. J Am Soc Echocardiogr. 1999;12:997-1000.

8. Lima CO, Sahn DJ, Valdes-Cruz LM, Goldberg SJ, Barron JV, Allen HD et al. Noninvasive prediction of transvalvular pressure gradient in patients with pulmonary stenosis by quantitative two-dimensional echocardiographic Doppler studies. Circulation. 1983;67:866-71.

9. Aldousany AW, DiSessa TG, Dubois R, Alpert BS, Willey ES, Birnbaum SE. Doppler estimation of pressure gradient in pulmonary stenosis: maximal instantaneous vs peak-to-peak, vs mean catheter gradient. Pediatr Cardiol. 1989;10:145-9.

10. Frantz EG, Silverman NH. Doppler ultrasound evaluation of valvar pulmonary stenosis from multiple transducer positions in children requiring pulmonary valvuloplasty. Am J Cardiol. 1988;61:844-9.

11. Johnson GL, Kwan OL, Handshoe S, Noonan JA, DeMaria AN. Accuracy of combined two-dimensional echocardiography and continuous wave Doppler recordings in the estimation of pressure gradient in right ventricular outlet obstruction. J Am Coll Cardiol. 1984;3:1013-8.

12. Silvilairat S, Cabalka AK, Cetta F, Hagler DJ, O'Leary PW. Echocardiographic assessment of isolated pulmonary valve stenosis: which outpatient Doppler gradient has the most clinical validity? J Am Soc Echocardiogr. 2005;18:1137-42.

13. Foale R, Nihoyannopoulos P, McKenna W, Kleinebenne A, Nadazdin A, Rowland E, et al. Echocardiographic measurement of the normal adult right ventricle. Br Heart J. 1986;56:33-44.

14. Matsukubo H, Matsuura T, Endo N, Asayama J, Watanabe T. Echocardiographic measurement of right ventricular wall thickness. A new application of subxiphoid echocardiography. Circulation. 1977;56:278- 84.

15. Lang RM, Bierig M, Devereux RB, Flachskampf FA, Foster E, Pellikka PA, et al. Recommendations for chamber quantification. Eur J Echocardiogr. 2006;7:79-108.

7 Pulmonary Regurgitation

Poonam Malhotra Kapoor, Suruchi Hasija

- Etiology of Pulmonic Regurgitation
- Etiology and Mechanisms of Pulmonary Regurgitation
- Other Etiologies of Pulmonary Regurgitation
- Pulmonary Regurgitation in Tetralogy of Fallot
- Pathophysiology of Pulmonary Regurgitation
- Clinical Presentation of Pulmonary Regurgitation
- Investigations for Pulmonary Regurgitation
- 2-Dimensional Echocardiography and M-Mode
- Color Flow Doppler
- Continuous-wave Doppler and Pulse Wave Doppler
- Vena Contracta Width
- Flow Convergence Method
- Pulsed Doppler
- Regurgitant Volume and Fraction
- 3-Dimensional TEE of Pulmonary Regurgitation
- Role of Exercise Echocardiography
- Integrating Indices of Severity
- Assessment of Pulmonary Regurgitation Severity
- Severity of the Pulmonary Regurgitation

INTRODUCTION

Pulmonary regurgitation is the flow of blood from the pulmonary artery back through the pulmonary valve during diastole. A trace amount of pulmonary regurgitation, in the absence of any structural heart disease, is a common finding in normal individuals. More significant pulmonary regurgitation can be a result of:

- Rheumatic valve disease
- Infective endocarditis
- Idiopathic dilatation (e.g. in pulmonary hypertension)
- Carcinoid syndrome
- Congenital absence of one or more cusps
- Pulmonary valvuloplasty.

Pulmonary regurgitation (PR) is common after surgical or percutaneous relief of pulmonary stenosis and following repair of tetralogy of Fallot. Pulmonary regurgitation is usually well-tolerated in childhood. However, recent long-term studies have demonstrated that PR leads to progressive right ventricular (RV) dilatation and, with time, to RV dysfunction, exercise intolerance, ventricular tachycardia, and sudden cardiac death (SCD).[1-5] In this chapter, we discuss the role of TEE as a diagnostic modalities in PR. Morphological spectrum PR is not usually found as an isolated congenital lesion, although physiological (mild) regurgitation is commonly detected by color Doppler echocardiography in otherwise normal hearts.

ETIOLOGY OF PULMONIC REGURGITATION

Most patients will have a small degree of PR, especially if the patient has a PA line. Significant PR is most often due to dilation of the pulmonary artery in patients with pulmonary hypertension. Endocarditis, carcinoid syndrome, and congenital heart disease (residual or unrepaired defects) can also cause PR. Estimation of the severity of PR typically relies on the size and depth of penetration of the PR jet. Although somewhat speculative, the use of the jet height relative to the RVOT height (similar to the method used to assess AI) as a means to assess the severity of PR makes intuitive sense (and that is what I use). Alternatively, if the CWD jet has high intensity and decays fast, then the PR is severe.

Pulmonic Regurgitation

CFD analysis is used to map the extent of PR jet into the RVOT.

Definitions:

- **Mild PR: PR jet < 1 cm.**
- **Pathologic PR: Pandiastolic jet > 1 to 2 cm.**
- **Significant PR: Jet extends > 2 cm in the RVOT or within 1 cm of TV and PWD velocity > 1.5 m/sec.**

Pulmonary insufficiency is commonly observed in cardiac surgical patients, especially if a PAC is in place. Severe pulmonary insufficiency is always pathologic and usually the result of dilation of the main pulmonary artery as seen in patients with pulmonary hypertension from any etiology.

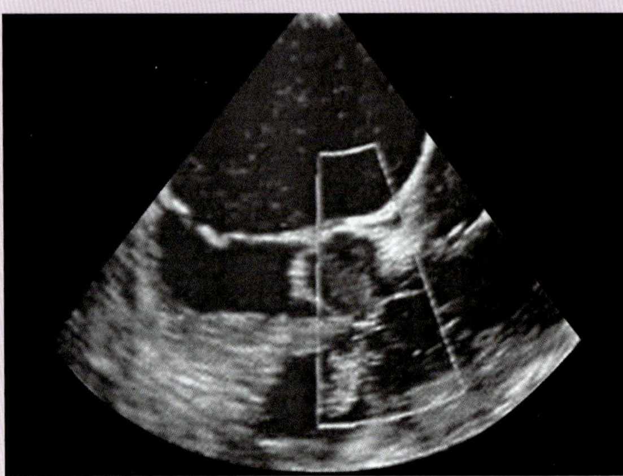

Figure 1

TEE showing PR in carcinoid syndrome

The causes of pulmonary insufficiency include fenfluramine-phentermine valvulopathy and carcinoid syndrome **(Fig. 1)**. These lesions result in short and thickened valves which fail to properly coapt. Infectious endocarditis can affects the tricuspid and pulmonic valves and presents as mobile masses attached to the valve leaflets.

Tetralogy of Fallot PR is extremely common in patients after repair of tetralogy of Fallot. While most of these patients carry an excellent prognosis,[6,7] there is a late morbidity and mortality related largely to RV dysfunction. Pulmonary regurgitation in these patients is shown to relate to the use of a transannular patch—more liberally performed in an earlier surgical era—to reconstruct the RV outflow tract (RVOT). Furthermore, transannular patching and/or aggressive infundibulectomy predispose to RVOT aneurysms or akinetic regions. The latter, combined with chronic PR, have an adverse effect on RV function and overall prognosis.[8] As a result, routine and generous transannular patch type of repair has now been abandoned and limited RVOT patching with preservation of pulmonary valve function have become key therapeutic goals during primary repair of tetralogy in infancy.

ETIOLOGY AND MECHANISMS OF PULMONARY REGURGITATION

Pulmonary regurgitation may be caused by congenital anomalies (quadricuspid or bicuspid valves), hypoplasia, post-repair of tetralogy of Fallot or prolapse of the pulmonary valve. Other causes include infective endocarditis, carcinoid syndrome, and rheumatic heart disease. Carcinoid syndrome results in shortening and thickening of the pulmonary valve leaflet. Similar to the involvement of the tricuspid valve, myxomatous valve is rare, resulting in thickening, redundancy, and sagging of the pulmonary valve leaflets. As for AR, examining the anatomic abnormalities associated with PR may help define the mechanisms of regurgitation and yield clues to its severity. TTE, TEE, 01′ 3D echo could provide useful information regarding anomalies of cusp number (bicuspid 01′ quadricuspid valves), motion (doming or prolapse), 01′ structure (hypoplasia, dysplasia, absence of pulmonary valve).

OTHER ETIOLOGIES OF PULMONARY REGURGITATION

It may follow some surgical or cath lab procedures as in following:

1. *Balloon valvuloplasty for pulmonary stenosis:* Balloon valvuloplasty has become the treatment of choice for patients with valvular pulmonary stenosis. Surgical valvotomy—widely employed in the 1960s and the 1970s—is now reserved for patients with supra- or sub-valvular stenosis. Variable degrees of PR are seen

in more than 70 percent of patients after either a surgical or transcatheter intervention,[9-13] although PR appears to be less frequent following balloon valvuloplasty.[14] In the Second Natural History Study of Congenital Heart Defects, 87 percent of the surgically operated patients had PR on echocardiography, being more than moderate in 28 percent.[11] A number of these patients now return requiring pulmonary valve replacement (PVR).

2. *Absent pulmonary valve syndrome:* Absent pulmonary valve syndrome is a rare manifestation comprising faulty development and dysplasia or complete absence of pulmonary valve cusps leading to PR. It is commonly associated with tetralogy of Fallot although occasionally it is seen in isolation. Its management and prognosis are often determined by the degree of pulmonary arterial dilatation, which can be excessive in some patients causing external bronchial compression.

PULMONARY REGURGITATION IN TETRALOGY OF FALLOT

Several congenital heart diseases involving the right ventricular outflow tract (RVOT) require surgical repair in early childhood. These procedures often require further revision of the RVOT at a later stage. Tetralogy of Fallot and its subtypes remain the most common defects in this category. Pulmonary regurgitation, patch aneurysm and valvular or conduit stenosis encompass many of the late complications seen following early intracardiac repair. Long-term follow-up has revealed the detrimental hemodynamic effects on regurgitation of the right and left ventricular function. Atrial arrhythmias, and sudden death are all linked to pulmonary regurgitation during late follow-up after tetralogy of Fallot repair. Preservation or restoration of pulmonary valve competence has resulted in improvement of right ventricular function, incidence of arrhythmias and exercise capacity.

PATHOPHYSIOLOGY OF PULMONARY REGURGITATION

The functional situation of a severely or freely regurgitant pulmonary valve is different from that of a severely regurgitant aortic valve for two reasons. First, as illustrated by the Fontan circulation, forward pulmonary blood flow can be maintained indirectly by the work of the left heart via the systemic venous return and by right atrial contraction. This occurs for part of each cycle in patients with severe PR and a 'restrictive right ventricle', in whom late diastolic forward flow in the pulmonary trunk coincident with atrial systole is seen and the right ventricle

Table 1 Pathophysiology of chronic pulmonary regurgitation	
Substrate	• Postrepair of tetralogy of Fallot • Postvalvotomy for pulmonary stenosis (balloon or surgical) • Absent pulmonary valve syndrome (rare) • Isolated congenital PR (rare)
Co-variables	• Peripheral pulmonary artery stenosis (–) • Pulmonary hypertension (–) • RVOT aneurysm/akinesia (–) • RV restrictive diastolic physiology (+ in the older patient)
Clinical progression	• RV dilatation (there is usually a long compensatory phase while RV systolic function is maintained) • QRS prolongation (associated with increased risk of sustained ventricular tachycardia and SCD) • Onset of tricuspid regurgitation • RV systolic dysfunction • Overt symptoms ensue
(–/+) indicates negative or positive effect on PR and/or RV function	

temporarily acts as a conduit (during late diastole) **(Table 1)**. The second difference between PR and aortic regurgitation is that the pulmonary microvascular bed, compared with the systemic, is of low resistance and located close to the heart. The importance of this is that with each RV systole blood moves readily forwards through the pulmonary microvessels whose slight resistance acts as a 'watershed' into the pulmonary veins, which in turn are maintained at low pressure by action of the left heart. Flow that passes forward through alveolar capillaries in systole is unlikely to pass back again in diastole, there being no significant reversal of gradient.

The pulmonary microvascular bed, therefore, has a valve-like effect in the setting of severe PR. This is borne out by the fact that severe or free PR is usually associated with a regurgitant fraction of only about 40 percent,[8,15] which is generally well-tolerated for a long period of time. Pulmonary regurgitation is, however, exacerbated by conditions that lead to elevated pulmonary artery pressure, e.g. branch pulmonary arterial stenosis, acquired bronchopulmonary disease, left ventricular dysfunction, or pulmonary vascular disease (uncommon in the setting of tetralogy).[16]

The adaptive RV response to volume overload resulting from PR depends on the degree and duration of the regurgitant flow[17] and the properties of the right ventricle and of the pulmonary arteries. More than moderate chronic PR produces RV volume overload, with increased end diastolic volumes followed in time by an

- **Consistent correlation between QRS prolongation and RV dilatation**
- **The pulmonary microvascular bed, therefore, has a valve-like effect in the setting of severe pulmonary regurgitation**

increase on end-systolic volumes, and progressive deterioration of myocardial function. It is of interest that immediate postoperative PR is well-tolerated after repair of tetralogy of Fallot in infancy. In contrast, postoperative PR is poorly tolerated in the adult following late primary repair. Adult patients, therefore, should be considered for pulmonary valve implantation at the time of repair if native pulmonary valve function cannot be preserved. It is speculated that this happens due to poor adaptation of a hypertrophied and relatively noncompliant right ventricle in the adult patient, further compromised by the acute volume overload of significant PR that can be induced following late repair of tetralogy of Fallot in adulthood. Significant tricuspid regurgitation, present in about 32 percent of adult patients with repaired tetralogy of Fallot in a recent report, appears to be the result of either progressive RV and tricuspid annulus dilatation or, occasionally, secondary to iatrogenic tricuspid valve injury during ventricular septal defect closure. Tricuspid regurgitation in turn contributes to additional dilatation of the right ventricle and right atrium.[18] Furthermore, RV dilatation and stretch slows interventricular conduction and creates a mechanoelectrical substrate for re-entry circuits, predisposing to sustained ventricular tachycardia. There has been a loose but consistent correlation between QRS prolongation and RV dilatation.[8,19] A QRS duration of 180 ms or more is shown to be a highly sensitive predictor of sustained ventricular tachycardia and SCD in patients with previous tetralogy repair. While QRS lengthening, seen immediately after repair, reflects surgical injury to the Myocardium and on the right bundle branch, late QRS prolongation almost universally reflects RV dilatation, mostly due to PR. Interval change in QRS duration, thus, may have a greater prognostic value for sustained ventricular tachycardia and SCD than absolute QRS measurements at any point in time.[5] This is particularly relevant to contemporary cohorts undergoing tetralogy repair via a transatrial/transpulmonary approach, where direct myocardial damage is limited, thus initial postoperative QRS prolongation is less compared with older cohorts who underwent tetralogy repair via a right ventriculotomy.[20]

CLINICAL PRESENTATION OF PULMONARY REGURGITATION

Pulmonary regurgitation is usually well-tolerated for many years. Patients often remain free of overt symptoms until marked RV dilatation and systolic dysfunction ensue.[21] Patients with early RV dysfunction are often New York Heart Association (NYHA) class 1, although variable degrees of exercise intolerance on exercise testing are to be expected.[1,2,22] When patients become symptomatic, RV dysfunction is usually well established and may have become irreversible.

In patients with isolated congenital PR, and otherwise normal hearts, symptoms are rare before the age of 30. After the age of 40, however, patients manifest symptoms of right heart failure[23] and may also present with sudden cardiac death (SCD). In contrast, symptoms in patients with repaired tetralogy of Fallot may appear at an earlier stage. Probably, this seen in a study by Shimazki et al.[23] that this relates largely to associated lesions and also to the adverse effects of early cyanosis, ventricular hypertrophy, and of previous operations, on myocardial function.

Clinical manifestations comprise exercise intolerance, congestive heart failure, atrial and ventricular arrhythmia, and SCD. Elevated jugular venous pressure, liver enlargement, and peripheral edema can all be present when there is RV dysfunction with clinical heart failure. However, this is uncommon. Severity of PR is notoriously difficult to assess by clinical examination. Nevertheless, patients with moderate to severe PR often have a RV heave with a single second heart sound and a to and fro murmur. The extent of the regurgitant murmur into diastole is important as early termination (i.e. a short diastolic murmur) suggests severe PR.[24]

INVESTIGATIONS FOR PULMONARY REGURGITATION

ECG

Most patients are in sinus rhythm although atrial arrhythmia can be present. In patients with isolated PR the presence of QRS prolongation, with rSr morphology in the right precordial leads, reflects volume overload of the RV. Right bundle branch block is extremely common in patients who underwent tetralogy repair via a right ventriculotomy and may mask RV hypertrophy. QRS duration in these patients increases with time, reflecting progressive RV enlargement and potentially RV dysfunction. As discussed above, QRS duration and QRS change have prognostic implications for malignant arrhythmia and SCD in these patients.

Chest X-ray

Patients with severe PR characteristically have dilatation of the pulmonary trunk and central pulmonary arteries. There is also RV enlargement, evident as filling of the retrosternal space on lateral projections.

- **More than moderate chronic PR produces RV volume overload, with increased end diastolic volumes followed in time by an increase on end-systolic volumes, and progressive deterioration of myocardial function.**
- **Tricuspid regurgitation in turn contributes to additional dilatation of the right ventricle and right atrium.**

Echocardiography

Evaluation of the pulmonary valve, RVOT morphology, and the presence and severity of PR can be performed with echocardiography. The complex RV geometry further distorted by previous surgery may limit complete assessment, however. The presence of retrograde color flow from the distal main pulmonary artery, or its branches, and a high regurgitant fraction calculated with pulsed Doppler[25] have been used until recently as echo markers of severe PR.

It was recently reported that good agreements exists between duration of pulmonary regurgitant flow (expressed as a percentage of the total diastolic time on continuous wave Doppler) and CMR-derived pulmonary regurgitant fraction[26,27] **(Fig. 2)**. The size and function of the right ventricle should also be evaluated. RV systolic function in the presence of severe PR can be maintained, but ultimately deterioration occurs following prolonged exposure to volume overload. Interventricular septal motion is usually paradoxical in these patients, again reflecting volume overload. Adult patients with repaired tetralogy may exhibit restrictive RV physiology. In these patients, a stiff right ventricle is acting as

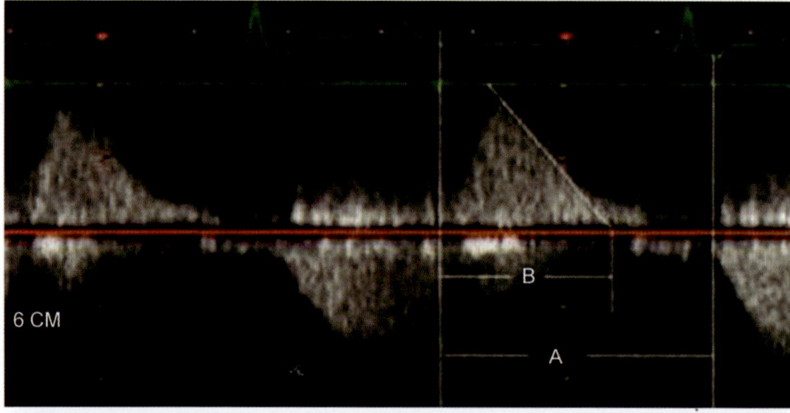

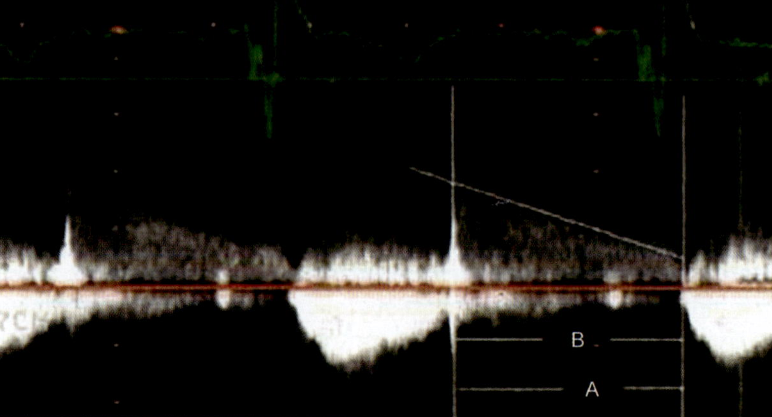

Figure 2

Severity of pulmonary regurgitation assessed by continuous wave Doppler. Continuous wave Doppler echocardiographic recordings of pulmonary flow from a patient with severe (top) and mild (bottom) PR. The duration of regurgitant flow (B) with respect to total diastole (A) is shorter in the patient with severe PR (top). *Source:* W Li, Am Heart J, 2004;147:165-72.

a conduit between the right atrium and the pulmonary artery at the end of diastole, counteracting the effects of PR and contributing to forward pulmonary flow, and thus, cardiac output (see Pathophysiology above). RV restriction can be detected with pulsed wave Doppler as a laminar diastolic pulmonary flow coincident with atrial systole, and seems to limit the degree of RV dilatation. Consequently, patients with RV restrictive physiology may have smaller RV volumes and better exercise tolerance.[28]

2-DIMENSIONAL ECHOCARDIOGRAPHY AND M-MODE

2D and M-mode echo are used to assess the structure of the valve. With 2D echo, typically only one or two leaflets can be simultaneously visualized. On occasion, the pulmonary valve can be seen in a short-axis view. In adults, visualization of the pulmonary valve is obtained from the parasternal short-axis view at the level of the aortic valve or from a subcostal approach. Evaluation of the pulmonary valve anatomy is however 98 more difficult than for other valves (limited by POOI-acoustic access). In pulmonary hypertension, the dilatation of pulmonary artery allows better assessment of the valve. The role of TEE in PR is limited since the pulmonary valve is more difficult to image with TEE (far from the probe). The views that maximize visualization of the pulmonary valve include horizontal (0 degrees) plane imaging at 25 to 30 cm from the incisors and a deep gastric view in 120° imaging plane.

COLOR FLOW DOPPLER

Color Flow Imaging

Detection of PR relies almost exclusively on color flow imaging. Pulmonary regurgitation is diagnosed by documenting a diastolic jet in the RV outflow tract directed towards the RV. Pathological PR is distinguished from physiological PR by a longer duration of flow (holodiastolic) and a wider jet as the regurgitant jet crosses the pulmonic valve. Functional PR jets are usually very)' small, central, and spindle-shaped. In severe PR, where equalization of diastolic pulmonary artery and RV pressures occurs early in diastole, the color jet area can be brief and inaccurate (dependency on the driving pressure).[29]

The assessment of PR severity is usually estimated by the diameter of the jet at its origin[30] The maximum color jet diameter (width) is measured in diastole immediately below the pulmonic valve (at the junction of the RV outflow tract and pulmonary annulus) in the parasternal short-axis view or from the subcostal view.

Although, this measurement suffers from a high inter-observer variability, a jet width that occupies > 65 percent of the RV outflow tract width measured in the same frame is in favor of severe PR.

CONTINUOUS-WAVE DOPPLER AND PULSE WAVE DOPPLER

Record a CW Doppler trace with the probe carefully aligned with the direction of the regurgitant jet **(Fig. 3)**. The CW Doppler trace is faint in mild pulmonary regurgitation, and denser in moderate or severe regurgitation. Look at the contour of the regurgitant jet—in mild pulmonary regurgitation the deceleration rate of the jet is slow, becoming steeper with more severe degrees of regurgitation. The density of the CW signal provides a qualitative measure of regurgitation.[31] In mild PR, there is a slow deceleration of the jet velocity. A rapid deceleration rate with termination of flow in mid to late diastole is not specific but compatible with severe regurgitation **(Fig. 4)**.

Use PW Doppler to assess the VTI of forward flow in the RVOT (in the parasternal view) and also in the LVOT (in the apical 5-chamber view). The ratio of RVOTVT/LVOTVT1 increases with increasing severity of pulmonary regurgitation.

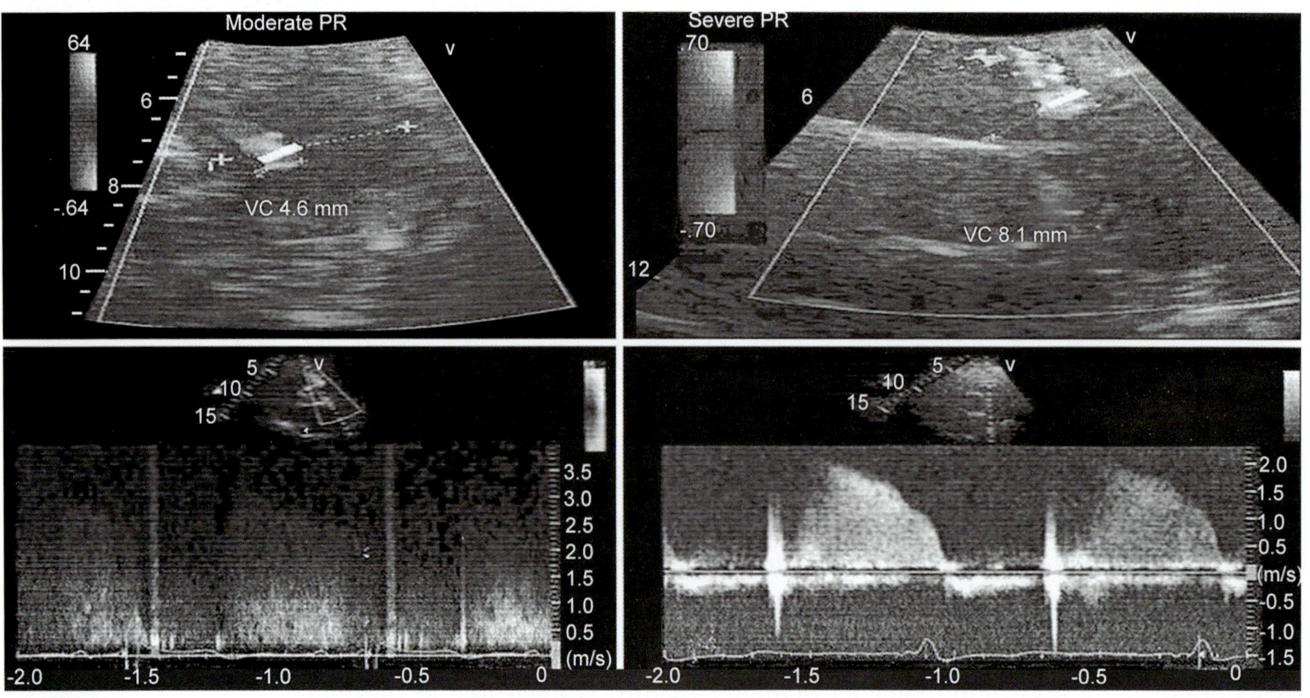

Figure 3

Assessment of pulmonary regurgitation (PR) severity by using color flow imaging. (Top) Measurement of the vena contracta width in two patients with PR (left: moderate and right: severe). (Bottom) Continuous-wave Doppler recordings.

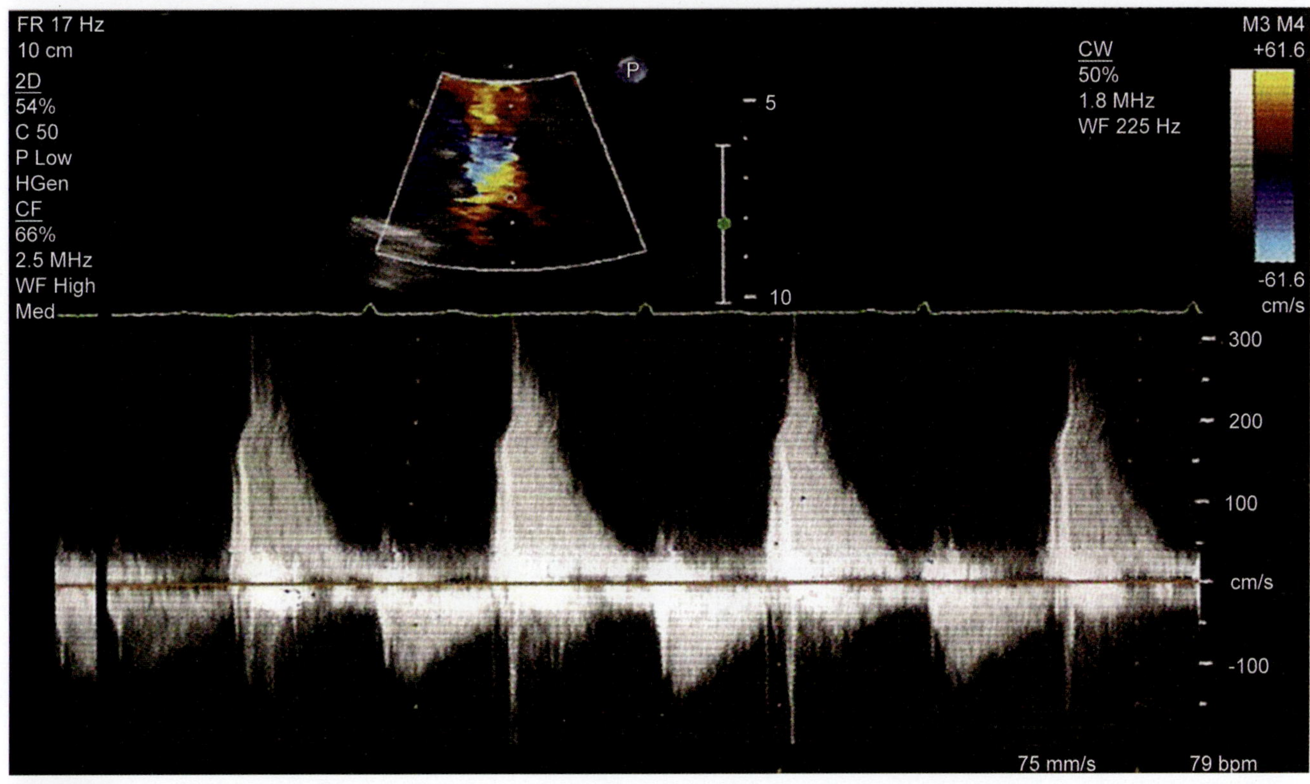

Figure 4

Severe pulmonary regurgitation following TOF in a 17-year-old, 2 years later, showed severe PR on CWD

Measurement of the peak velocity of the jet of pulmonary regurgitation allows calculation of pulmonary artery diastolic pressure.

VENA CONTRACTA WIDTH

Although the vena contracta width is probably a more accurate method than the jet width to evaluate PR severity by color Doppler, it lacks validation studies **(Figs 4 and 5)**. As for other regurgitations, the same limitations are applicable. The shape of the vena contracta is complex in most cases. The 3D vena contracta is correlated with the 20 vena contracta but provides more quantitative assessment of PR.[32] The EROA values of < 20, 21 to 115, and > 115 mm^2 have been proposed to serve as cut-offs for PR grade mild, moderate, and severe. By multiplying the 3D vena contracta with the spectral Doppler-derived velocity integral of the PR jet, the regurgitant volume (R Vol) can be obtained. The regurgitant volume values of < 15, 15 to 115, and > 115 mL have also been proposed to serve as cut-offs for PR grade mild moderate and severe. These values require further validation since they are coming from a single study. Values are relatively high and could reflect some technical drawbacks.

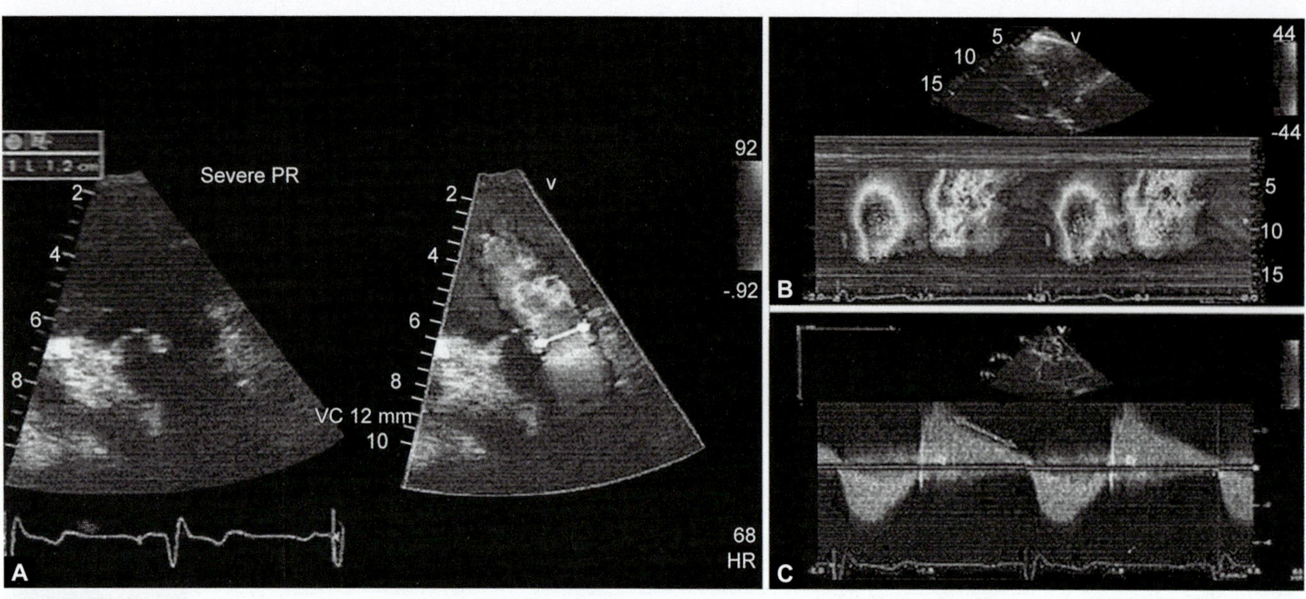

Figures 5A to C

Example of a patient with a severe pulmonary regurgitation (PR). (A) Complete lack of valve coaptation (left) and measurement of the vena contracta width (VC) (right); (B) Color-coded M-mode depicting the time dependency of flow signal during the heart cycle; (C) Continuous Doppler recording of PR showing a rapid flow deceleration during the diastole and increased systolic flow velocity (not related to concomitant pulmonary stenosis)

FLOW CONVERGENCE METHOD

In some patients the flow convergence zone can be assessed **(Figs 6A and B)**. However, no studies have examined the clinical accuracy of this method in quantifying the severity of PR.

PULSED DOPPLER

Theoretically, PW Doppler assessment of the forward and the reverse flows at the pulmonary annulus and in the pulmonary artery can been used to calculate regurgitant volume (R Vol) and regurgitant fraction.

The pulmonary annulus should be measured carefully during early ejection (2–3 frames after the R wave on the ECG), just below the valve. This technique is subject to errors in measurement and is not well validated.[33]

REGURGITANT VOLUME AND FRACTION

The volume of blood entering the RV via the tricuspid valve during diastole normally equals the volume of blood leaving it via the RVOT (stroke volume) during systole.

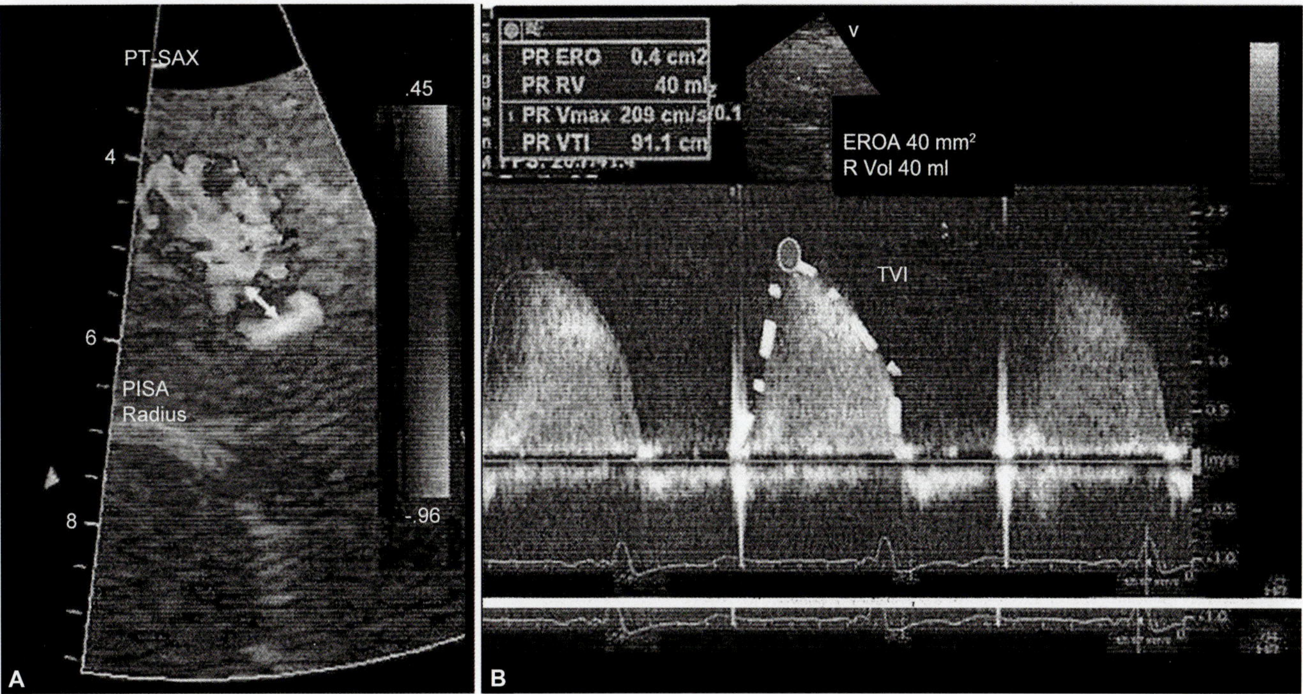

Figures 6A and B

Assessment of pulmonary regurgitation by the proximal isovelocity surface area (PISA) method. PT-SAX—parasternal short-axis view. *Abbreviations:* EROA, effective regurgitant orifice area; R Vol, regurgitant volume.

In the presence of pulmonary regurgitation, RVOT outflow will be greater than tricuspid valve inflow as the systolic RVOT outflow will consist of the blood that has entered via the tricuspid valve plus the blood that entered the ventricle via pulmonary regurgitation during diastole. The difference between RVOT outflow and tricuspid valve inflow gives the regurgitant volume:

1. In the modified apical 4-chamber view, measure the diameter of the tricuspid annulus in cm, and then use this to calculate the CSA of the tricuspid valve in cm. This calculation makes the assumption that the tricuspid orifice is circular:

$$CSA_{TV} = 0.785 \times (\text{tricuspid annulus diameter})^2$$

2. In the modified bicaval view, measure the VTI of tricuspid valve inflow (using PW Doppler) to give VTI_{TV} in cm. It is generally easiest to place the sample volume at the valve tips (some place it at the level of the tricuspid valve annulus).
3. The stroke volume of the tricuspid valve (SV_{TV}) in mL/beat, can then be calculated from:

$$SV_{TV} = CSA_{TV} \times VTI_{TV}$$

4. In the MEAV short-axis view (aortic valve level), measure the diameter of the RVOT at the level of the pulmonary valve annulus ($RVOT^2$) in cm, and then use this to calculate the cross-sectional area (CSA) of the RVOT in cm:

$$CSA_{RVOT} = 0.785 \times (\text{RVOT diameter})^2$$

5. At the same point in the aortic valve short-axis view, measure the VTI of RVOT outflow (using PW Doppler) to give VTI_{RVOT} in cm.
6. The stroke volume of the RVOT (SV_{RVOT}) in mL/beat, can then be calculated from:

$$SV_{RVOT} = CSA_{RVOT} \times VTI_{RVOT}$$

7. Pulmonary regurgitant volume (RV) can be calculated from:

$$RV = SV_{RVAR} - SV_{TV}$$

8. Pulmonary regurgitant fraction (RF) can be calculated from:

$RF = \frac{RV}{SVIV}$ (×100 to express as a percentage)

This measurement is not valid if there is significant tricuspid regurgitation, and any error in measurement of tricuspid valve orifice area or RVOT diameter can have a large impact on the result.

Associated Features

If pulmonary regurgitation is present:

- Assess any co-existent pulmonary stenosis
- Assess any co-existent disease affecting the other valves
- Assess RV dimensions and function—the RV may become dilated due to volume overload if pulmonary regurgitation is severe
- Assess flow in the pulmonary artery (diastolic flow reversal indicates severe pulmonary regurgitation)
- Calculate pulmonary artery systolic and diastolic pressure **(Figs 7 to 10)** to assess if there is pulmonary hypertension.

3-DIMENSIONAL TEE OF PULMONARY REGURGITATION

Consequences of Pulmonary Regurgitation

Evaluation of the size and function of the RV in the absence of pulmonary hypertension provides indirect clues to the severity of PR. Evidence of RV dilatation are however not for severe PR. Nevertheless, its absence suggests milder degree of PR. As for TR, the RV function is classically evaluated by the RV ejection fraction.

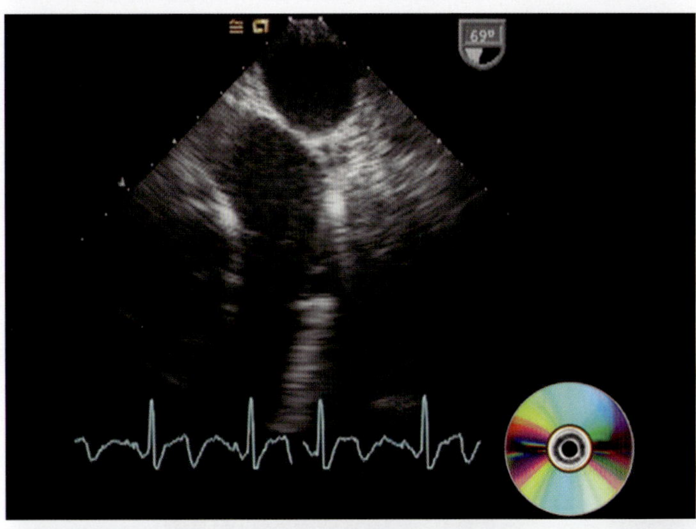

Figure 7 (VIDEO 1)

Pulmonic valve and RVOT at 70. At this angle, the pulmonary valve is well visualized, especially for interrogation of the gradient in case of pulmonary stenosis

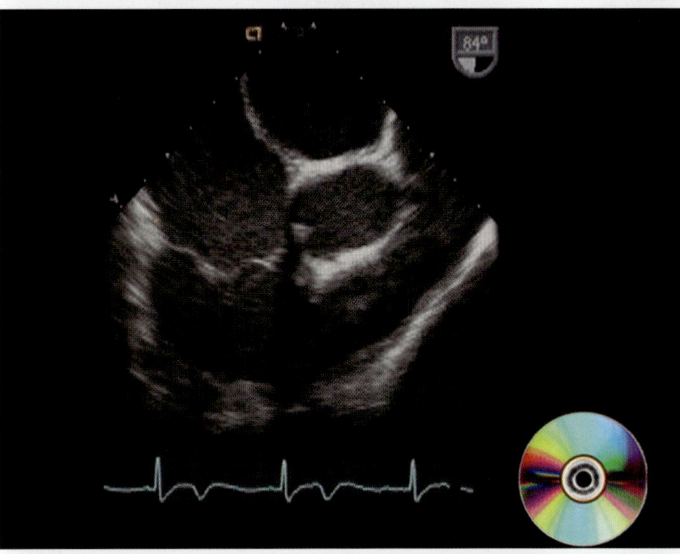

Figure 8 (VIDEO 2)

Pulmonary valve in right sided inflow-outflow view. The aortic valve is seen in short axis view. Both the RV inflow (TV) and outflow (PV) are nicely seen in this view and is the best view for right ventricle interrogation

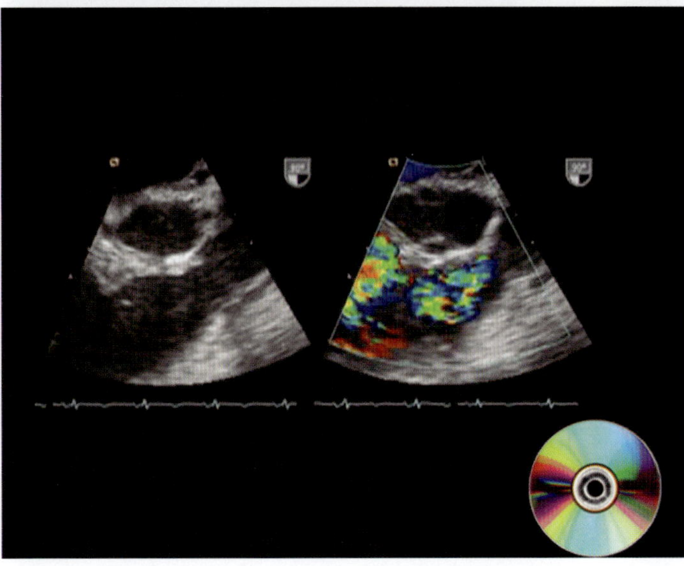

Figure 9 (VIDEO 3)

Tricuspid inflow and pulmonic regurgitation in diastole. PR is rarely observed vena contracta width can be best measured in this view, to quantify PR severity

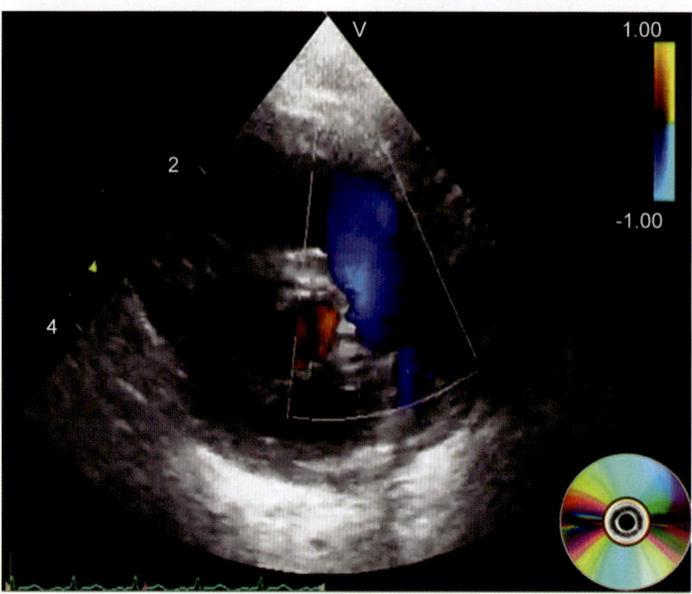

Figure 10 (VIDEO 4)

PPHN, pulmonary regurgitation

The utility of the new indices deriving from tissue Doppler imaging has not been extensively examined in the context of PR unrelated to congenital heart disease. In the tetralogy of Fallot, the severity of PR has a negative influence on RV functional parameters and there is significant relation between RV functions and exercise capacity. In this disease, the myocardial acceleration during the isovolumic contraction is a new emerging index of RV function. The assessment of RV function in the setting of congenital heart disease is not the scope of this document.

ROLE OF EXERCISE ECHOCARDIOGRAPHY

Latent RV dysfunction and impaired functional response to stress can be unmasked by exercise echocardiography. Except in the setting of congenital heart disease, the value of exercise testing in patients with PR has not been examined.[34]

INTEGRATING INDICES OF SEVERITY

Echocardiographic assessment of PR includes integration of data from 20/30 imaging of the pulmonary valve and RV as well as Doppler measures of regurgitant severity. In the absence of extensive data on quantitation of PR, the experts recommend to assess the PR severity by using the different approaches available and to corroborate each other. Advantages and limitations of the various echo Doppler parameters used in assessing PR severity are detailed in **Table 2**.

Table 2: Grading the severity of pulmonary regurgitation			
Parameters	*Mild*	*Moderate*	*Severe*
Qualitative pulmonic valve morphology	Normal	Normal/abnormal	Abnormal
Color flow PR jet	Small, usually < 10 mm in length with a narrow origin	Intermediate	Large, with a wide origin; may be brief in duration
CW signal of PR jet	Faint/slow deceleration	Dense/variable	Dense/steep deceleration, early termination of diastolic flow
Pulmonic vs aortic flow by PW	Normal or slightly increased	Intermediate	Greatly increased
Semiquantitative VC width (mm)	Not defined	Not defined	Not defined
Quantitative EROA (mm^2)	Not defined	Not defined	Not defined
R Vol (mL) + RV size	Not defined	Not defined	Not defined
Abbreviations: PR, pulmonic regurgitation; CW, continuous wave; EROA, effective regurgitant orifice area; PW, pulse wave; RV, right ventricle; R Vol., regurgitant volume; VC, vena contracta			

ASSESSMENT OF PULMONARY REGURGITATION SEVERITY

Determination of the PR severity has been less validated than determination of AR degree.

SEVERITY OF THE PULMONARY REGURGITATION

Severity of pulmonary regurgitation can be assessed by:

- Jet size
- RF
- CW Doppler jet density
- CW Doppler jet deceleration rate
- $RVOT_{VTI}/LVOT_{VTI}$ ratio.

KEY POINT

Grading of PR severity remains difficult since standards for quantification of PR are less robust than for AR. The vena contracta is probably the most accurate approach. If possible the PISA method could provide quantitative evaluation of PR. In all cases, the experts recommend corroborating the results of these methods with the other available parameters.

REFERENCES

1. Wessel HU, Cunningham WJ, Paul MH, et al. Exercise performance in tetralogy of Fallot after intracardiac repair. J Thorac Cardiovasc Surg. 1980;80:582-93.
2. Carvalho JS, Shinebourne EA, Busst C, et al. Exercise capacity after complete repair of tetralogy of Fallot: deleterious effects of residual pulmonary regurgitation. Br Heart J. 1992;67:470-3.
3. Redington AN, Oldershaw PJ, Shinebourne EA, et al. A new technique for the assessment of pulmonary regurgitation and its application to the assessment of right ventricular function before and after repair of tetralogy of Fallot. Br Heart J. 1988;60:57-65.
4. Marie PY, Marcon F, Brunotte F, et al. Right ventricular overload and induced sustained ventricular tachycardia in operatively "repaired" tetralogy of Fallot. Am J Cardiol. 1992;69:785-9.
5. Gatzoulis MA, Balaji S, Webber SA, et al. Risk factors for arrhythmia and sudden cardiac death late after repair of tetralogy of Fallot: a multicentre study. Lancet. 2000;356:975-81.
6. Murphy JG, Gersh BJ, Mair DD, et al. Long-term outcome in patients undergoing surgical repair of tetralogy of Fallot. N Engl J Med. 1993;329:593-9.
7. Nollert G, Fischlein T, Bouterwek S, et al. Long-term survival in patients with repair of tetralogy of Fallot: 36-year follow-up of 490 survivors of the first year after surgical repair. J Am Coll Cardiol. 1997;30:1374-83.
8. Davlouros PA, Kilner PJ, Hornung TS, et al. Right ventricular function in adults with repaired tetralogy of Fallot assessed with cardiovascular magnetic resonance imaging: detrimental role of right ventricular outflow aneurysms or akinesia and adverse right-to-left ventricular interaction. J Am Coll Cardiol. 2002;40:2044-52.
9. Chen CR, Cheng TO, Huang T, et al. Percutaneous balloon valvuloplasty for pulmonic stenosis in adolescents and adults. N Engl J Med. 1996;335:21-5.
10. Griffith BP, Hardesty RL, Siewers RD, et al. Pulmonary valvulotomy alone for pulmonary stenosis: results in children with and without muscular infundibular hypertrophy. J Thorac Cardiovasc Surg. 1982;83:577-83.
11. Hayes CJ, Gersony WM, Driscoll DJ, et al. Second Natural History Study of Congenital Heart Defects. Results of treatment of patients with pulmonary valvar stenosis. Circulation. 1993;87(Suppl.):I28-I37.
12. McCrindle BW. Independent predictors of long-term results after balloon pulmonary valvuloplasty. Valvuloplasty and Angioplasty of Congenital Anomalies (VACA) Registry Investigators. Circulation. 1994;89:1751-9.
13. McCrindle BW, Kan JS. Long-term results after balloon pulmonary valvuloplasty. Circulation. 1991;83:1915-22.
14. O'Connor BK, Beekman RH, Lindauer A, et al. Intermediate term outcome after pulmonary balloon valvuloplasty: comparison with a matched surgical control group. J Am Coll Cardiol. 1992;20:169-73.
15. Rebergen SA, Chin JG, Ottenkamp J, et al. Pulmonary regurgitation in the late postoperative follow-up of tetralogy of Fallot. Volumetric quantitation by nuclear magnetic resonance velocity mapping. Circulation. 1993;88:2257-66.

16. Ilbawi MN, Idriss FS, DeLeon SY, et al. Factors that exaggerate the deleterious effects of pulmonary insufficiency on the right ventricle after tetralogy repair. Surgical implications. J Thorac Cardiovasc Surg. 1987;93:36-44.

17. Laneve S, Uesu, CT, Taguchi, JT. Isolated pulmonary valvular regurgitation. Am J Med Sci. 1962;244:446.

18. Mahle WT, Parks WJ, Fyfe DA, et al. Tricuspid regurgitation in patients with repaired Tetralogy of Fallot and its relation to right ventricular dilatation. Am J Cardiol. 2003;92: 643-5.

19. Gatzoulis MA, Till JA, Somerville J, et al. Mechanoelectrical interaction in tetralogy of Fallot. QRS prolongation relates to right ventricular size and predicts malignant ventricular arrhythmias and suddendeath. Circulation. 1995;92:231-7.

20. Atallah-Yunes NH, Kavey RE, Bove EL, et al. Postoperative assessment of a modified surgical approach to repair of tetralogy of Fallot. Long-term follow-up. Circulation. 1996; 94(Suppl.):II22-26.

21. Geva T, Sandweiss BM, Gauvreau K, et al. Factors associated with impaired clinical status in long-term survivors of tetralogy of Fallot repair evaluated by magnetic resonance imaging. J Am Coll Cardiol. 2004;43:1068-74.

22. Davlouros PA, Wensel R, Bayne S, et al. Reduced cardiopulmonary exercise performance after tetralogy of Fallot repair is not related to resting central haemodynamics assessed with MRI. Eur Heart J. 2002;23(Suppl.):314.

23. Shimazaki Y, Blackstone EH, Kirklin JW. The natural history of isolated congenital pulmonary valve incompetence: surgical implications. Thorac Cardiovasc Surg. 1984;32:257-9.

24. Bousvaros C, Deuchar DC. The murmur of pulmonary regurgitation which is not associated with pulmonary hypertension. Lancet. 1961;2:962.

25. Goldberg SJ, Allen HD. Quantitative assessment by Doppler echocardiography of pulmonary or aortic regurgitation. Am J Cardiol. 1985;56:131-5.

26. Li W, Davlouros PA, Kilner PJ, et al. Doppler-echocardiographic assessment of pulmonary regurgitation in adults with repaired tetralogy of Fallot: comparison with cardiovascular magnetic resonance imaging. Am Heart J. 2004;147:165-72.

27. Silversides CK, Veldtman GR, Crossin J, et al. Pressure half-time predicts hemodynamically significant pulmonary regurgitation in adult patients with repaired tetralogy of Fallot. J Am Soc Echocardiogr. 2003;16:1057-62.

28. Gatzoulis MA, Clark AL, Cullen S, et al. Right ventricular diastolic function 15 to 35 years after repair of tetralogy of Fallot. Restrictive physiology predicts superior exercise performance. Circulation. 1995;91:1775-81.

29. Kobayashi J, Akaoo S, Matsuda H, Arisawa J, Kawashima Y. Quantitative evaluation of pulmonary regurgitation after repair of tetralogy of Fallot using real-rime flow imaging system. Jpn Cric J. 1989:53:721-7.

30. Williams RV, Minich LL, Shaddy RE. Pagotto LT, Tani LY. Comparison of Doppler echocardiography with angiography for determining the severity of pulmonary regurgitation. Am J Cardrol. 2002;89:1438-41.

31. Lei MH, Chen JJ, Ko YL, Cheng JJ, Kuan P, Lien WP. Reappraisal of quantitative evaluation of pulmonary regurgitation and estimation of pulmonary artery pressure by continuous wave Doppler echocardiography. Cardiology. 1995;86:249-56.

32. Pothineni KR, Wells BJ, Hsiung MC, Nanda NC, Yelamanchili P, Suwanjutah T, et al. Real time three-dimensional transthoracic echocardiographic assessment of pulmonary regurgitation. Echocordiography. 2008:25:911-7.

33. Goldberg SJ, Allen HD. Quantitative assessment by Doppler echocardiography of pulmonary or aortic regurgitation. Am J Cardiol. 1985;56:131-5.

34. Marx GR, Hicks RW, Allen HD, Goldberg SJ. Noninvasive assessment of hemodynamic responses to exercise in pulmonary regurgitation after operations to correct pulmonary outflow obstruction. Am J Cardia. 1988;61:595-601.

8 Pulmonary Artery Hypertension

Poonam Malhotra Kapoor, Vishwas Malik, Usha Kiran

INTRODUCTION AND DEFINITION

Pulmonary hypertension refers to an increase in blood pressure within the pulmonary vasculature. It is defined hemodynamically as a mean pulmonary artery pressure ≥25 mm Hg at rest. It can be subdivided into:

- **Precapillary pulmonary hypertension** (in which the pulmonary capillary wedge pressure is ≤15 mm Hg).
- **Postcapillary pulmonary hypertension** (in which the pulmonary capillary wedge pressure is >15 mm Hg).
- **Echocardiography** especially transesophageal echocardiography is an excellent non-invasive tool to detect pulmonary artery hypertension (PAH), as mild, moderate or severe, details of which are given in **Table 1** echocardiography.
- Allows the differential diagnosis of possible **causes of PAH**
  - Valvular heart disease
  - Myocardial disease
  - Congenital heart disease (CHD) with systemic to pulmonary shunt

Postcapillary pulmonary hypertension is seen in pulmonary hypertension due to left heart disease (see the classification scheme below). Precapillary pulmonary hypertension is seen in all the other causes.

Table 1: Indicators of pulmonary regurgitation severity			
	Mild	*Moderate*	*Severe*
Jet size	Narrow, <1.0 cm	Intermediate	Wide, large
Regurgitant fraction (%)	<40	40–60	>60
CW jet density	Soft	Dense	Dense
CW jet deceleration rate	Slow	Variable	Steep
$RVOT_{VTI}/LVOT_{VTI}$	↑	↑↑	↑↑↑
Abbreviations: CW, continuous wave; LVOT, left ventricular outflow tract; RVOT, right ventricular outflow tract; VTI, velocity time integral. References ranges reproduced with permission of the British Society of Echocardiography and British Heart Foundation.			

Note that the hemodynamic definitions refer to mean pulmonary artery pressure, not the pulmonary artery systolic pressure, and are based on cardiac catheter studies.

CAUSES OF PULMONARY HYPERTENSION

Pulmonary hypertension results from an increased resistance to blood flow through the pulmonary vasculature. The World Health Organization (WHO) categorizes the causes of pulmonary hypertension into a number of groups:

- Pulmonary arterial hypertension (e.g. idiopathic, heritable, drug or toxin induced, connective tissue disease, persistent pulmonary hypertension of the newborn)
- Pulmonary veno-occlusive disease and/or pulmonary capillary hemangiomatosis
- Pulmonary hypertension due to left heart disease (e.g. valvular disease, LV systolic or diastolic dysfunction)
- Lung diseases and/or hypoxemia (e.g. chronic obstructive pulmonary disease, interstitial lung disease, sleep-disordered breathing)
- Chronic thromboembolic disease (e.g. pulmonary embolism)
- Miscellaneous causes (e.g. sarcoidosis, lymphangiomatosis).

It is important to be aware of the potential causes of pulmonary hypertension, so that a search can be made for any clues to the underlying cause whenever pulmonary hypertension is detected on echo.

CLINICAL FEATURES OF PULMONARY HYPERTENSION

The clinical features of pulmonary hypertension are summarized in **Table 2**. As well as symptoms and signs relating to the pulmonary hypertension itself, the patient may also have clinical features specific to the underlying cause and therefore a detailed history and clinical examination are necessary in every case.

Table 2: Clinical features of pulmonary hypertension	
Symptoms	*Signs*
• Symptoms are often of very gradual onset breathlessness	• Elevated jugular venous pressure
• Fatigue	• Parasternal heave
• Cough	• Loud pulmonary component to second heart sound (P2)
• Dizziness and syncope	• Tricuspid regurgitation
• Peripheral edema	• Peripheral edema
	• Ascites

ECHO ASSESSMENT OF PULMONARY HYPERTENSION

Echo provides a valuable noninvasive method for estimating pulmonary artery pressure.

PULMONARY ARTERY SYSTOLIC PRESSURE MEASUREMENT ON TEE

The technique that is commonly used for measuring pulmonary artery systolic pressure (PASP) relies upon the presence of tricuspid regurgitation. Fortunately, at least two-thirds of normal individuals have a detectable degree of tricuspid regurgitation (and it is even common in those with pulmonary hypertension). We can assess tricuspid regurgitation using CW Doppler in:

- ME RV inflow-outflow view **(Fig. 1A)**
- ME aortic valve short axis view **(Fig. 2)**
- TG RV inflow view **(Fig. 3)**.
- IVC LE view **(Fig. 4)**
- Hepatic view LE view **(Fig. 5)**

Using CW Doppler, measure the peak velocity of regurgitant flow through the tricuspid valve (TR V_{max}) in m/s. It is a good idea to assess the tricuspid regurgitation in as many of the above views as possible, and to use the highest value (or, if atrial fibrillation is present, to calculate the mean of five consecutive values). If it is difficult to obtain a clear spectral Doppler trace using CW Doppler, the use of agitated saline bubble contrast can enhance the tricuspid regurgitation jet.

Figure 1B shows a CW Doppler trace of a tricuspid regurgitation jet with a V_{max} of 4.26 m/s **(Fig. 6)**. The tricuspid regurgitation reflects, the pressure gradient between right ventricular systolic pressure (RVSP) and RAP, and this pressure gradient can be calculated using the simplified Bernoulli equation:

$$RVSP - RAP = 4^2$$

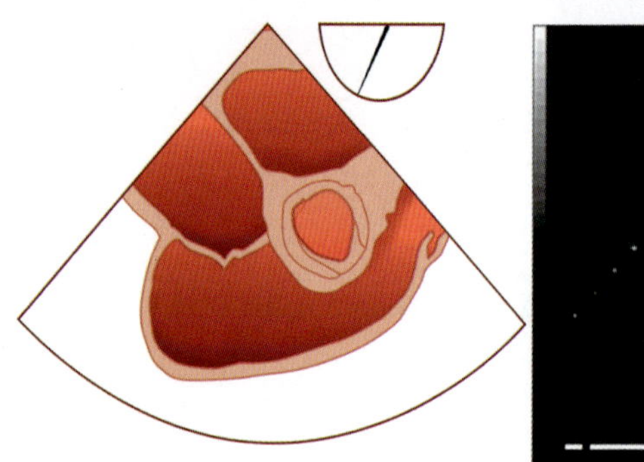

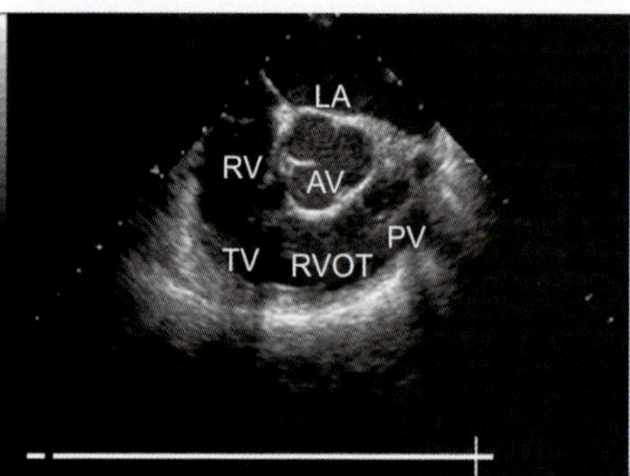

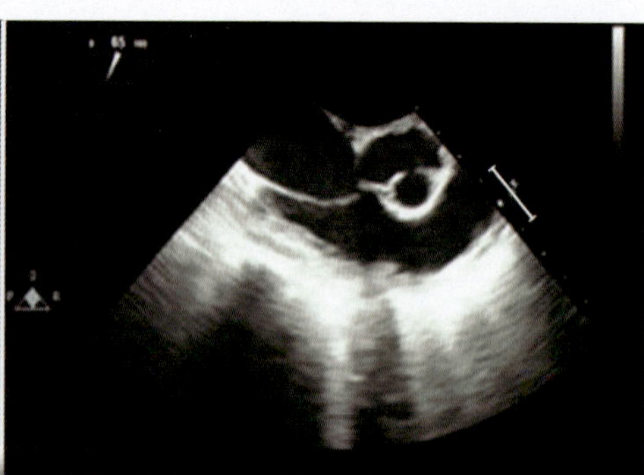

Figure 1A

Midesophageal right ventricular inflow-outflow view

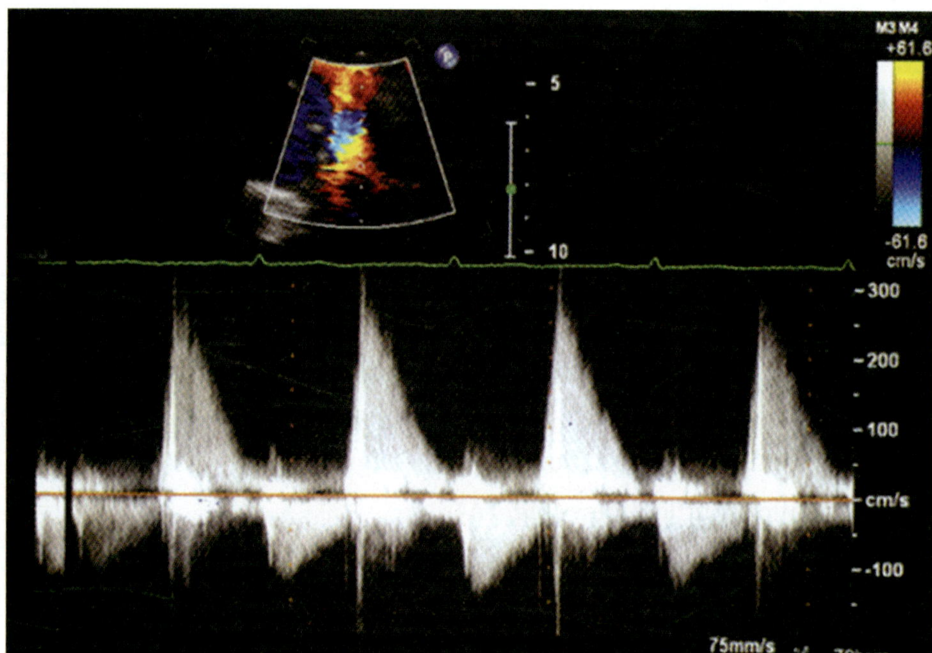

Figure 1B

Gradient measurement in RV inflow-outflow view showing severe PAH

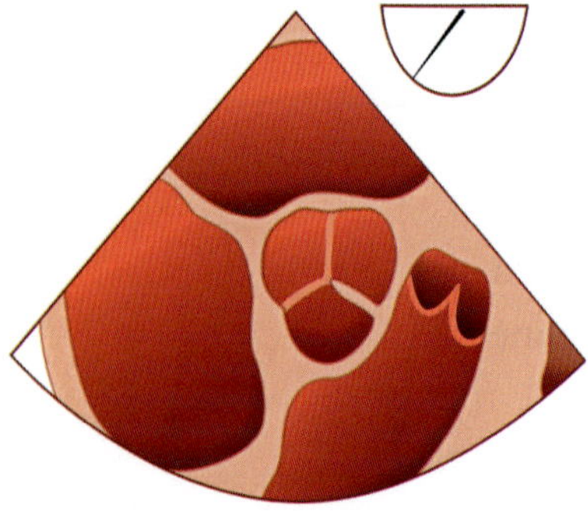

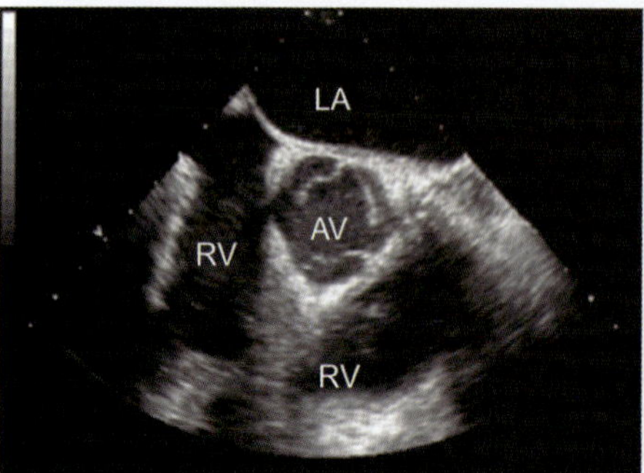

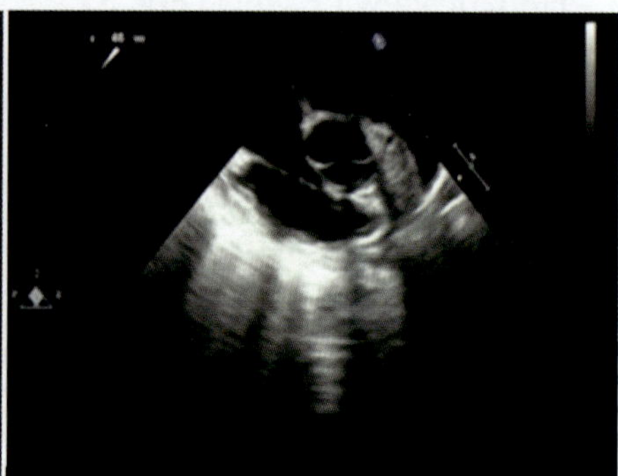

Figure 2

Midesophageal aortic valve short-axis view

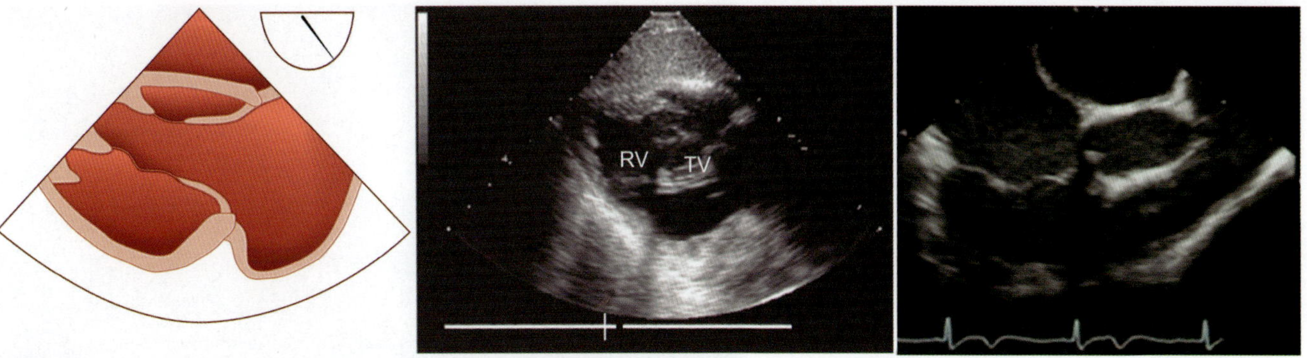

Figure 3

Transgastric right ventricular inflow view. PAP can be measured well in this view which is easily obtainable at 110° to 120° as transgastric view

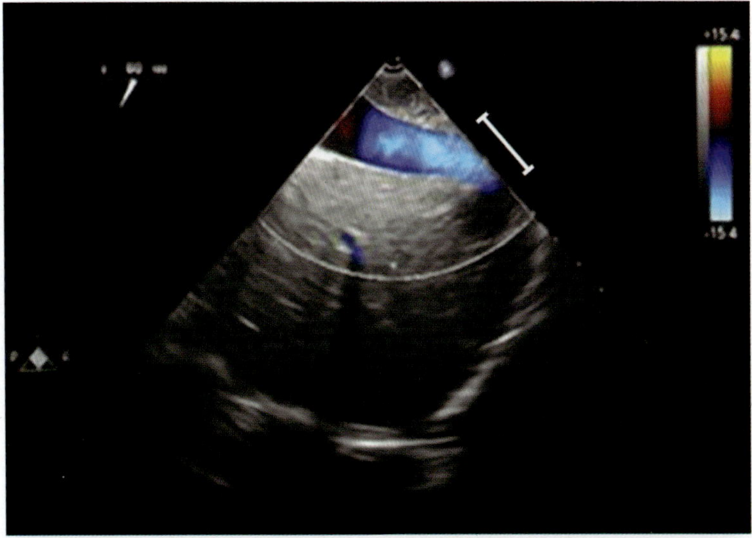

Figure 4

Inferior vena cava LE view. Doppler evaluation can best be interrogated here and IVC diameter measured after confirmation of IVC flow on Doppler

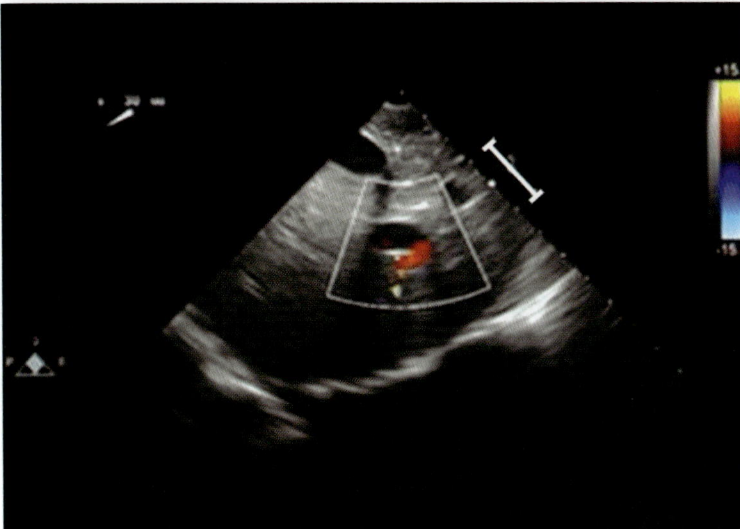

Figure 5

Hepatic vein LE view where again IVC diameter can be measured to obtain RA pressures

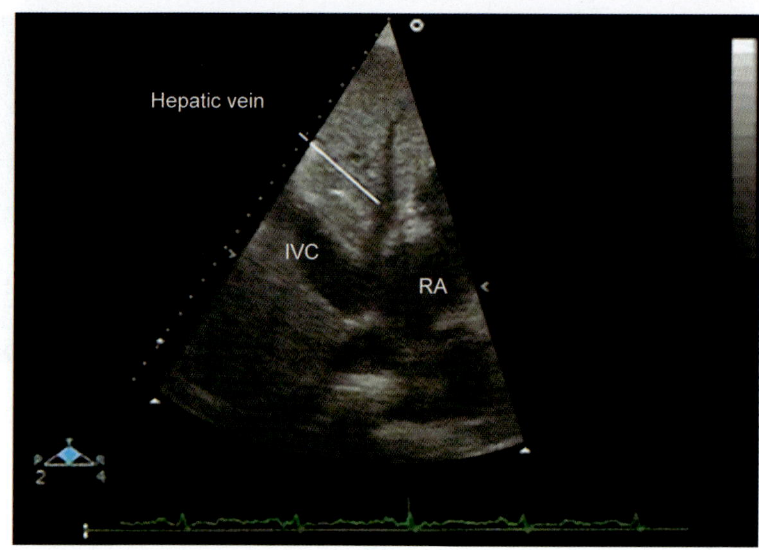

Figure 6

Moderate tricuspid regurgitation showing measurement of peak velocity (TR V_{max}). *Abbreviation:* PG, pressure gradient

For example, if the peak velocity of the TR jet is 4.26 m/s then:

$$RVSP - RAP = 4 \times (4.26)^2$$

$$RVSP - RAP = 4 \times 18.15$$

$$RVSP - RAP = 73 \text{ mm Hg.}$$

Now we know the pressure difference between the RV and the RA. The next step is to estimate the actual systolic pressure in the RV, and to do that we need to know what the RAP is. The estimation of RAP from IVC diameter has been described earlier in Doppler evaluation. If assessment of the IVC gives an estimated RAP of 15 mm Hg (using the principle outlined by the American Society of Echocardiography), then, continuing with our example from above:

$$RVSP - RAP = 73 \text{ mm Hg}$$

$$RVSP - RAP = 73 \text{ mm Hg} + RAP$$

$$RVSP = 73 + 15 \text{ mm Hg}$$

$$RVSP = 88 \text{ mm Hg.}$$

The patient therefore has an estimated RVSP of approximately 88 mm Hg. Assuming there is no significant pulmonary stenosis, the RVSP is approximately equal to the pulmonary artery systolic pressure (PASP):

$$PASP = RVSP$$

$$PASP = 88 \text{ mm Hg}$$

Table 3: Transesophageal echocardiography (TEE) estimates pulmonary artery systolic pressure (PASP) using tricuspid jet velocity PASP = RVSP = $4V^2$ + RAP	
IVC findings	*Estimated RAP*
Small and collapse	00–05 mm Hg
Normal and normal ↓ in size	05–10 mm Hg
Normal and abnormal ↓ in size	10–15 mm Hg
Dilated and abnormal ↓ in size	15–20 mm Hg
Dilated and no change in size	>20 mm Hg

Table 4: Pulmonary artery hypertension grading and criteria based on TR V_{max}		
	TR V_{max}	*PASP*
Unlikely PAH	≤2.8 m/s	≤36 mm Hg (additional echo variables)
Possible PAH	≤2.8 m/s	≤36 mm Hg (additional echo variables)
	2.9–3.4 m/s	37–50 mm Hg (no additional echo variables)
Likely PAH	>3.4 m/s	>50 mm Hg (no additional echo variables)

(If there is coexistent pulmonary stenosis, then the RVSP will be higher than PASP, and the difference will be equal to the peak pressure gradient across the stenosis). **Table 3** shows how PASP and RVSP can be got from IVC diameter and RAP.

However, although it is widely used, a number of studies have questioned the accuracy of estimating PASP using this method. This method should not therefore be used to decide when to initiate treatment for pulmonary hypertension, nor to assess the effectiveness of therapy.

TR V_{MAX} FOR PULMONARY ARTERY HYPERTENSION DIAGNOSIS

Recent guidelines have placed more of an emphasis on using the value of TR V_{max} itself to identify individuals with pulmonary hypertension, rather than trying to calculate the PASP. The BSE defines the normal upper limit of TR V_{max} as 2.6 m/s (or 2.8 m/s in obese patients, or 2.9 m/s in individuals aged >60 years) **(Fig. 7)**. Remember that these figures only apply in the absence of pulmonary stenosis. The European Society of Cardiology has similarly advised that **(Table 4)**.

- *Pulmonary hypertension is 'unlikely' if:* TR V_{max} is ≤2.8 m/s, PASP is ≤36 mm Hg, and there are no additional echo variables suggestive of pulmonary hypertension
- *Pulmonary hypertension is 'possible' if:*
  - TR V_{max} is ≤2.8 m/s, PASP is ≤36 mm Hg, and there are additional echo variables suggestive of pulmonary hypertension, or

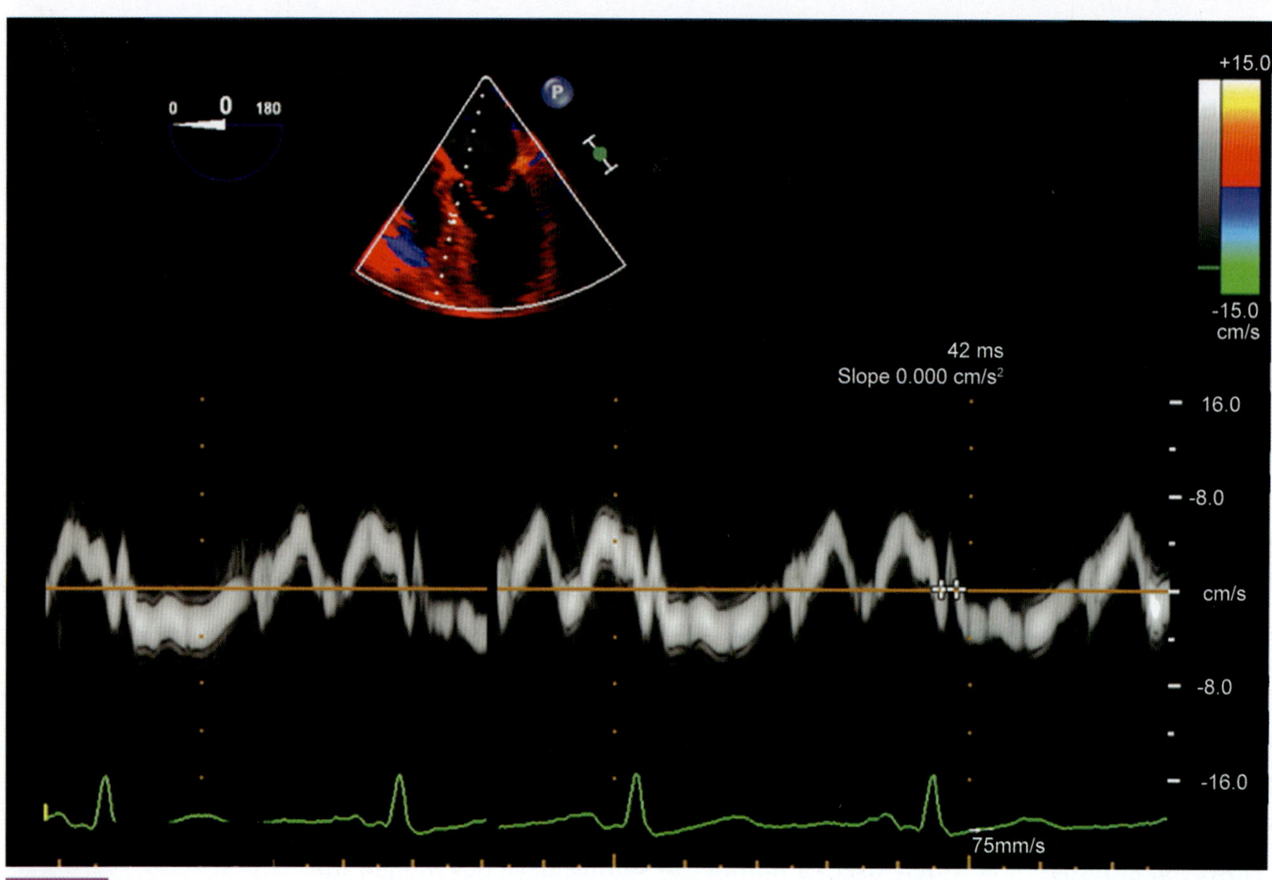

Figure 7

Inferior vena cava diameter showing the TR V_{max} in M-mode 2D TEE

- TR V_{max} is 2.9 to 3.4 m/s, PASP is 37 to 50 mm Hg, whether or not there are additional echo variables suggestive of pulmonary hypertension

- PASP is >50 mm Hg, and there are no additional echo variables suggestive of pulmonary hypertension.

Assuming there is no significant pulmonary stenosis, the RVSP is approximately equal to the pulmonary artery systolic pressure (PASP):

The 'additional echo variables' that can be used to look for evidence of pulmonary hypertension include:

- RV and RA dilatation
- RV hypertrophy
- Dilatation of the pulmonary artery

- Reduced RVOT acceleration time—use PW Doppler to measure flow in the RVOT in the ME RV inflow-outflow or wraparound view, with the patient holding their breath at end-expiration. Measure the time from the onset of RVOT flow to the peak velocity. An acceleration time < 105 ms is supportive of a diagnosis of pulmonary hypertension.

PULMONARY ARTERY DIASTOLIC PRESSURE

Estimation of pulmonary artery diastolic pressure (PADP) relies on the presence of pulmonary regurgitation. You can assess pulmonary regurgitation using CW Doppler in:

- TG RV outflow view
- ME RV inflow-outflow view.

Using CW Doppler, measure the peak velocity of regurgitant flow through the pulmonary valve (PR velocity) in m/s. The pulmonary regurgitation is driven by, and therefore reflects, the diastolic pressure gradient between the pulmonary artery (PADP) and the right ventricle (RVDP), and this pressure gradient can be calculated using the simplified Bernoulli equation:

$$\text{PADP} - \text{RVDP} = 4 \times (\text{PR velocity})^2$$

For example, if the peak velocity of the pulmonary regurgitation jet is 1.1 m/s then:

$$\text{PADP} - \text{RVDP} = 4 \times (1.1)^2$$

$$\text{PADP} - \text{RVDP} = 4 \times 1.2$$

$$\text{PADP} - \text{RVDP} = 4.8 \text{ mm Hg.}$$

Now we know the diastolic pressure difference between the pulmonary artery and the RV. The next step is to estimate the actual diastolic pressure in the RV, and this is taken to be the same as RA pressure (estimated using the IVC technique, as outlined above). For example, if the IVC is normal then the RAP would be estimated at 3 mm Hg, and so the RVDP would be 3 mm Hg too. Continuing with our example:

$$\text{PADP} - \text{RVDP} = 4.8 \text{ mm Hg}$$

$$\text{PADP} = 4.8 \text{ mm Hg} + \text{RVDP}$$

$$\text{PADP} = 4.8 + 3 \text{ mm Hg}$$

$$\text{PADP} = 7.8 \text{ mm Hg.}$$

The patient therefore has a PADP of approximately 8 mm Hg.

ASSOCIATED FEATURES

If pulmonary hypertension is present, we must include a careful search for potential causes in our echo study, for example:

- Mitral and/or aortic valve disease
- Left-to-right shunts (e.g. ASD, VSD)
- LV dysfunction
- Pulmonary emboli.

You must also look for, and report upon, any consequences of pulmonary hypertension:

- Pulmonary artery dilatation
- Pulmonary and/or tricuspid regurgitation
- RV dilatation and impairment
- RA dilatation.

SAMPLE REPORT AS A SUMMARY OF PULMONARY ARTERIAL HYPERTENSION ECHO MEASUREMENT

The RV is severely dilated and impaired, and there is moderate functional tricuspid regurgitation into a dilated right atrium. The tricuspid regurgitation peak velocity is 4.1 m/s, giving a regurgitation gradient of 67 mm Hg. The RVOT acceleration time is 88 ms. There is moderate pulmonary regurgitation with a regurgitation gradient of 10 mm Hg. The IVC is dilated at 2.8 cm and decreases to 1.8 cm on inspiration, giving an estimated right atrial pressure of 15 mm Hg, estmated pulmonary artery pressure is therefore 82/25 mm Hg, indicating severe pulmonary hypertension. The patient also has severe mitral stenosis.

SUMMARY

Pulmonary artery hypertension can be best measured on echo using:

- Tricuspid regurgitation peak velocity regurgitation gradient
- RVOT acceleration time
- IVC diameter
- Estimate RAP.

- **An acceleration time a 105 MS is supportive of a diagnosis of pulmonary hypertension.**

BIBLIOGRAPHY

1. Galie N, Hoeper MM, Humbert M, et al. Guidelines for the diagnosis and treatment of pulmonary hypertension. Eur Heart J. 2009;30:2493-537.
2. Lancellotti P, Moura L, Pierard LA, et al. European Association of Echocardiography recommendations for the assessment of valvular regurgitation. Part 2: mitral and tricuspid regurgitation (native valve disease). Eur J Echocardiogr. 2010;2:307-32.
3. Lancellotti P, Tribouilloye C, Hagendorff A, et al. European Association of Echocardiography recommendations for the assessment of valvular regurgitation. Part 1: aortic and pulmonary regurgitation (native valve disease). Eur J Echocardiogr. 2010;11:223-44.
4. Lang RM, Bierig M, Devereux RB, et al. Recommendations for chamber quantification: a report from the American Society of Echocardiography's Guidelines and Standards Committee and the Chamber Quantification Writing Group, developed in conjunction with the European Association of Echocardiography, a branch of the European Society of Cardiology. J Am Soc Echocardiogr. 2005;18:1440-63.
5. Milan A, Magnino C, Veglio F. Echocardiographic indexes for the non-invasive evaluation of pulmonary hemodynamics. J Am Soc Echocardiogr. 2010;23:225-39.
6. Nef HM, Mollmann H, Hamm C, et al. Pulmonary hypertension: updated classification and management of pulmonary hypertension. Heart. 2010;96:552-9.
7. Rudski LG, Lai WW, Afilalo J, et al. Guidelines for the echocardiographic assessment of the right heart in adults: a report from the American Society of Echocardiography. J Am Soc Echocardiogr. 2010;23:685-713.
8. Tei C, Dujardin KS, Hodge DO, et al. Doppler index combining systolic and diastolic myocardial performance: clinical value in cardiac amyloidosis. J Am Coll Cardiol. 1996; 28:658-64.

9 Ebstein's Anomaly

Navin C Nanda, Poonam Malhotra Kapoor, Arun Subramaniam

- Anatomy of Ebstein's Anomaly
- Clinical Presentation in Ebstein's Anomaly
- Congenital Abnormalities of Tricuspid Valve: Ebstein's Anomaly
- Jugular Venous Pressure in Ebstein Anomaly
- Cathlab of Ebstein's Anomaly
- Electrocardiogram in Ebstein's Anomaly
- Echocardiography of Ebstein's Anomaly
- Management of Ebstein's Anomaly
- Three-Dimensional Transesophageal Echocardiographic (TEE) Ebstein's Anomaly

ANATOMY OF EBSTEIN'S ANOMALY

Ebstein's malformation is one of the most common congenital abnormalities of the tricuspid valve in adults. Ebstein's anomaly consists of downward displacement of fused malformed portions of tricuspid valvular tissue into the right ventricular cavity.[1,2] *Ebstein's anomaly and the right heart* is characterized by apical displacement of all or part of the TV into the RV. It is diagnosed when the distance from the level of the mitral annulus to the septal leaflet exceeds 11 mm.[3] The RA therefore appears larger and the RV, smaller. The leaflets are attached in part to the tricuspid annulus and in part to the right ventricular wall below the annulus. In general, the anterior leaflet is enlarged at times, forming a large curtain across the right ventricular cavity.[4] The posterior leaflet may be rudimentary or entirely absent.[5] The right atrium is enlarged. The right ventricular portion that is above the abnormal insertion of the tricuspid valve is said to be 'atrialized' **(Fig. 1)**.

- Isolated congenital malformation characterized by downward displacement of leaflets towards the RV apex.
- Posterior, septal and a portion of the anterior leaflets arise from RV free wall.
- 'Atrialized' RV- portion of the RV above the valve is thin and severly hypokinetic.

Figures 2A and B shows the Ebstein's anomaly.

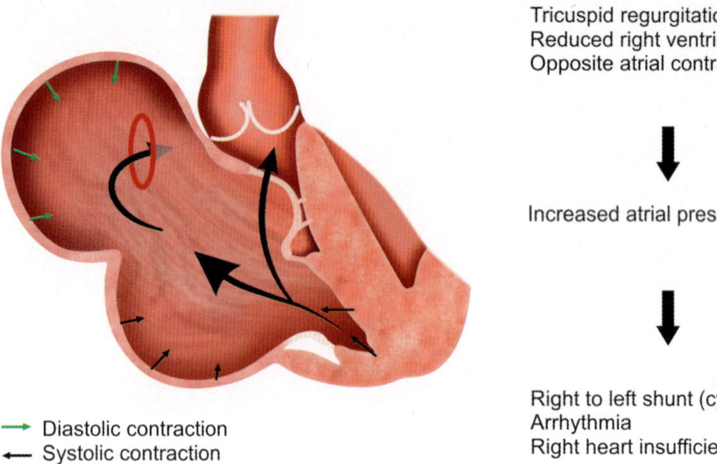

Figure 1

Etiology of tricuspid regurgitation

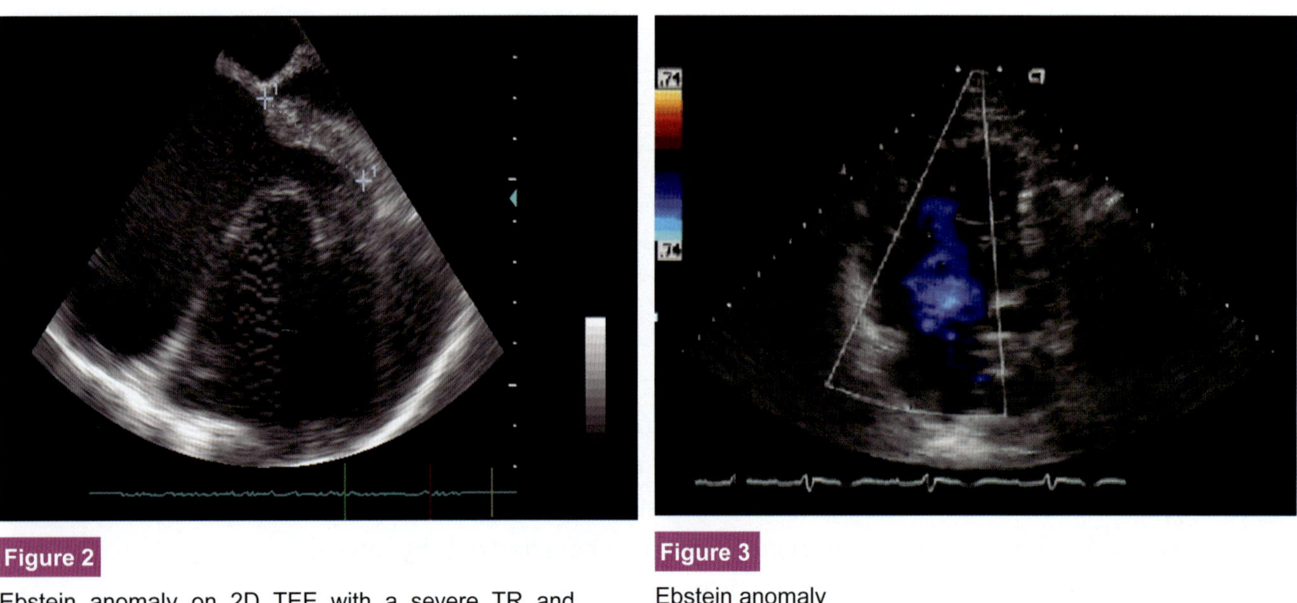

Figure 2

Ebstein anomaly on 2D TEE with a severe TR and decreased RV volume

Figure 3

Ebstein anomaly

CLINICAL PRESENTATION IN EBSTEIN'S ANOMALY

Clinical presentation is highly variable and dependent on the degree of apical displacement of the TV and distortion of RV anatomy and function. The cardinal symptoms of the disease include cyanosis, right ventricular failure, and arrhythmias.[6] Generally, greater degrees of valvular displacement and smaller portions of residual normal RV cavity result in more severe symptoms and a worse prognosis. Tricuspid dysplasia may sometimes be seen in Ebstein's anomaly and is defined as irregularity, thickening, and nodularity of the TV leaflets. The valve may be described as tethered when three or more accessory attachments of the leaflet to the RV wall exist and restrict leaflet motion **(Fig. 3)**.

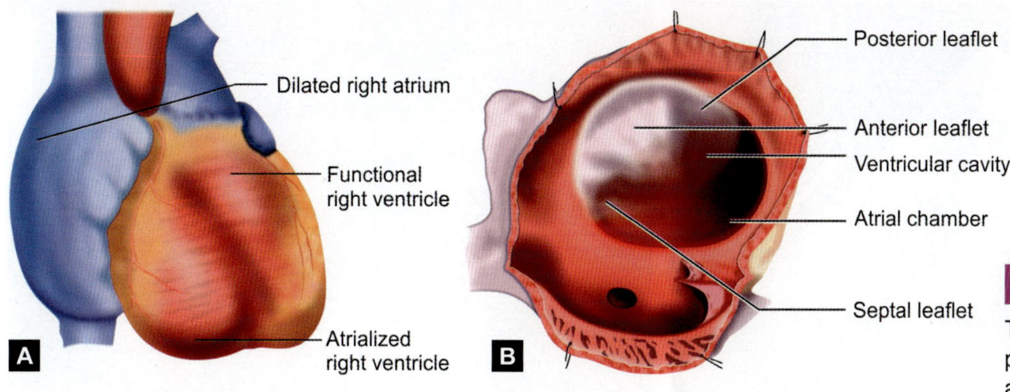

Figures 4A and B

Tricuspid anomaly and tricuspid regurgitation in Ebstein's anomaly

When the pulmonary pressure drops to normal, the burden on the right heart is relieved; the right atrial pressure declines, the right to left shunt diminishes or disappears and with it the cyanosis.

As time goes on cyanosis may reappear since the inadequate right ventricle, burdened by tricuspid regurgitation, ultimately fails again. Right ventricular end-diastolic pressure rises together with right atrial pressure and a right to left shunt is re-established. The degree of cyanosis does not always coincide with the patient's symptoms.[7,8] In fact, a history of relatively good effort tolerance despite cyanosis favors the diagnosis of Ebstein's anomaly **(Figs 4A and B)**.[9]

CONGENITAL ABNORMALITIES OF TRICUSPID VALVE: EBSTEIN'S ANOMALY

The hemodynamic alterations of Ebstein's anomaly are related to the malformed tricuspid valve and the dysfunction of the right ventricle.[9] All gradations of severity exist, and thus this abnormality may be compatible with a relatively long and active life. When symptoms appear, dyspnea, fatigue, and weakness are most common. Palpitations are usually due to atrial dysrhythmias. Death is due to congestive heart failure, hypoxia, and dysrhythmias. Cyanosis occurs in 50 to 80 percent of patients. Perloff [9] emphasized the chronologie sequence of cyanosis as a useful diagnostic feature of the history. Neonatal cyanosis may regress or disappear and' then return at a later date, He states, "The functionally inadequate right ventricle copes poorly with the high pulmonary vascular resistance in the newborn". The right atrial pressure rises and a right to left shunt develops through an interatrial communication.

Ebstein's anomaly of the TV is a rare congenital disorder that occurs in approximately 1 per 210,000 live births.[10] Echocardiography is the diagnostic test of choice for this heterogeneous condition, in which there is inadequate delamination

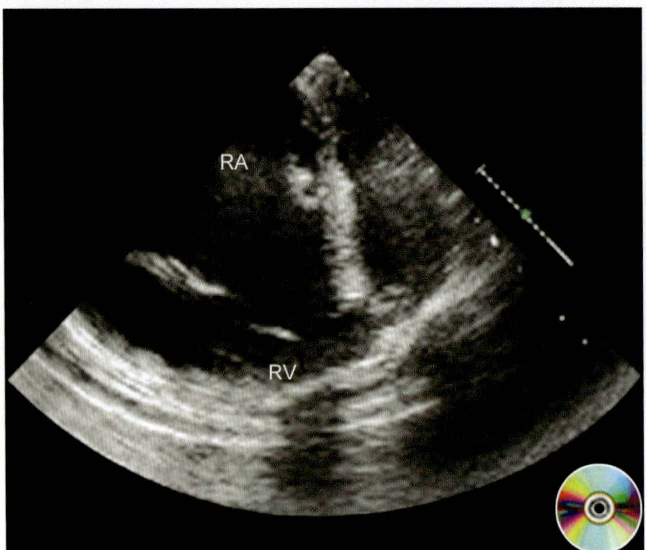

Figure 5 (VIDEO 1)

The marked distortion of right ventricular and right atrial geometry. The approx position of the mitral annulus is noted by the broad arrow at the lower right

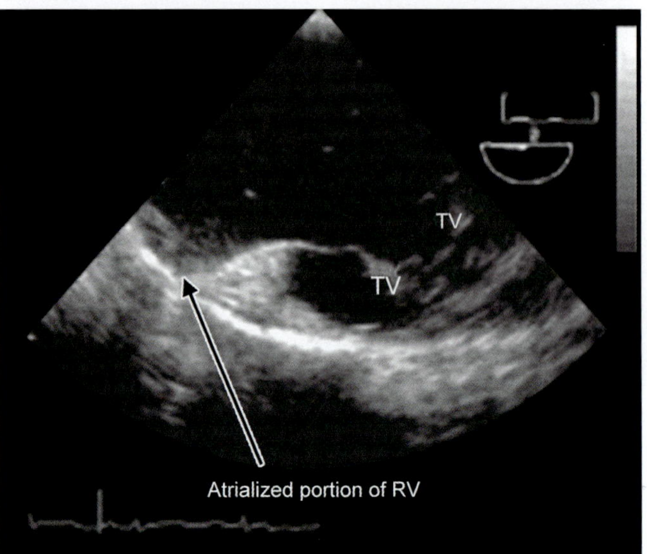

Figure 6

Transesophageal echocardiography image of a patient with Ebstein's anomaly showing apical displacement of the TV leaflet and the thin, 'atrialized' portion of the affected right ventricular wall. *Abbreviation:* TV, tricuspid valve

of the TV leaflets from the endocardium of the RV. This results in features that are characteristic of this anomaly, which include apical displacement of the leaflets, particularly the septal leaflet, with associated TR and right ventricular dysfunction **(Fig. 5)**.

Figure 6 shows the marked distortion of right ventricular and right atrial geometry. The approx position of the mitral annulus is noted by the broad arrow at the lower right.

The cardinal echocardiographic feature is apical displacement of the insertion point of the septal leaflet of the TV relative to the insertion of the anterior leaflet of the MV by at least 8 mm/m^2 body surface area.[11] Other features include dilation of the 'atrialized' portion of the RV, redundancy, fenestrations and tethering of the anterior TV leaflet, and dilation of the true tricuspid annulus.[12-14] An atrial septal defect or patent foramen ovale is commonly seen in these patients, most likely due to increased right atrial pressures.[15] Other associated findings in patients with Ebstein's anomaly include MV prolapse, bicuspid AV, coarctation of the aorta, ventricular septal defects, pulmonary stenosis, and hypoplastic PA.

Other features include RV dysplasia (thinning, dilation, and hypokinesis or dyskinesis) and marked enlargement of the RA.[6] The characteristics of the anterior leaflet of the TV and the size of the RV relative to the remaining three-chambers

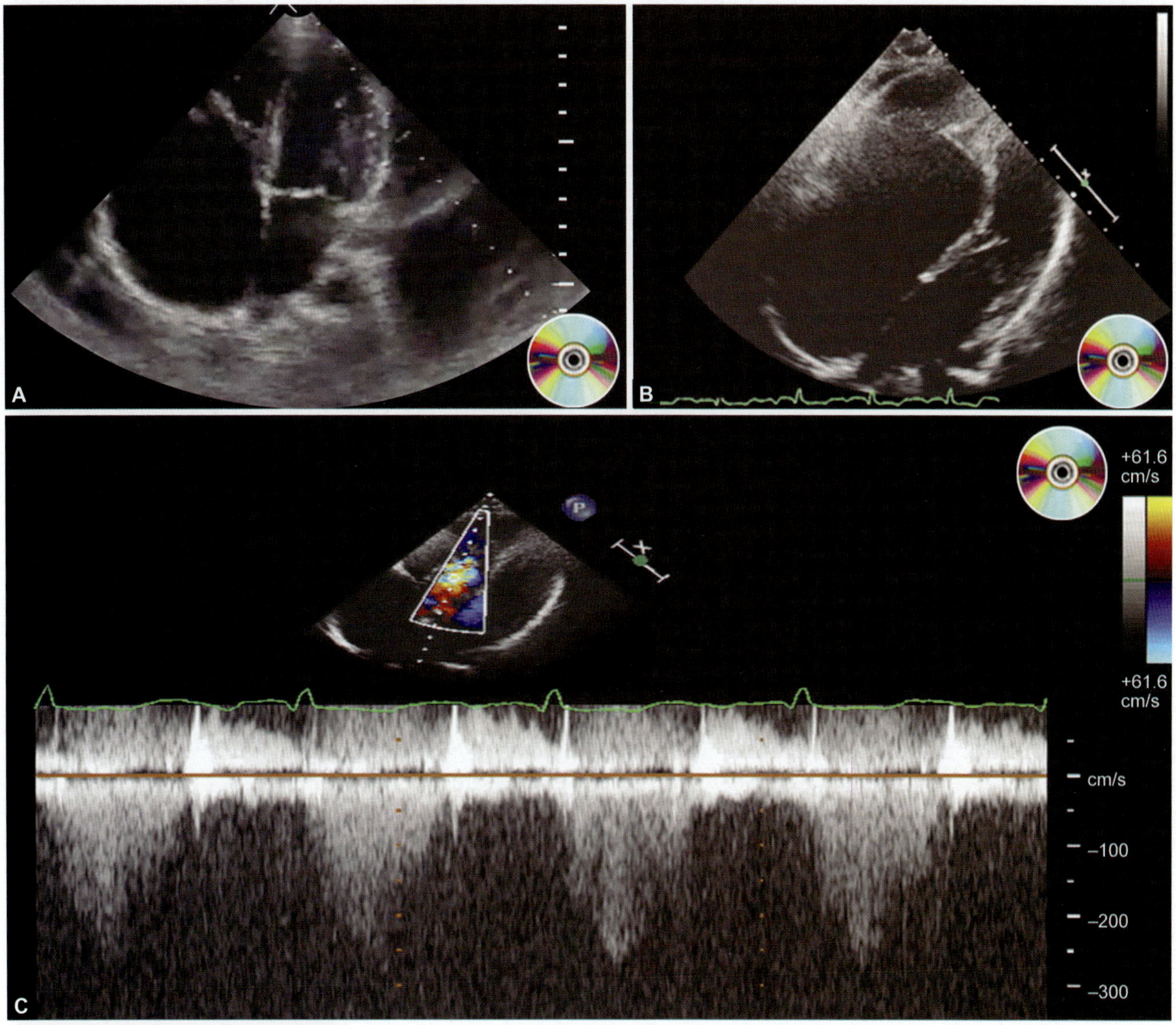

Figures 7A to C (VIDEOS 2 TO 4)

Ebstein anomaly in adult patient with continuous wave Doppler

are especially important to note during the echocardiographic assessment of Ebstein's anomaly. A tethered anterior leaflet with restricted motion and a small functional RV (ratio of functional to total RV cavity dimension <35 percent in the ME four-chamber view) are indications for valve replacement. Plastic repair may be considered if the anterior TV leaflet is elongated, has no fenestrations, and shows large excursion.[16] Limitations of 2D echocardiography include inability to adequately characterize the posterior TV leaflet and identify fenestrations or perforations in the anterior TV leaflet.[17] By allowing an *en face* view of the entire valve, real-time 3D TEE overcomes some of these difficulties and may provide a more precise description of the anomalies present in this condition[16] **(Figs 7A to C)**.

JUGULAR VENOUS PRESSURE IN EBSTEIN ANOMALY

In Ebstein's anomaly, the jugular venous pressure may be normal despite tricuspid incompetence because of the commodious right atrium. On auscultation, the first heart sound is widely split due to the delay in closure of the tricuspid valve. The smaller and poorly contracting right ventricle and the increased excursion of the large anterior leaflet results in a delayed tricuspid component of the first heart sound.[18]

This early systolic sound is prominent and is due to the large sail-like tricuspid valve reaching the limits of its systolic excursion. Referred to as the 'sail sound,' this may Q~ most specific auscultatory finding in Ebstein's 'anomaly.[18] The second heart-sound splitting 'is variable. Systolic murmurs are also quite variable; they may be totally absent' or quite prominent. They are best heard along the lower left sternal border. The murmur of tricuspid regurgitation is not necessarily pansystolic. In the absence of pulmonary hypertension, the end-systolic pressure difference between the right ventricle and the V wave of the right atrium is small, and flow is decreased in late systole. In Ebstein's anomaly the murmur of tricuspid regurgitation does not necessarily increase with inspiration. This may be due to the inability of the small right ventricle to increase its stroke volume.[9]

Early diastolic sounds have been described and are attributed to the 'opening snap' of the large anterior tricuspid leaflet or to the rapid filling of a small nondistensible right ventricle. The cadence created by the first heart sound (mitral valve closure), the early systolic sound (tricuspid valve closure), the second heart sound, and the early diastolic sound has been likened to the chugging of a steam locomotive.[9]

CATHLAB OF EBSTEIN'S ANOMALY

Before the advent of echocardiography, the diagnosis of Ebstein's anomaly was made at cardiac catheterization by using a catheter that had an electrode near the opening of the lumen in the pressure—recording catheter. In the right atrium, atrial pressure and an intra-atrial electrocardiogram are recorded, but the atrialized portion of the right ventricle generates an intracavitary right ventricular electrogram while registering an atrial pressure pulse. As the catheter tip is advances across the tricuspid valve, a right ventricular pressure tracing and an intracavitary right ventricular electrocardiogram are recorded.[9]

ELECTROCARDIOGRAM IN EBSTEIN'S ANOMALY

The electrocardiogram (ECG) is usually abnormal in the adult with Ebstein's anomaly. The P waves may be prominent and the PR interval prolonged. Pre-excitation (Wolff-Parkinson-White) has been described in as many as 20 to 25 percent of patients with Ebstein's anomaly, and, as would be anticipated, the atrioventricular bypass tracts are usually located on the right.[9] Although paroxysmal supraventricular tachycardia occurs from reentry over the bypass tract, other atrial dysrhythmias, such as atrial flutter and fibrillation, are also common because of the enlarged right atrium.

ECHOCARDIOGRAPHY OF EBSTEIN'S ANOMALY

Views for Ebstein Anomaly

- ME four-chamber view
- RV inflow outflow view
- TG RV inflow view
- TG RV outflow view.

M-mode

The echocardiographic features of Ebstein's anomalies are characteristic. The M-mode recording shows an increased excursion of the tricuspid valve when the echo beam traverses the large anterior leaflet. The most characteristic M-mode feature is delayed closure (50 ms of more) of the tricuspid valve when compared with that of the mitral valve. The two-dimensional echocardiogram is also diagnostic. In the apical four-chamber view, the right ventricular displacement of the leaflet and right atrial enlargement can be visualized.

2D in Ebstein Anomaly

Use 2D echo to assess the structure of the tricuspid valve:

- Is the tricuspid valve position normal or is it displaced apically? In Ebstein's anomaly the septal or posterior tricuspid leaflet is displaced towards the RV apex by at least 0.8 cm/m^2 (in adults, the displacement should be indexed for body surface area), in comparison with the mitral valve plane.
- Are the tricuspid valve leaflets morphologically normal or abnormal? Do the leaflets coapt normally or eccentrically?
- Is the RA dilated?
- Is the RV dilated? Is RV function impaired?

Color Doppler

Use color Doppler to:

- Assess the severity of tricuspid regurgitation
- Look for shunts (*See* 'Associated features' below).

Continuous Wave and Pulse Wave Doppler

Use continuous wave (CW) Doppler to obtain a trace of regurgitant flow through the tricuspid valve. Obtain traces from the apex and from at least one other position, such as the parasternal short axis or RV inflow views. Assess the severity of tricuspid regurgitation and calculate pulmonary artery systolic pressure.

Associated Features

A number of conditions can be associated with Ebstein's anomaly, so perform a complete echo study to look for them:

- ASD
- PFO (as a consequence of RA dilatation)
- VSD
- Pulmonary stenosis.

MANAGEMENT OF EBSTEIN'S ANOMALY

The management of Ebstein's anomaly includes the treatment of any RV failure and arrhythmias. Surgical options include tricuspid valve repair (or sometimes replacement), resection of the atrialized portion of the RV, and correction of any shunts.

In light of the right-sided heart failure and the findings of EA with tricuspid stenosis, surgical repair is recommended. Intraoperative transesophageal echocardiography confirms the displacement of the tricuspid valve into the right ventricular outflow tract with associated tricuspid stenosis as noted by color flow Doppler. The pulmonary and aortic valves are normal. Surgical repair consists of resection of the stenotic anterior tricuspid leaflet in the right ventricular outflow and removal of a large amount of organized thrombus from the right ventricle **(Figs 8A and B)**. A porcine bioprosthetic tricuspid valve may be placed, and a right atrial reduction performed. Furthermore, a bidirectional Glenn shunt may be placed to offload the right ventricle.

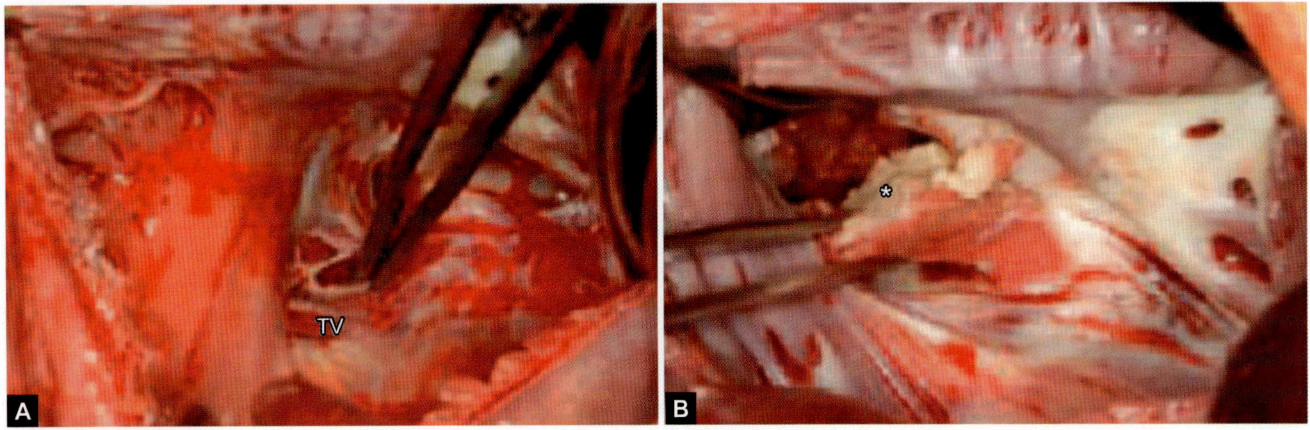

Figures 8A and B

(A) Surgical view of the tricuspid valve (TV) stenosis; (B) Surgical view of thrombus (*) in the atrialized right ventricle and outflow tract

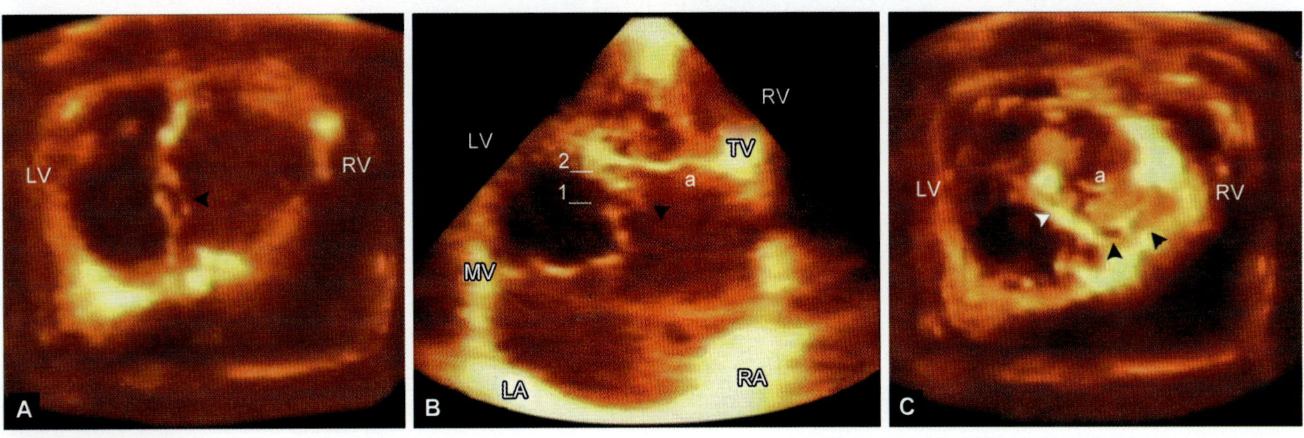

Figures 9A to C

Shows Ebstein's anomaly in a 2 year old where the septal TV leaflet is towards the apex, which may be tethered (A) and (C) shows same towards the base of the heart. Showing the tethered septal and posterior leaflets

THREE-DIMENSIONAL TRANSESOPHAGEAL ECHOCARDIOGRAPHIC (TEE) OF EBSTEIN'S ANOMALY

Live/real time 3D transthoracic echocardiography in Ebstein's anomaly associated with transposition of the great vessels **(Fig. 9A)**. Four-chamber view shows apparent displacement of the attachment of the septal leaflet of the tricuspid valve (TV) toward the apex **(Fig. 9B)**. Tethering of the septal leaflet of the TV results in a bubble-like appearance (white arrowhead) in the middle portion of the ventricular septum as the non tethered portion moves toward closure during systole. This transverse section was taken at a level denoted by #1 in **(Figs 9A and C)**. Transverse section taken at a more inferior level (#2 in

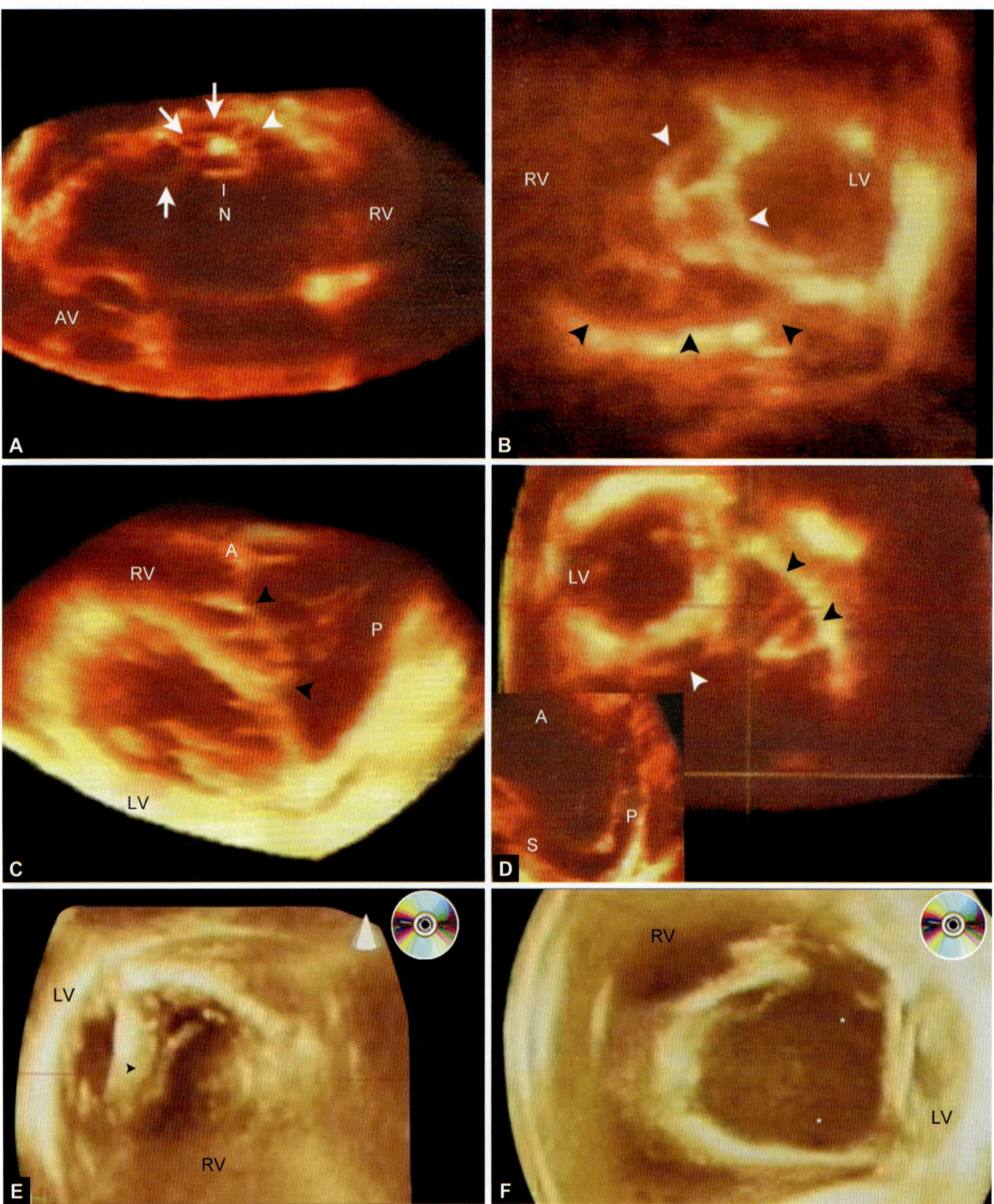

Figures 10A to F (VIDEOS 5 AND 6)

(A) Transverse section in 3D echo taken at the apex of tricuspid valve (TV) shows a large area of noncoaptation (N) as well as tethering and bubble-like appearance. (A, white arrowhead) and posterior (P, black arrowhead) TV leaflets (B and D) show all three leaflets on the TV in the open position. A long snake-like posterior leaflet (E–F)

(Fig. 9A)) demonstrates bubble-like appearance of both septal (white arrowhead) and posterior (black arrowheads) TV leaflets produced by tethering.[19]

Live/real time 3D transthoracic echocardiography in isolated Ebstein's anomaly **(Fig. 10A)**. Transverse section taken at the apex of tricuspid valve (TV) shows a large area of noncoaptation (N) as well as tethering and bubble-like appearance of anterior (A; white arrows) and posterior (P; black arrowhead) TV **(Fig. 10B)** (4D) leaflets **(Figs 10B to D)**. Transverse sections taken more basally demonstrate multiple 'bubbles' in the septal (5; white arrowheads) and posterior (P; black arrowheads) TV leaflets. Inset in **(Fig. 10D)** shows all three leaflets of the TV in the open position.

Oblique section shows multiple 'bubbles' (black arrowheads) in the posterior (P) TV leaflet produced by tethering to right ventricular (RV) inferior wall. In **Figure 10E** shows a long snake-like posterior (P) TV leaflet **(Fig. 10F)**. The oblique section shown in **Figure 10E** has been rotated to more optimally view the attachment of posterior (P) TV leaflet to the RV inferior wall.[20]

Isolated Ebstein's anomaly **(Fig. 11)**. Shows tethering of all three tricuspid valve (TV) leaflets. The resulting 'bubbles' are denoted by arrowheads for the septal (white) and posterior (P; black) TV leaflets and an arrow for the anterior (A) TV leaflet[21] **(Figs 12 and 13)**.

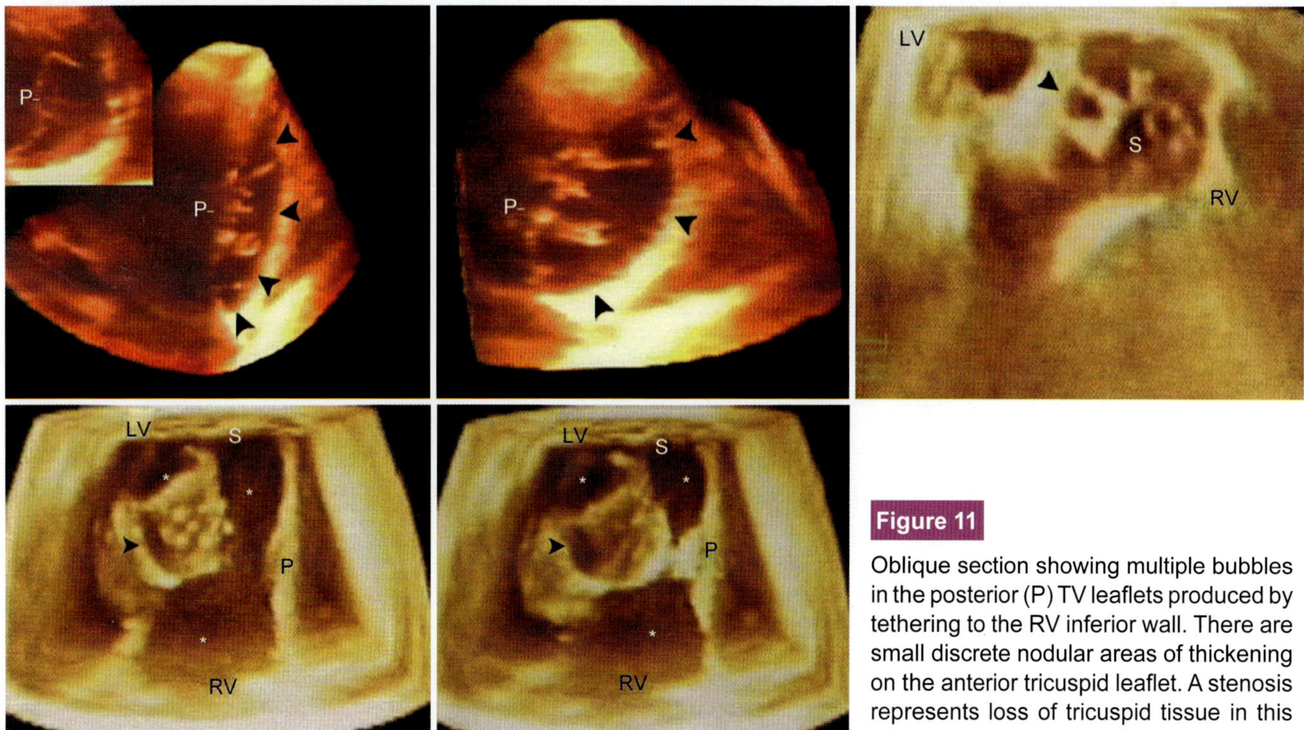

Figure 11

Oblique section showing multiple bubbles in the posterior (P) TV leaflets produced by tethering to the RV inferior wall. There are small discrete nodular areas of thickening on the anterior tricuspid leaflet. A stenosis represents loss of tricuspid tissue in this patient of Ebstein anomaly

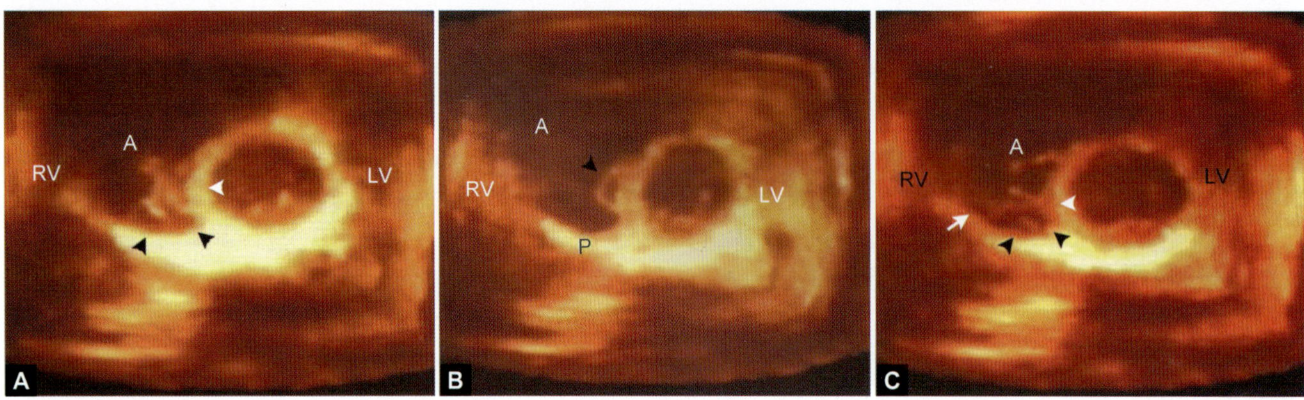

Figures 12A to C

Isolated Ebstein anomaly (A, C) showing tethering of all the three tricuspid valve leaflets and bubbles as shown by arrowheads

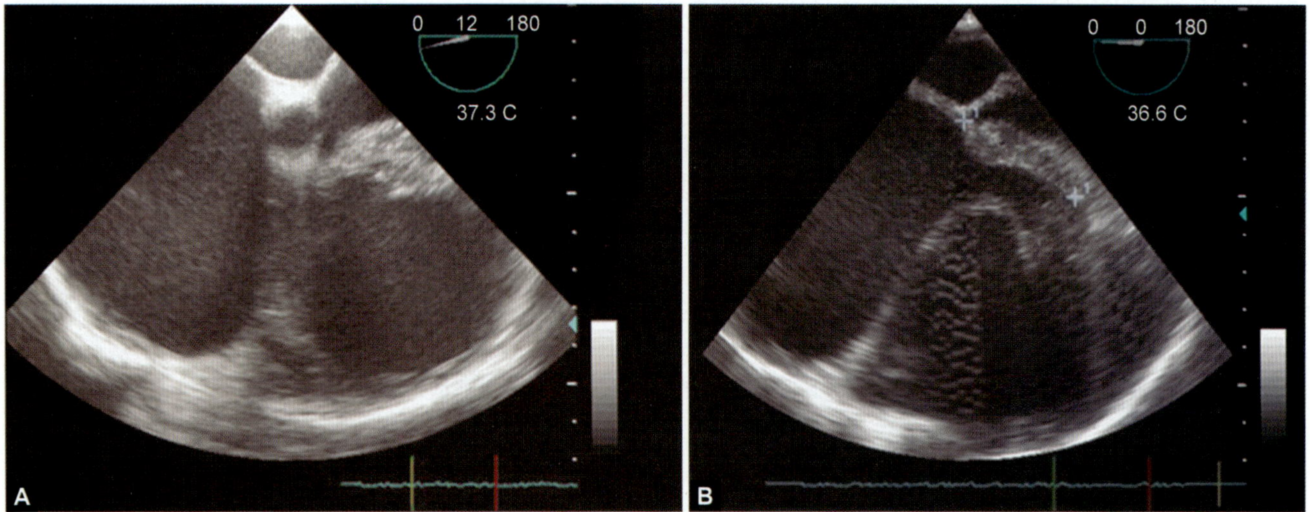

Figures 13A and B

The atrialized RV portion of the RV above the valve is thin and severely hypokinetic

SUMMARY

- Isolated congenital malformation characterized by downward displacement of leaflets towards the RV apex.
- Posterior, septal and a portion of the anterior leaflets arise from RV free wall.
- 'Atrialized' RV-portion of the RV above the valve is thin and severly hypokinetic.
- Tricuspid regurgitation is the predominant lesion.

REFERENCES

1. Ebstein W. On a very rare case of insufficiency of the tricuspid valve caused by severe congenital malformation of the same. Arch Anat Physiol Wissensch Med Leipz 1866;238. [Translated by Schiebler GL, Gravenstein JS, Van Mierop LHS. Am J CardioI 1968;22:867.

2. Vacca JB, Bussman DW, Mudd JG. Ebstein's anomaly: complete review of 108 cases. Am J Cardiol. 1958;2:210.
3. Weyman AE. The Principles and Practice of Echocardiography, 2nd edn. Philadelphia, Lippincott Williams, 1994.
4. Goodwin JF, Wynn A, Steiner RE. Ebstein's anomaly of the tricuspid valve. Am Heart J. 1953;45:144.
5. Edwards JE. Pathologic features of Ebstein's malformation of the tricuspid valve. Proc Staff Meet Mayo Clin. 1953;28:89.
6. Attenhofer Jost CH, Connolly HM, Dearani JA, et al. Ebstein's anomaly. Circulation. 2007;115:277-85.
7. Genton E, Blount SG Jr. The spectrum of Ebstein's anomaly. Am Heart J. 1967;73:395.
8. Kumar AE, Flyer DC, Miettinsen OS, et al. Ebstein's anomaly: clinical profile and natural history. Am J Cardiol. 1971;28:84.
9. Perloff JK. Ebstein's anomaly of the tricuspid valve. In: Perloff JK (Ed). The Clinical Recognition of Congenital Heart Disease, 2nd edn. Philadelphia: WB Saunders, 1978;184-200.
10. Boston US, Dearani JA, O'Leary PW, et al. Tricuspid valve repair for Ebstein's anomaly in young children: a 30-year experience. Ann Thorac Surg. 2006;81:690-5; discussion 695-6.
11. Oechslin E, Buchholz S, Jenni R. Ebstein's anomaly in adults: Doppler-echocardiographic evaluation. Thorac Cardiovasc Surg. 2000;48:209-13.
12. Netter F. Atria and ventricles. In: Yonkman F (Ed). The Heart. New York: CIBA-GEIGY Corporation, 1981:8.
13. Zaroff JG, Picard MH. Transesophageal echocardiographic (TEE) evaluation of the mitral and tricuspid valves. Cardiol Clin. 2000;18:731-50.
14. Watson H. Natural history of Ebstein's anomaly of tricus-pid valve in childhood and adolescence. An international co-operative study of 505 cases. Br Heart J. 1974;36:417-27.
15. Attenhofer Jost CH, Connolly HM, Edwards WD, et al. Ebstein's anomaly—review of a multifaceted congenital cardiac condition. Swiss Med Wkly. 2005;135:269-81.
16. Parranon S, Abadir S, Acar P. New insight into the tricuspid valve in Ebstein anomaly using three-dimensional echocardiography. Heart. 2006;92:1627.
17. Shiina A, Seward JB, Tajik AJ, et al. Two-dimensional echocardiographic—surgical correlation in Ebstein's anomaly: preoperative determination of patients requiring tricuspid valve plication versus replacement. Circulation. 1983;68:534-44.
18. Fontana ME, Wooley CF. Sail sound in Ebstein's anomaly of the tricuspid valve. Circulation. 1972;46:155.
19. Patel V, Nanda NC, Arellano I. Cortriatriatum sinistrum: assessment by live/real time 3D transthoracic echocardiography. Echocardiography. 23:801-2.
20. Pothineni KR, Webb G. Clinical update on adults with congenital heart disease. Lancet 2003;26:1095-104.
21. Patel V, Nanda NC, Rajdev S. Live/real time three-dimensional transthoracic echocardiographic assessment of Ebstein's anomaly. Echocardiography. 2005;22:847-54.

10 Cardiac Masses Across Tricuspid and Pulmonary Valves

Ramchandran Gopinath, Poonam Malhotra Kapoor, Suruchi Ladha

- Tumors
- Myxoma
- Thrombus
- Vegetations
- Endocarditis
- Abscesses
- Bioprosthetic Valve Endocarditis

INTRODUCTION

Cardiac masses are well-recognized on echo. Some normal structures in the right atrium (RA) (crista terminalis/Eustachian valve) or in the right ventricle (RV) (moderator band) may appear like a mass or vegetation. Thus, it is important to do a detailed transesophageal echocardiogram (TEE) examination in various views and correlate it clinically, before making a mass appear pathological.

Cardiac masses on echo can result from:

- Tumors
  - Primary cardiac tumors
    - Benign
    - Malignant
- Thrombus
- Vegetations
- Normal variants and other conditions
  - Moderator band
  - Lambl's excrescences
  - Eustachian valve
  - Chiari network

- Lipomatous hypertrophy of the interatrial septum
- Dilated vessels
- Cysts
- Implanted devices.

TUMORS

A detailed TEE assessment of a cardiac tumor should include a description of its:

- Size (measure its dimensions)
- Location
- Shape (e.g. spherical, pedunculated, papillary, flat)
- Surface appearance (e.g. regular, irregular, multilobular)
- Texture (e.g. solid, layered, cystic, calcified, heterogeneous)
- Mobility (mobile or fixed)
- Associated features (local invasion, pericardial effusion).

Because echo does not allow for a precise diagnosis, it is generally more appropriate to report a cardiac mass as being, e.g. 'suggestive of a myxoma' than as a 'definite' myxoma.

The characteristics of the most common tumors and the features that distinguish them from other cardiac masses are described below.

Primary Cardiac Tumors

Primary cardiac tumors are those that arise from the heart itself. They are rare (1 in 2000 autopsies) and 75 percent are benign **(Table 1)**.

Primary cardiac tumors can present with systemic features such as fever and weight loss, or more specifically with:

- Embolism—either of part the tumor itself or adherent thrombus
- Obstruction—usually of a valve orifice or outflow tract
- Arrhythmias—either tachyarrhythmias, such as ventricular tachycardia, or atrioventricular block.

However, cardiac tumors are most commonly discovered incidentally during echo studies for other indications.

MYXOMA

Myxoma is the most common primary cardiac tumor, accounting for 50 percent of cases, and is most common in women. It is typically diagnosed between the ages of

Table 1: Primary cardiac tumors	
Benign (75 percent)	Malignant (25 percent)
Myxoma	Angiosarcoma
Papillary fibroelastoma	Rhabdomyosarcoma
Lipoma	
Hemangioma	
Teratoma	
Rhabdomyoma	
Fibroma	

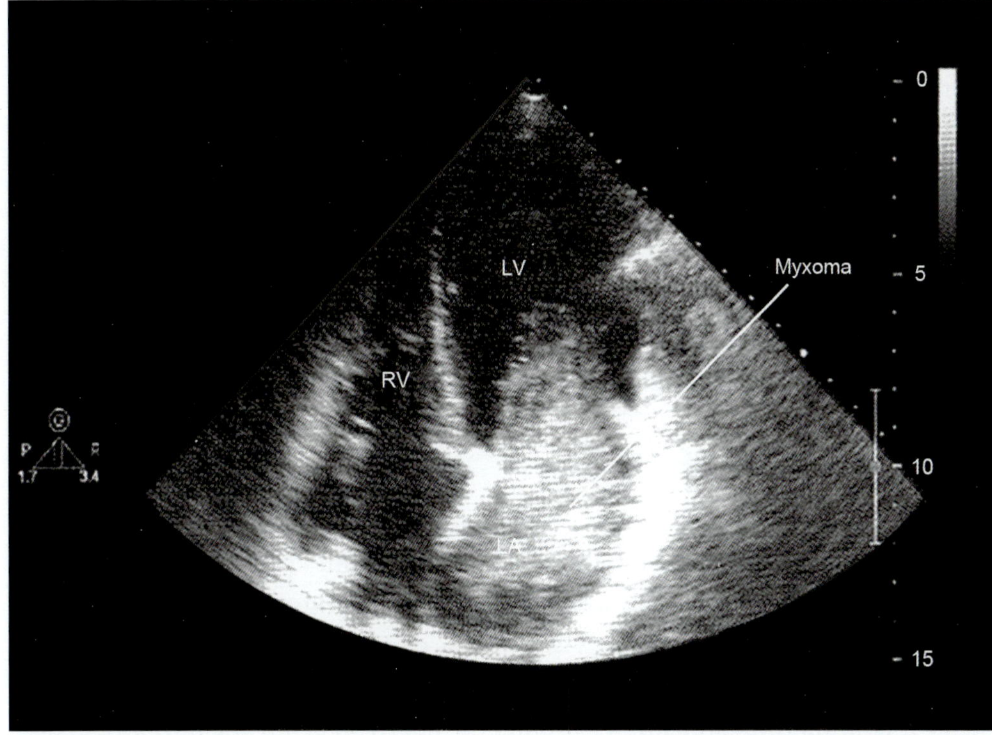

Figure 1

Large left atrial myxoma on TEE, prolapsing through the mitral valve during diastole. *Abbreviations:* LA, left atrium; LV, left ventricle; RA, right atrium; RV, right ventricle

30 and 60 years. Myxomas are usually (but not always) solitary: 75 to 80 percent are found in the left atrium (LA, **Fig. 1**), 15 to 20 percent in the right atrium (RA), and rarely in the ventricles.

Around 7 percent of myxomas are familial (autosomal dominant), and these are more commonly multiple and found in the ventricles. Familial myxomas tend to present at, a younger age. There can be associated abnormalities such as facial freckling and endocrine tumors, and such syndromes are grouped together as a 'Carney complex'. Other myxoma syndromes include NAME syndrome and LAMB syndrome. Screening of first-degree relatives is appropriate in suspected familial cases.

Myxomas are attached to the heart by a pedunculated stalk—in the case of atrial myxomas, they attach to the interatrial septum at the fossa ovalis. The echo appearances of a myxoma are of a well-defined mass, which is often mobile, and the pedicle may be visible. The tumor itself appears heterogeneous and may contain small areas of lucency and occasionally speckles of calcium. Transthoracic echo (TTE) is usually adequate for making the diagnosis, but transesophageal echo (TEE) has a greater sensitivity and specificity and provides a more detailed assessment of the myxoma.

Sample Report

The left atrium contains a mass attached to the interatrial atrial septum via a pedicle. The mass is approximately spherical, measuring 1.6 cm by 1.4 cm, and has an irregular surface and a heterogeneous texture with areas of lucency and of calcification. The mass is mobile but is not causing any obstruction to mitral valve flow. No other intracardiac masses are seen. The appearances are suggestive of a left atrial myxoma.

Surgical resection of the myxoma is the treatment of choice. Following resection, longer-term follow-up is appropriate to monitor for tumor recurrence (particularly in familial cases, where the recurrence rate is 20 percent).

Other Benign Cardiac Tumors

Papillary fibroelastoma is a small (< 1.5 em) is a benign tumor and is most commonly found attached to the aortic or mitral valve. They account for 10 percent of primary cardiac tumors. They are usually found incidentally during echo, cardiac surgery or post mortem, and their similarity to vegetations can lead to a mistaken diagnosis of infective endocarditis. They are usually highly mobile and have been described as having a 'shimmering' appearance around the edges on echo. The tumors can be a source of thrombotic emboli, or fragments of the fibroelastoma itself can embolize, and surgical resection should therefore be considered, particularly if they are large (> 1.0 em), mobile and present in the left heart.

Lipomas are usually seen beneath the epicardium. Cardiac magnetic resonance imaging (MRI) is a useful technique to confirm the diagnosis. Lipomas are distinct from lipomatous hypertrophy of the interatrial septum.

Hemangioma is a rare benign vascular tumor which can occur in any chamber.

Rhabdomyoma is the most common cardiac tumor seen in infants and children. It is usually multiple and found in the ventricles. It is commonly associated with tuberous sclerosis.

Fibromas are also most common in infants and children, are usually solitary and mainly affect the interventricular septum. Fibromas are up to 10 cm in diameter

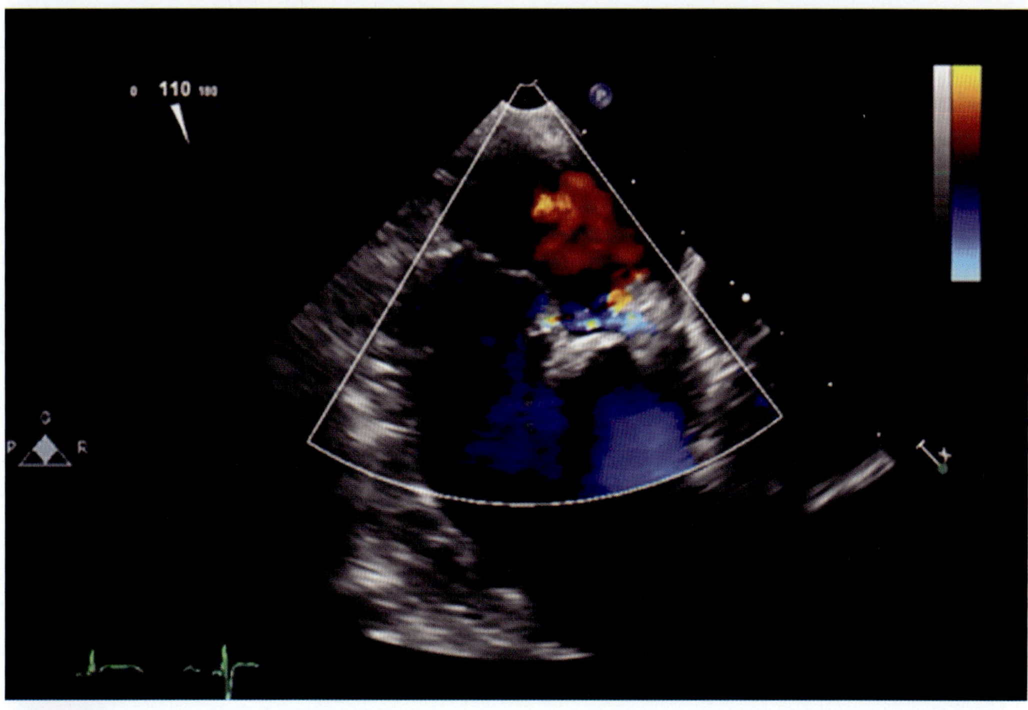

Figure 2

RV fibroelastoma of the tricuspid valve

and appear heterogeneous with multifocal calcification on echo. They often cause obstruction and arrhythmias **(Fig. 2)**.

Teratomas are germ cell tumors found in infants and children that usually affect the pericardium and are associated with a pericardial effusion. Echo shows a complex cystic mass within the pericardium and usually on the right side of the heart.

Malignant Primary Cardiac Tumors

Malignant tumors make up 25 percent of primary cardiac tumors and the vast majority is sarcomas. There are various types of cardiac sarcoma, including angiosarcoma (the most common), rhabdomyosarcoma, malignant fibrous histiocytoma and osteosarcoma.

Angiosarcomas almost always affect the right atrium (in contrast to the other sarcomas which can arise anywhere in the heart, but most commonly on the left) and they occur more commonly in men, usually in the age range 30 to 50 years. Patients often present with symptoms of right heart obstruction and, because pericardial involvement is common, cardiac tamponade. On echo the mass is broad based often arises near the junction of the inferior cava with the right atrium, and may be invasive.

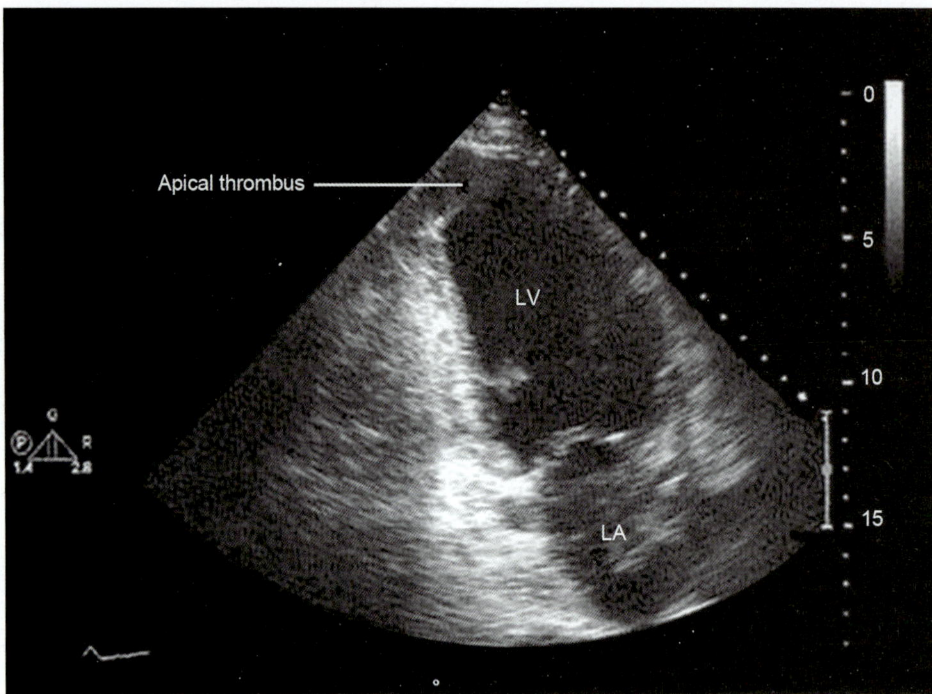

Figure 3

Left ventricular apical thrombus on TEE. *Abbreviations:* LA, left atrium; LV, left ventricle

THROMBUS

Cardiac thrombus is more likely to form when:

- There is stasis (or slow flow) of blood
- There is abnormal endocardium (allowing thrombus to attach)
- The blood is hypercoagulable (making it more likely to clot).

Thrombus formation is therefore more likely in the left atrium in atrial fibrillation (AF), when there is a loss of normal atrial contraction, and in the left ventricle (LV) following myocardial infarction, when reduced contractility predisposes to thrombus formation (particularly if there is aneurysm formation). The presence of an intracardiac device, such as a prosthetic valve or a pacing wire, can also act as a focus for thrombosis. Where there is a high risk of thrombosis (or where a thrombus has already formed) anticoagulation with a drug such as warfarin is used **(Fig. 3)**.

Echo Assessment of Thrombus

The echo assessment of a cardiac thrombus should include a description of its:

- Size (measure its dimensions)
- Location
- Shape (e.g. flat, protruding, spherical)
- Surface appearance (e.g. regular, irregular)
- Texture (e.g. solid, layered, calcified)

- Mobility (mobile or fixed)
- Associated features (e.g. dilated left atrium, left ventricle aneurysm).

Compared with a myxoma, a thrombus usually has a more irregular shape. Thrombus usually attaches to the endocardium via a broad base rather than a pedicle, and is consequently less mobile. A large proportion of left artrium thrombi are within the left artrium appendage, which can be difficult to inspect fully on TTE. The appendage is, however, clearly seen on TOE. It is important to try to distinguish between thrombus and the pectinate muscles, the normal muscle ridges found on the walls of both atria and the appendage. Pectinate muscles are immobile and run in bands; thrombus is usually more rounded and mobile.

Thrombus in the right heart is less commonly found, and may represent a thromboembolism that has arisen in the peripheral veins and is 'in transit' to becoming a pulmonary embolism. Another cause of right heart thrombi is the presence of devices such as pacing/defibrillator leads or intravascular catheters, which can act as a focus for thrombus formation.

VEGETATIONS

Vegetations are usually irregular in shape, mobile and attached to valve leaflets on the upstream side (in contrast with papillary fibroelastoma, which attaches downstream). Infective endocarditis can also cause abscesses, which also have the appearance of cardiac masses. As well as the echo features, the clinical context is important in distinguishing between vegetations and other causes of cardiac masses.

ENDOCARDITIS

Endocarditis of right-sided valves has become a common problem with the advent of intravenous access used in various forms of therapy and especially with individuals who use contaminated needles for intravenous drug abuse. The agents most often involved in right-sided endocarditis come from the skin flora, in particular staphylococci. Structural heart disease is not a prerequisite but is often present. Vegetations classically appear as a chaotically mobile echo dense mass attached on the low pressure aspect of a valve leaflet **(Figs 4A and B)**.

Vegetations

The characteristics echo appearance of vegetation is of an echogenic mass, irregular in shape, attached to the 'upstream' side of a valve leaflet (i.e. the atrial side in the case of the mitral and tricuspid valves, the ventricular side for the aortic and pulmonary valves). Vegetations can be attached to any part of the valves, but most commonly at the coaptation line. Vegetations move with the leaflet but in a more

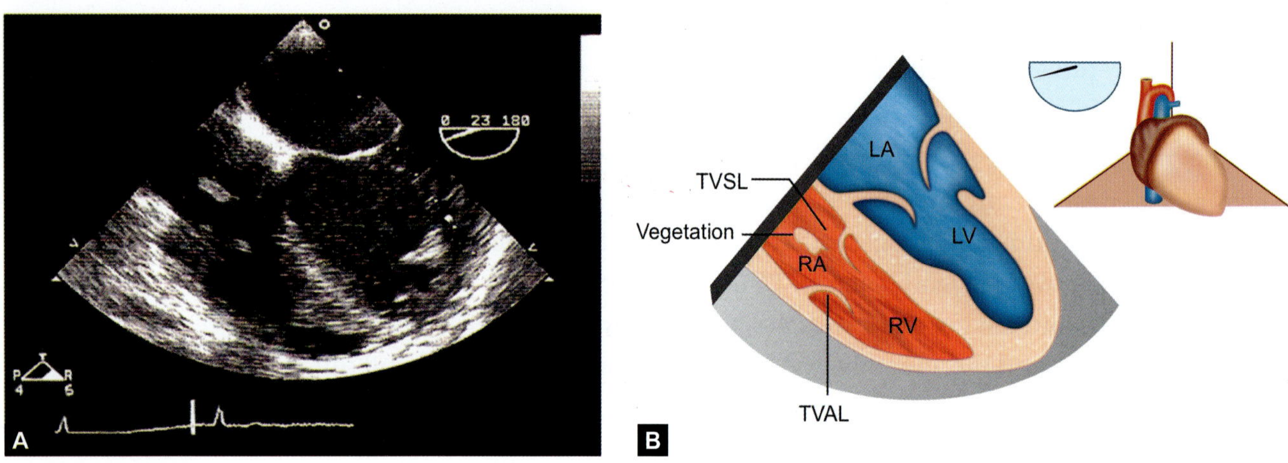

Figures 4A and B

In midesophageal, the four chamber view of a patient with endocarditis of the tricuspid valve. An echogenic mobile mass is seen between the tricuspid valve septal leaflet moving into the RA (TVSL). *Abbreviations:* LV, left ventricle; LA, left atrium; RA, right atrium; RV, right ventricle

chaotic ('oscillating') manner. It is common for a vegetation to prolapse through the valve as it opens.

Vegetations vary in size, often being just a few millimeter in diameter but sometimes reaching 2 to 3 cm. Vegetations resulting from fungal infections (e.g. *Candida, Aspergillus*) are usually much bigger than bacterial vegetations and can be so big that they are mistaken for a cardiac tumor. Fungal endocarditis is rare and is more likely to occur in patients who are immunosuppressed **(Table 2)**.

Thus tricuspid valve vegetations are typically found on the atrial aspect of the valve, while PV vegetations are seen on the ventricular aspect of the valve. Most investigators found that the sensitivity of TTE and TEE for right-sided endocarditis and TR were similar. Transesophageal echocardiography provides a superior characterization of vegetation size and extent as well as a greater specificity for endocarditis.[1,2]

If vegetations are present, describe their:

- Location [which valve(s) and which parts of the valve, are affected]
- Mobility (e.g. immobile, oscillating)
- Size.

The mechanisms of tricuspid regurgitation (TR) causing endocarditis include leaflet destruction or perforation, abnormal coaptation from chordal or papillary muscle rupture. A vegetation size >10 mm is associated with an increased likelihood of pulmonary emboli.[3]

Infection of indwelling central venous catheters and permanent pacemakers also occasionally leads to right-sided endocarditis, which occurs in the face

Table 2: Common causes of infective endocarditis	
Bacterial	*Staphylococcus aureus* *Streptococcus viridans* *Streptococcus intermedius* *Pseudomonas aeruginosa* HACEK organisms *Bartonella* *Coxiella burnetii*
Fungal	*Candida* *Aspergillus* *Histoplasma*

of valvular microtrauma caused by catheters, followed by bacteremia.[4] The identification of vegetation on foreign surface can be challenging with TTE, as catheters often produce reverberations.[5,6] Transesophageal echocardiography offers the advantage of a higher resolution to differentiate vegetation attachment to indwelling catheters or wires vs. attachment to valves.[5] Vegetations on pacemaker wires typically appear as sleeve like with satellite vegetations on the TV associated in more than 2/3 of cases of pacemaker wire infections **(Figs 5A to D)**.[5,7] Transesophageal echocardiography also offers the ability to visualize a greater catheter length including the superior vena cava using the sagittal 90° to 120° bicaval view. Importantly, the site of pacemaker or defibrillator infection may be in the pulse generator pocket, remote from the imaging capabilities of TEE and sometimes even missed by clinical examination.[8]

Thus, a negative TEE does not preclude the diagnosis of cardiac device infection. In case with a high level of suspicion, evaluation of the pacemaker generator pocket with a computed tomography (CT) scan can complement the TEE, especially in febrile patients soon after device implantation (< 12 weeks).[8] Almost all patients with proven or strongly suspected endocarditis on permanent pacemaker or defibrillator wires must have these surgically removed.[4,5,8] The imaging specialist in the operating room is in a privileged position to confirm the diagnosis and rule out the presence of TV and right heart injury following the pacemaker lead extraction.

ABSCESSES

An abscess is an encapsulated collection of necrotic and infected debris. The most common site of a cardiac abscess is the aortic root in association with an AoV infection.[9,10]

Left and especially right AV groove abscesses are uncommon, insidious and associated with fistulous tracts and false aneurysm. They are more common in drug addiction-related endocarditis.[10] A cardiac abscess appears typically as an oval

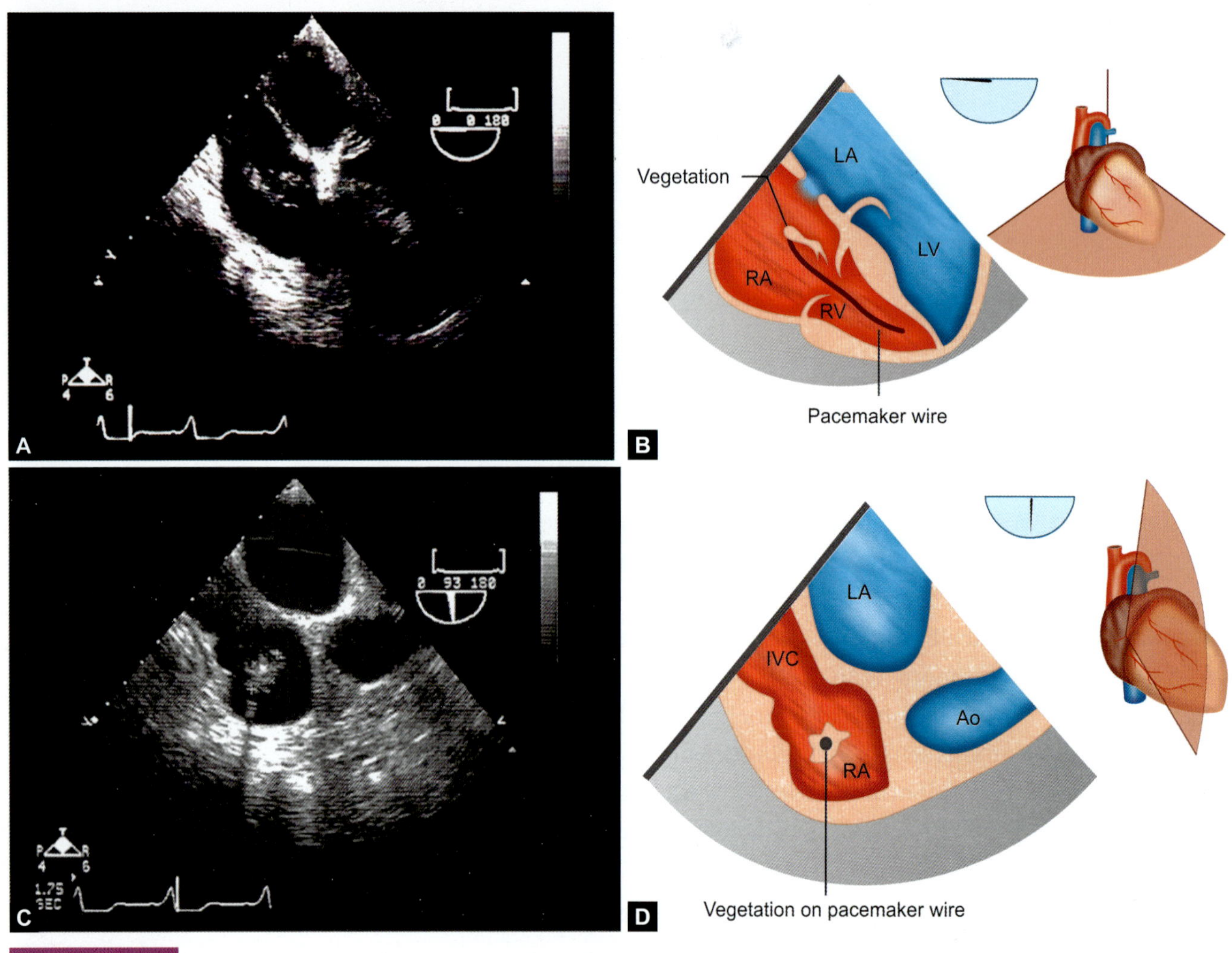

Figures 5A to D

Echogenic material attached to a pacemaker wire seen in a midesophageal four-chamber (A and B) and 90° view (C and D). *Abbreviations:* Ao, aorta; IVC, inferior vena cava; LA, left atrium; LV, left ventricle; RA, right atrium; RV, right ventricle

or circular lesion containing different echo densities, reflecting solid, liquid, and gaseous necrotic cintents. Transesophageal echocardiography has been shown to be superior to TTE in disclosing perivalvular abscess.[10] One should bear in mind that the right coronary artery is surrounded by adipose tissue in the right AV groove and may appears as a small echo free space. This should not be mistaken for an abscess or tumor. Adipose tissue appears more homogeneous, echo dence, and speckled, while a tricuspid abscess is usually associated with significant tricuspid leaflet infection, with a right-ventricular to right atrial flow seen within an annular perforation by color flow imaging. The presence of a pulmonary root abscess is usually associated with a prosthetic valve or conduit and is extremely rare. The diagnosis is generally difficult to establish by TEE because of the anterior location of the pulmonary trunk in the far field from the esophagus. Often, CT or magnetic resonance imaging (MRI) is required to confirm the diagnosis **(Fig. 6)**.

On echo, an abscess appears as an echolucent or echo dense area in the valve annulus or surroundings tissues. TOE has a much greater sensitivity for detecting perivalvular abscesses than TTE.

In abscess is present, describe its:

- Location (which valve is affected and where the abscess lies in relation to the valve)
- Size.

BIOPROSTHETIC VALVE ENDOCARDITIS

Tricuspid stenosis in prosthetic valve endocarditis has been reported in literature upon echocardiographic examination which revealed a large tricuspid valve vegetation and dilatation of the right ventricle and right atrium.[11] Unlike infective endocarditis involving native valves, prosthetic valve infections are not uncommonly associated with stenosis of the valve orifice and they may be recurrent requiring excision of the prosthetic valve as in the case described by Nunez et al.[12]

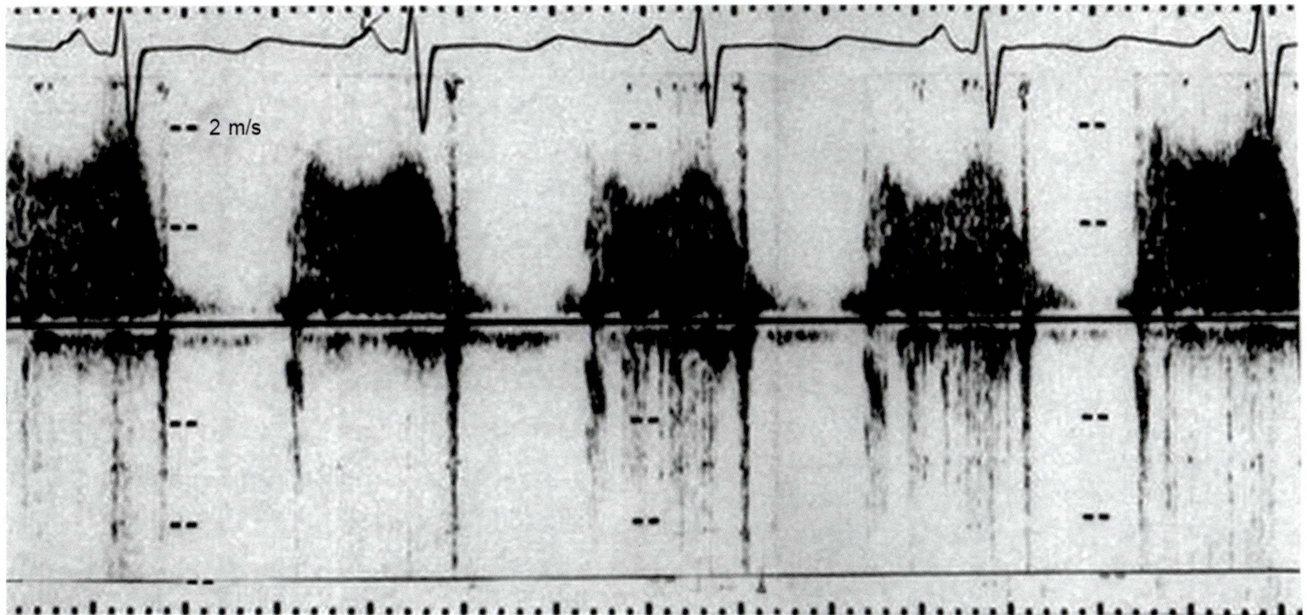

Figure 6

Continuous wave Doppler is tracing from the apex through tricuspid valve. There is marked increase in the velocity of inflow (m/s = meters per second) with distortion of the tricuspid inflow pattern. No tricuspid regurgitation is seen. The calculated mean gradient is 11 mm Hg

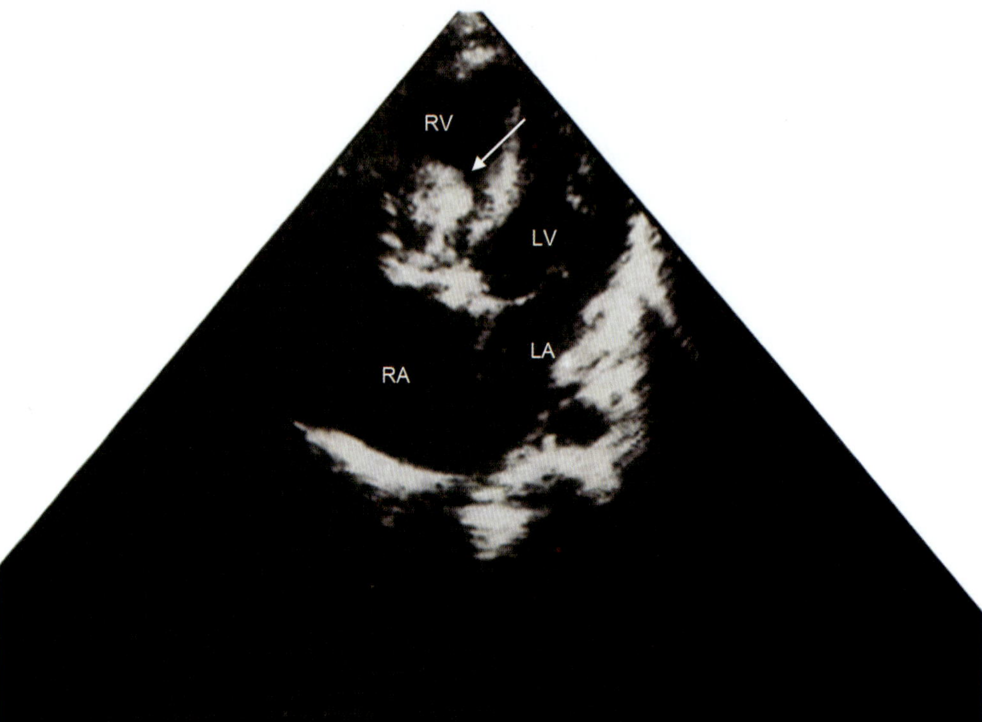

Figure 7

Apical four chamber on TEE view the tricuspid vegetation occupies much of the RV chamber (white arrow). *Abbreviations:* LA, left atrium; LV, left ventricle; RV, right ventricle

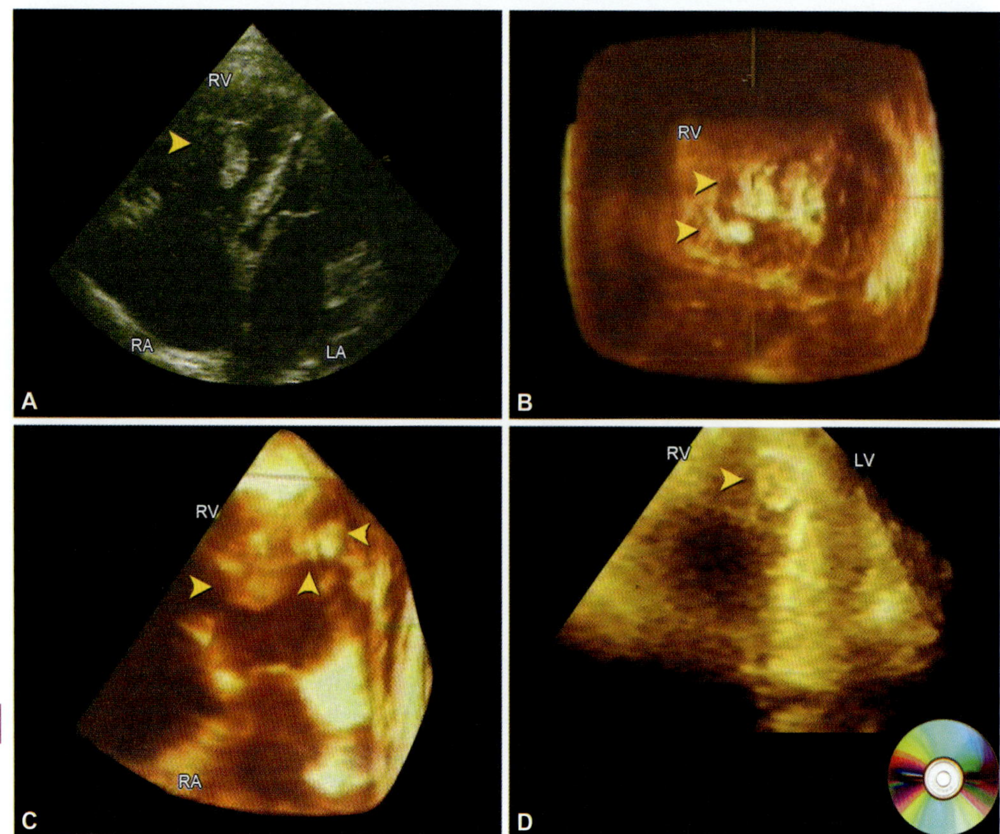

Figures 8A to D (VIDEO 1)

Real time 2D and 3D transthoracic echocardiography in right ventricular thrombus

In patients with prosthetic valve endocarditis, the presence of a murmur consistent with "increased flow velocity" across the involved valve and/or the finding by echocardiography of large vegetations should raise the suspicion of valvular obstruction **(Fig. 7)**. Doppler echocardiography can confirm the presence of obstruction and quantitate its severity. Although the need for operative intervention should still be guided by the clinical course, the experience by most patients suggest that medical therapy alone in these cases is likely to be unsuccessful and reoperations are essential for survival **(Figs 8A to D)**.

REFERENCES

1. San Roman JA, Vilacosta I, Zamorano JL, et al. Transesophageal echocardiography in right-sided endocarditis. J Am Coli Cardiol. 1993;21(5):1226-30.
2. Herrera CJ, Mehlman DJ, Hartz RS, et al. Comparison of transesophageal and transthoracic echocardiography for diagnosis of right-sided cardiac lesions. Am J Cardiol. 1992;70(9):964-6.
3. Robbins MJ, Frater RW, Soeiro R, et al. Influence of vegetation size on clinical outcome of right-sided infective endocarditis. Am J Med. 1986;80(2):165-71.
4. Rowley KM, Clubb KS, Smith GJ, et al. Right-sided infective endocarditis as a consequence of flow-directed pulmonary-artery catheterization. A clinicopathological study of 55 autopsied patients. N Engl J Med. 1984;311(18):1152-6.
5. Klug D, Lacroix D, Savoye C, Goullard L, Grandmougin D, Hennequin JL, et al. Systemic infection related to endocarditis on pacemaker leads: clinical presentation and management. Circulation. 1997;95(8):2098-107.
6. Vilacosta I, Sarria C, San Roman JA, Jimenez J, Castillo JA, Iturralde E, et al. Usefulness of transesophageal echocardiography for diagnosis of infected transvenous permanent pacemakers. Circulation. 1994;89(6):2684-7.
7. Tighe DA, Tejada LA, Kirchhoffer JB, Gilmette P, Rifkin RD, Estes NA. Pacemaker lead infection: detection by multi-plane transesophageal echocardiography. Am Heart J. 1996;131(3):616-8.
8. Victor F, De Place C, Camus C, Le Breton H, Leclercq C, Pavin D, et al. Pacemaker lead infection: echocardiographic features, management, and outcome. Heart. 1999; 81(1):82-7.
9. Arnett EN, Roberts WC. Valve ring abscess in active infective endocarditis. Frequency, location, and clues to clinical diagnosis from the study of 95 necropsy patients. Circulation. 1976;54(1):140-5.
10. Baumgartner FJ, Omari BO, Robertson JM, Nelson RJ, Pandya A, Pandya A, et al. Annular abscesses in surgical endocarditis: anatomic, clinical, and operative features. Ann Thorac Surg. 2000;70(2):442-7.
11. Arnett EN, Roberts WC. Prosthetic valve endocarditis. Clinicopathologic analysis of 22 necropsy patients with comparison of observations in 74 necropsy patients with 12 active infective endocarditis involving natural left-sided cardiac valves. Am J Cardiol. 1976; 38:281-92.
12. Nunez L, De Ia Llana R, Aguado MG, Iglesias A, Larrea JL, Celemin D. Bioprosthetic valve endocarditis. Indicators for surgical intervention. Ann Thorac Surg. 1983;35:262-70.

11 Miscellaneous Lesions Affecting Tricuspid and Pulmonary Valves

Poonam Malhotra Kapoor, Kalpana Irpachi

TRANSESOPHAGEAL ECHOCARDIOGRAPHY IN CARCINOID DISEASE AFFECTING THE HEART

The most common manifestation of carcinoid heart disease is valvular heart disease. It typically affects the right heart and generally occurs in patients with hepatic metastases where large amounts of serotonin and other vasoactive hormones can reach the heart directly before being inactivated by monoamine oxidases in the lungs.

Therefore, echocardiographic evaluation of a patient with carcinoid heart disease typically reveals involvement of the tricuspid and pulmonic valves with sparing of the mitral and aortic valves. Left-sided involvement can be seen in the setting of intracardiac shunts, extensive primary bronchial carcinoid or when high overall tumor secretions or poorly controlled disease overwhelm the metabolic capacity of the lungs. It is usually seen in conjunction with right-sided involvement **(Figs 1A and B)**.

Absence of the Tricuspid Valve Due to Severe Carcinoid Heart Disease

On intraoperative transesophageal echocardiography (TEE), 55-year-old man with carcinoid and dyspnea on exertion (DOE), he showed dilation of the right chambers and a severely affected tricuspid valve **(Fig. 2A)**. The tricuspid had a diseased appearance with marked echolucency, and thickening, retraction, and immobility

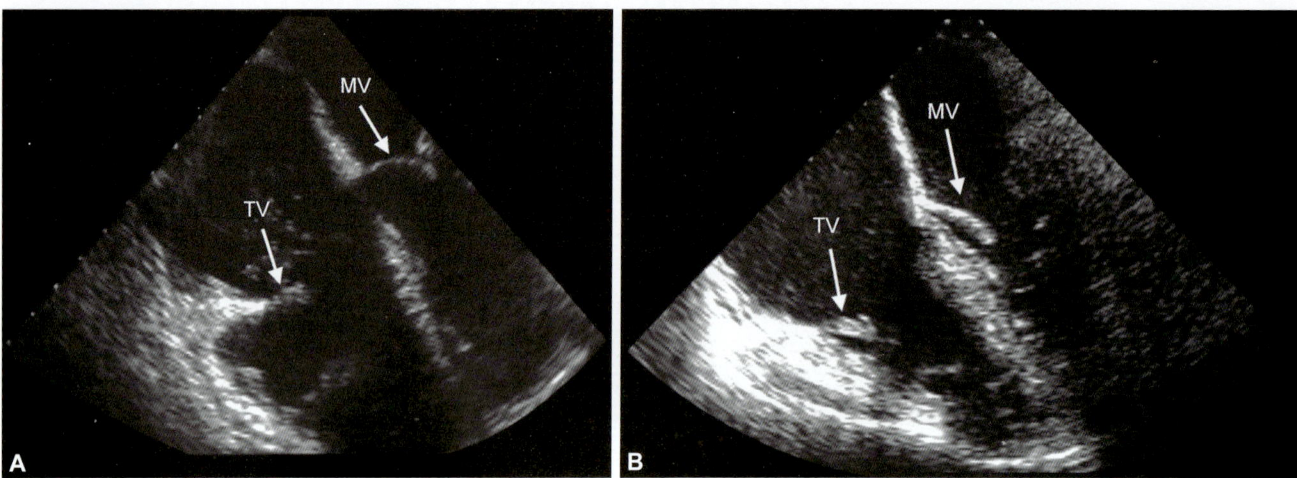

Figures 1A and B

Midesophageal transesophageal echocardiographic four-chamber view shows the tricuspid carcinoid valve. Figure A is the systolic frame and Figure B is the diastolic frame. Note the thickened, rigid carcinoid tricuspid valve leaflets that appear to be in a semi-open, "funnel-shaped" position. A comparison between the systolic and diastolic frames emphasizes the immobility of the leaflets: they appear to be the same in systolic and diastolic frames

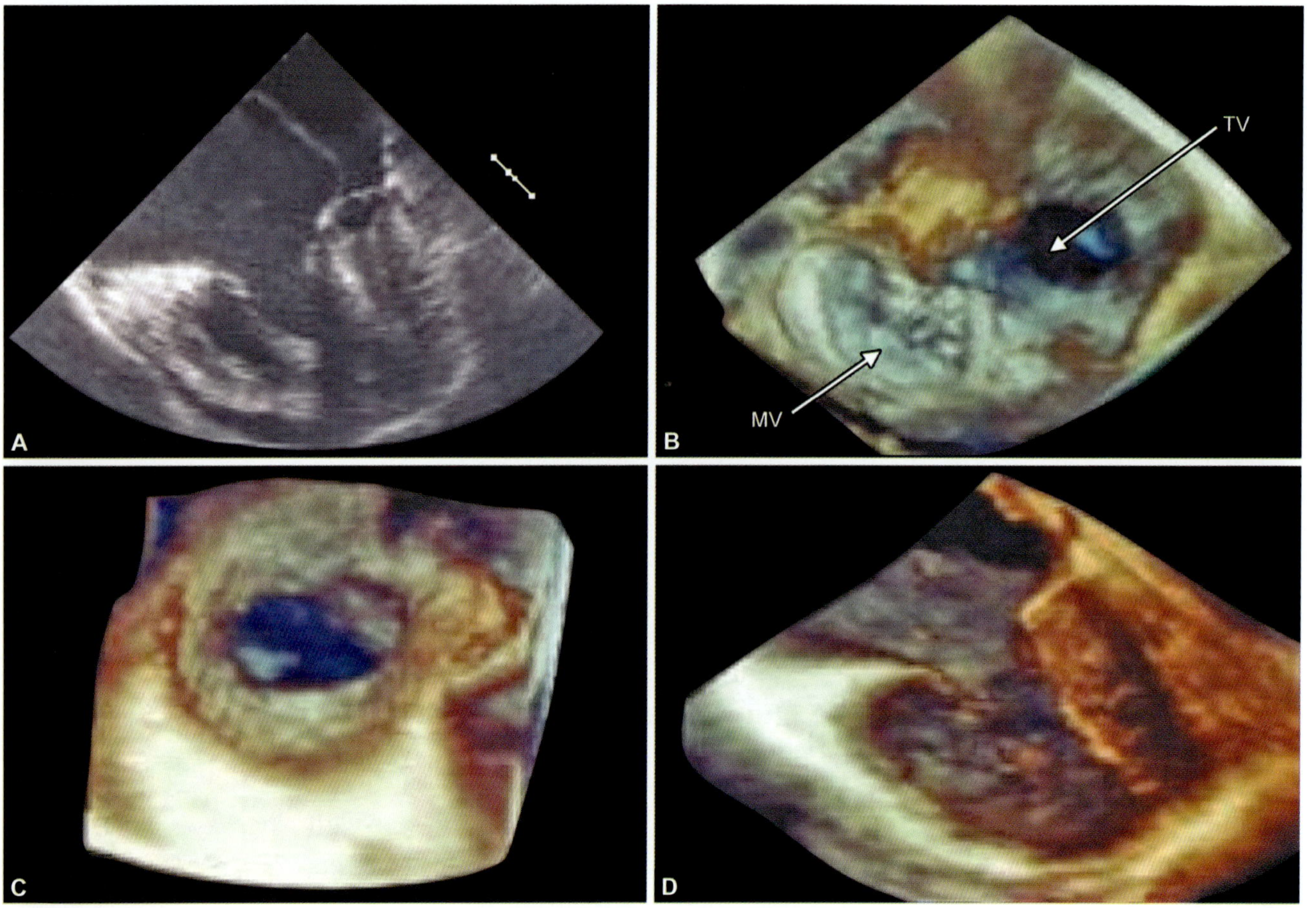

Figures 2A to D

3D TEE of carcinoid disease of tricuspid valve

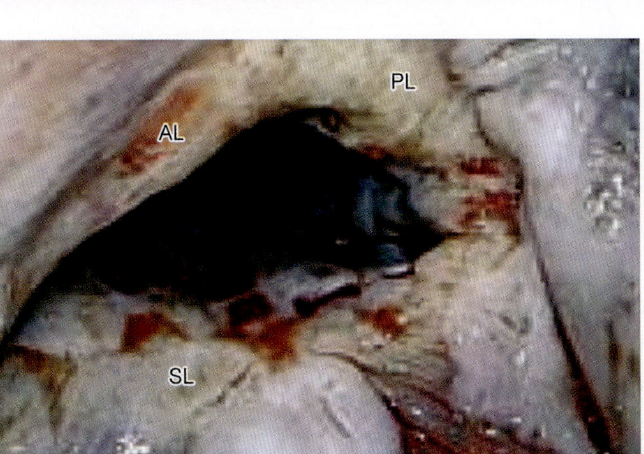

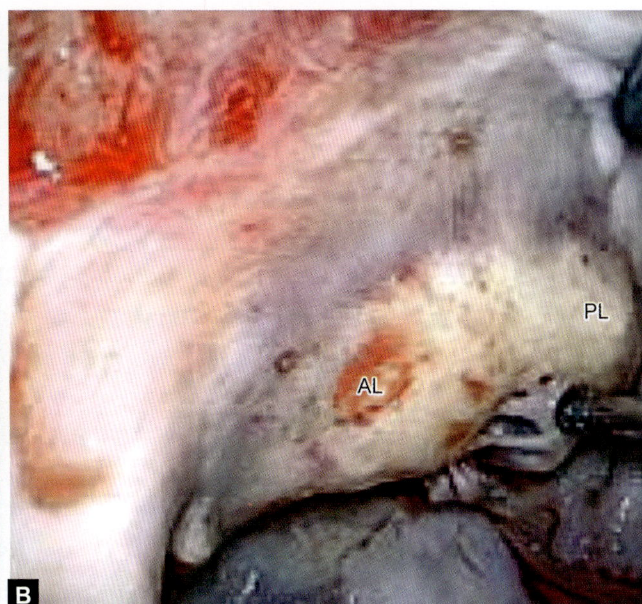

Figures 3A and B

Characteristic of carcinoid heart disease with anterior, posterior and septal leaflet (SL)

of the leaflets, which were fixed in the diastolic position, resulting in a complete "absence" of the valve structure. Real-time 3-dimensional TEE (3D TEE) confirmed the "absence" of tricuspid leaflets due to fibrosis and fusion with the ventricular tissue.

Evaluation from the right atrium **(Fig. 2B)** mitral valve (MV); tricuspid valve (TV), from the right ventricle **(Fig. 2C)** and lastly, a lateral view after off-line subtraction of the anterolateral wall of the right ventricle **(Fig. 2D)**. The surgical analysis confirmed the 3D echocardiographic findings and additionally disclosed severe involvement of the subvalvular apparatus and endocardial deposit of pearly fibrous plaques, a characteristic of carcinoid heart disease (**Figs 3A and B**) anterior leaflet (AL); posterior leaflet (PL); septal leaflet (SL). The patient underwent multivalvular surgery, with mitral repair, tricuspid valve and pulmonary valve replacement, and reconstruction of the right ventricular outflow tract.[1]

Tricuspid Valve in Carcinoid Disease

In the carcinoid tricuspid valve, regurgitation is more prominent than stenosis and septal and anterior leaflets are predominantly affected severity of tricuspid regurgitation can be assessed by evaluating color flow Doppler jet area, vena contracta width, proximal isovelocity surface area, and hepatic venous flow reversal with pulse wave Doppler. Continuous-wave Doppler spectral profile of severe tricuspid regurgitation typically appears dagger-shaped, with an early peak velocity and steep decline, indicating rapid equalization of right atrial and ventricular pressures, as opposed to a rounded envelope seen in patients with mild-to-moderate tricuspid regurgitation. Because the valve leaflets are rigid and fixed in the semi-open "funnel-shaped" position, some degree of tricuspid stenosis is commonly present in conjunction with tricuspid regurgitation. Severity of stenosis can be evaluated by two-dimensional imaging and quantified by calculating the mean pressure gradient across the valve.

OTHER INFLAMMATORY VALVULOPATHIES

Another form of characteristically right-sided inflammatory valve disease is carcinoid heart disease. Carcinoid valvulitis is more commonly seen with small bowel carcinoid complicated by liver metastases, which produce high levels of circulating serotonin and systemic symptoms (e.g. flushing, bronchospasm and diarrhea). Serotonin stimulates plaque development on the TV and PV, leading to leaflet thickening and rigidity. Tricuspid regurgitation occurs in >90 percent of cases. Less commonly, ~20 to 30 percent of carcinoid heart disease cases are associated to TS, PV regurgitation, and stenosis. Unless an intracardiac right-to-left shunt is present, it is unusual for the left heart to be involved in carcinoid disease as serotonin and its metabolites are inactivated in the lung. The short-term prognosis of this disease was formally quite grim but as a result of disease control by chemotherapy and with medium—term survival increasingly achieved, patients with significant right heart failure symptoms are occasionally referred for valve surgery.

Connolly et al.[2] reported a nonrandomized series of 26 patients operated on for carcinoid valve disease. All had severe TR and significant mixed PV disease with: (1) severe right heart failure symptoms; (2) controlled systemic disease; and (3) no current severe medical problems. All patients underwent TV replacement, most had pulmonic valvectomy and in five, removal of endomyocardial metastases was carried out. The perioperative mortality was 35 percent, with a substantial number of deaths occurring as a result of right heart failure or uncontrolled patients was 40 percent at two years compared with 8 percent for medically treated patients. Furthermore, when PV disease was present, data from the same institution supports the use of PV replacement over simple valvectomy in reducing right ventricular dilatation.[3] However, it is possible that carcinoid disease may accelerate bioprosthetic tissue valve degeneration in the tricuspid and pulmonary positions.[3]

Myxoid Degeneration

Degenerative myxoid or myxomatous valvular disease typically affects the mitral valve and tricuspid involvement most often consists of functional TR secondary to pulmonary hypertension. However, myxomatous tricuspid degeneration is rarely seen and is usually encountered in the setting of concomitant mitral valve disease. Inheritable disorders of connective tissue such as Marfan's as disease may be a common link. Less is known about the three-dimensional geometry of the TV than that of the saddle-shaped mitral valve. The typical appearance of tricuspid leaflet prolapsed is midsystolic coaptation. Chordal rupture is usually easily identified and causes significant leaflet malcoaptation with the leaflet up typically pointing towards the RA, in association with severe eccentric TR directed opposite the diseased leaflet.

Pulmonic Valve Disease

Pulmonic valve assessment remains challenged by TEE, because of its anterior location relative to the esophagus in the far field **(Figs 4 and 5)**. In most cases

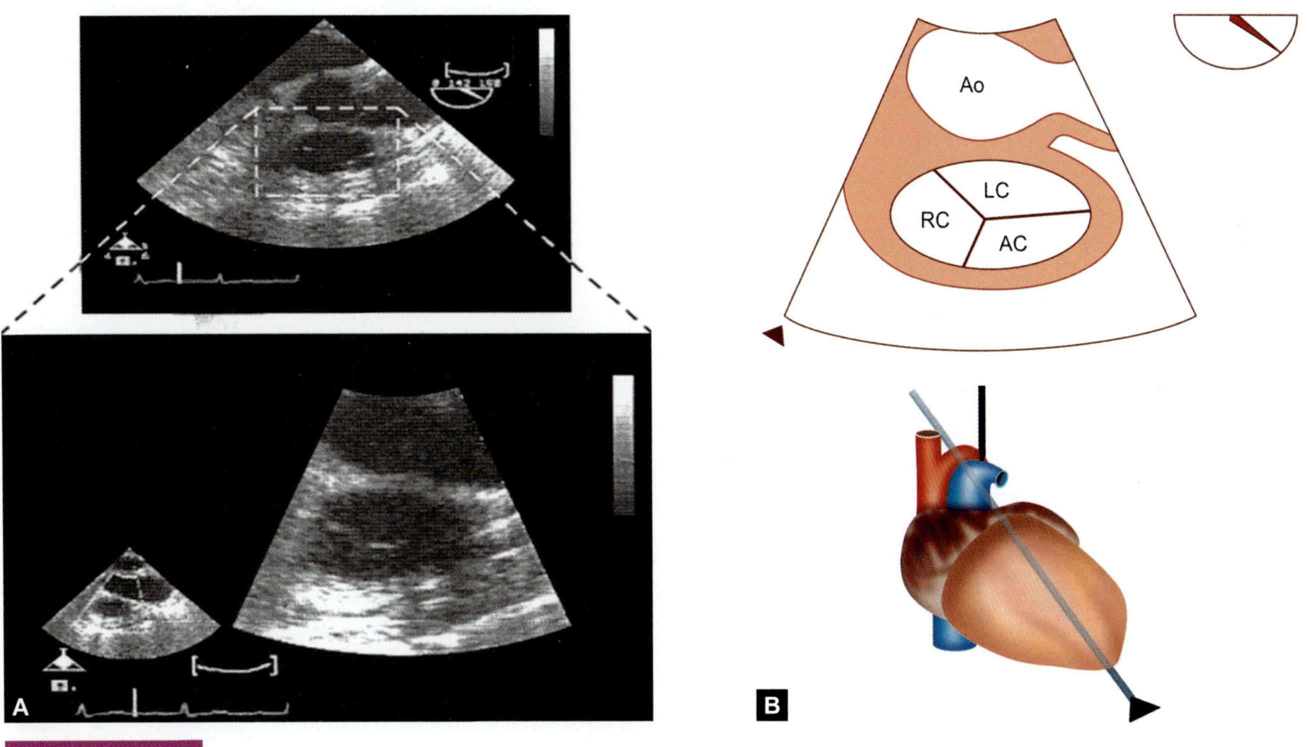

Figures 4A and B

Midesophageal long axis view at 142° showing a transverse view of a normal pulmonic valve. *Abbreviations:* AC, anterior cusp; Ao, aorta; LC, left cusp; RC, right cusp

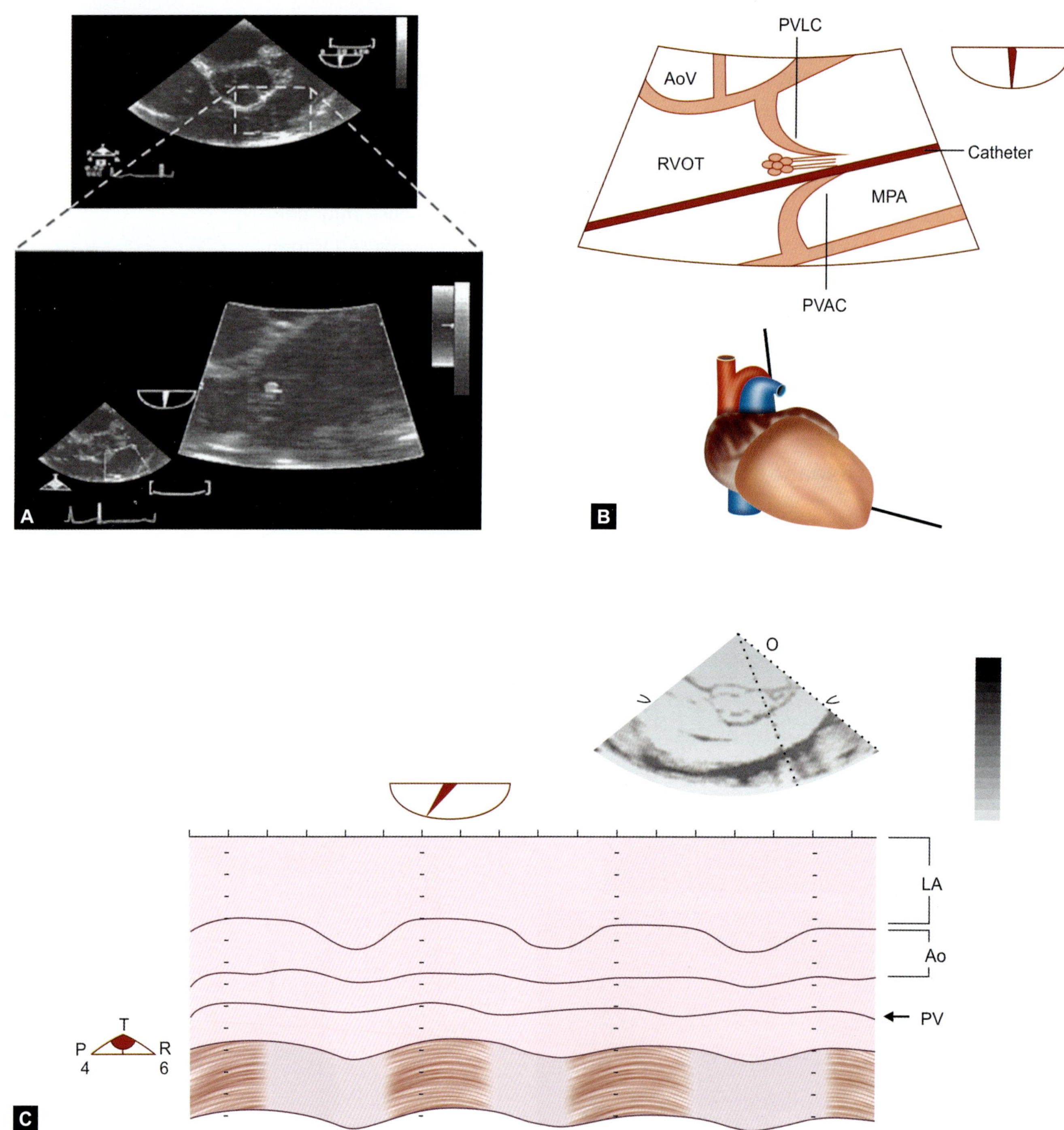

Figures 5A to C

Normal pulmonic valve (PV) in a 23-year-old man undergoing mitral valve replacement (A to C) midesophageal 85° view. A small jet of PV regurgitation was present around the pulmonary artery catheter. (C) m-mode of a normal PV. *Abbreviations:* Ao, aorta; AoV, aortic valve; LA, left atrium; MPA, main pulmonary artery; PVAC, pulmonic valve anterior cusp; PVLC, pulmonic valve left cusp; RVOT, right ventricular outflow tract

other than endocarditis or inflammatory disease, PV disease is congenital in origin. Dome-shaped or bicuspid PV stenosis is a common entity with good survival.[3] Most individuals with severe PV stenosis are treated in childhood by either percutaneous valvuloplasty or surgical valvotomy. Variable degrees of residual regurgitation may ensue, producing right ventricular dilatation when moderate or severe. The natural history of mild-to-moderate PV stenosis is benign and intervention is seldom required.[4]

Pulmonic valve regurgitation can occur as a result of valvular abnormalities or annular dilation, the latter being either due to increased flow through the valve (e.g. by an intracardiac systemic—to pulmonary hypertension. The use of short axis and sagittal views is helpful to visualize native or prosthetic PVs. Demonstration of PV stenosis and regurgitation by Doppler and color flow is more easily done in the sagittal view at 90 to 100° where pulmonary flow is nearly parallel to the ultrasound beam. Pulmonary regurgitation appears as a blue, anteriorly directed color jet from the posteriorly situated pulmonary artery to the RV. Most jets are monochromic unless pulmonary hypertension is present. Severe PV regurgitant leads to right ventricular volume overload with dilatation and paradoxical septal motion and may ultimately cause right ventricular systolic dysfunction. This may, in turn, lead to symptoms like dyspnea and atrial or ventricular arrhythmias.[5] The ASE published guidelines on the evaluation of PV regurgitation.[6] They are summarized in **Tables 1 and 2**.

Table 1: Echocardiographic and Doppler parameters used in the evaluation of pulmonary regurgitation severity: Utility, advantages, and limitations

Parameter	*Utility/advantages*	*Disadvantages*
RV size	RV enlargement sensitive for chromic significant PR Normal size virtually excludes significant PR	Enlargement seen in other condition
Paradoxical septal motion (volume overload pattern)	Simple sign of severe PR	Not specific for PR
Jet length-color flow	Simple	Poor correlation with severity or PR
Vena contracta width	Simple quantitative method that works well for other valves	More difficult to perform; requires good images of pulmonary valve; lacks published validation
Jet declaration rate-CWD	Simple	Steep deceleration not specific for severe PR
Flow quantitation-PWD	Quantitates regurgitant flow and fraction	Subject to significant errors due to difficulties of measurement of pulmonic annulus and a dynamic RVOT; not well validated

Abbreviations: CWD, continuous wave Doppler; PWD, pulsed wave Doppler; RV, right ventricle; PR, pulmonary regurgitation; RVOT, right ventricular outflow tract. With permission of Zoghbi WA

Table 2: Echocardiographic and Doppler parameters used in grading pulmonary regurgitation severity			
Parameters	*Mild*	*Moderate*	*Severe*
Pulmonic valve	Normal	Normal or abnormal	Abnormal
RV size	Normal[a]	Normal or dilated	Dilated[b]
Jet size by color Doppler[c]	Thin (usually <10 mm in length) with a narrow origin	Intermediate	Usually large, with a wide origin; may be brief in duration
Jet density and deceleration rate CWD[d]	Soft; slow deceleration	Dense; variable deceleration	Dense; steep deceleration early termination of diastolic flow
Pulmonary systolic flow compared to systemic flow-PWD[e]	Slightly increased	Intermediate	Greatly increased

[a]Unless there are other reasons for RV enlargement. Normal 2D measurements from the apical four chamber view; RV mediolateral end-diastolic dimention <4.3 cm, RV end-diastolic area <35.5 cm^2
[b]Exception: acute PR
[c]At a Nyquist limit of 50-60 cm/second
[d]Steep deceleration is not specific for severe PR.
[e]Cut-off values for regurgitant volume and fraction are not well validated.
Abbreviations: CWD, continuous wave Doppler; PR, pulmonary regurgitation; PWD, pulsed wave Doppler; RA, right atrium; RF, regurgitant fraction; RV, right ventricle. With permission of Zoghbi WA

Valve Repair, Tricuspid Indications and Methods of Repair

The principal indication for TV repair is isolated moderate to severe TR, generally in the face of left sided heart disease.[7] For pure TV disease, surgery is generally performed for significant TR associated with right-sided heart failure. Tricuspid valve surgical repair, using an annuloplasty ring or a suture annuloplasty (by the technique of De Vega), is the technique of choice as it retains the valve leaflets and provides adequate coaptation by reducing the diameter of the TV annulus.[8] Tricuspid valve replacement is the alternative and is performed when severe valve destruction has occurred or when previous TV repair has failed to relieve significant TR. Residual TR of moderated to severe magnitude on the postoperative TEE should probably be addressed by replacement of the valve or re-repair, if the patient is stable enough.

Predictors of adverse survival following TV surgery include: severe TR as assessed echocardiographically, high preoperative New York Heart Association (NYHA) functional class, left ventricular systolic dysfunction, need for coronary revascularization and need for TV replacement. Transesophageal echocardiography plays an important role in evaluating the success of surgical repair and was found to influence the surgical plan in 10 percent of cases in a large single-center study of 401 patients. The presence of residual TR (10-15%) disclosed by intraoperative TEE has a controversial ability in predicting long-term mortality following valve surgery but predicts at least a reduced event—free survival.

Suture Annuloplasty, Complications, Failed Repair

The TV suture annuloplasty by the technique of De Vega is done with a 2.0 propylene suture button stressed with Teflon. A first suture line is started at the anteroseptal commissure and proceeds clockwise to a point just beyond the posteroseptal commissure (**Fig. 6**).[9] A second suture line is similarly run 2 to 3 mm above the first one. The suture are then tied with Teflon over a 27 valve size in the annulus to prevent valvular stenosis.[10]

Significant residual TR following repair usually becomes clinically evident with symptoms of fatigue and signs of right-sided heart failure on long-term follows-up. Perioperative TEE may be useful in detecting residual problems following cardiac surgery. Indeed, right ventricular dimensions and systolic function remain important predictors of long-term success as the annuloplasty rapair alone may not correct incomplete tricuspid leaflet closure in the setting of choronic right ventricular remodeling. Dehiscence of a De Vega suture annuloplasty may appear on TEE as a horizontal linear echo-density running across the TV plane.

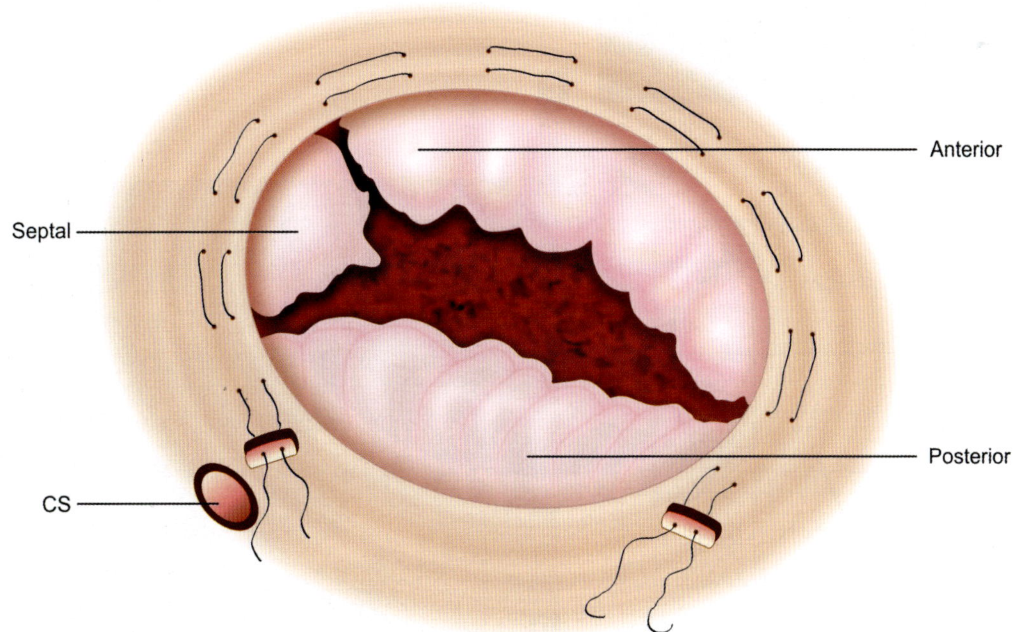

Figure 6

Double purse string suture technique in De Vega's annuloplasty of the tricuspid valve. *Abbreviations:* CS, coronary sinus, with permission of Rabago et al.

Annuloplasty Rings

Tricuspid annuloplasty rings appear in tomographic echo planes as two echodense annular structures located at the base of opposite leaflets in the atrial side of the valve, with variable acoustic shadowing **(Figs 7A to D).**

Tricuspid leaflet mobility is expected to be somewhat reduced but stenosis is rare as the annular dimensions remain large. Tricuspid regurgitation or vegetation are usually easily demonstrated at 30 to 90° **(Figs 8A to D)**, in the midesophageal, the transitional gastroesophageal, and the sagittal transgastric views.

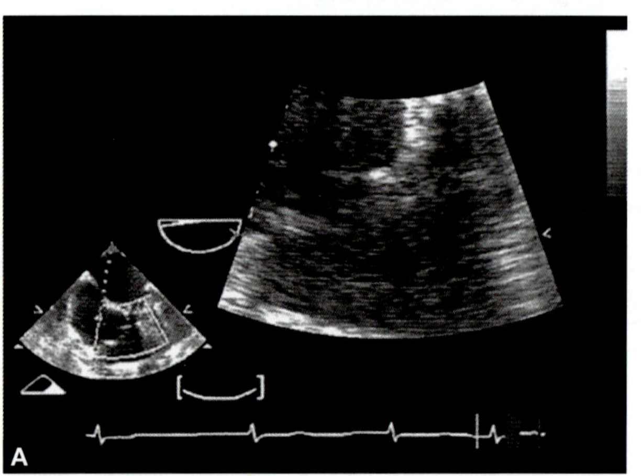

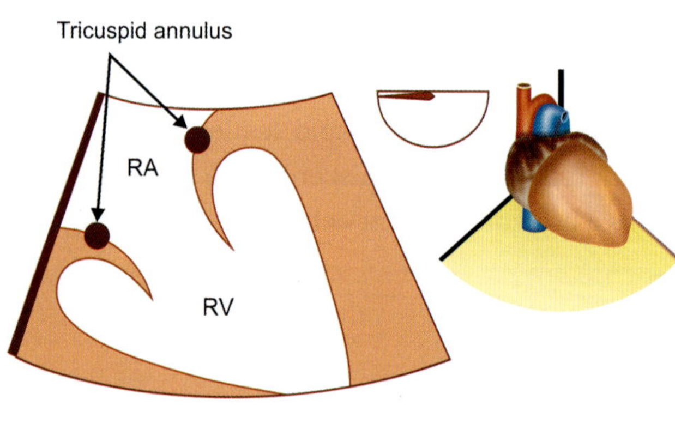

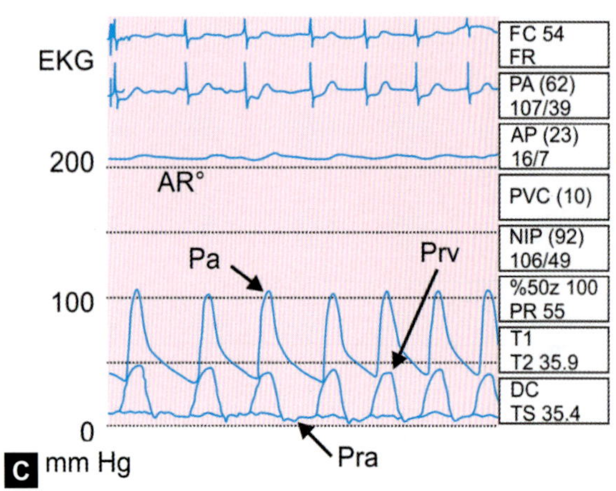

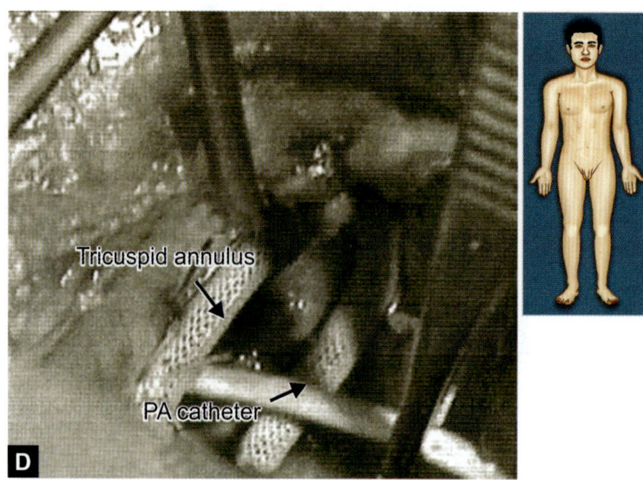

Figures 7A to D

(A and B) Echocardiographic appearance of a tricuspid valve prosthetic annulus; (C) After the procedure no significant stenosis is present as demonstrated by the absence of a diastolic gradient across the tricuspid valve is confirmed on the simultaneous right atrial pressure (Pra) and right ventricular pressure (Prv) tracings obtained through the paceport of the pulmonary artery catheter; (D) intraoperative findings. *Abbreviations:* ECG, electrocardiogram; Pa, atrial pressure; RA, right atrium (*Source:* Dr Denis Boachard)

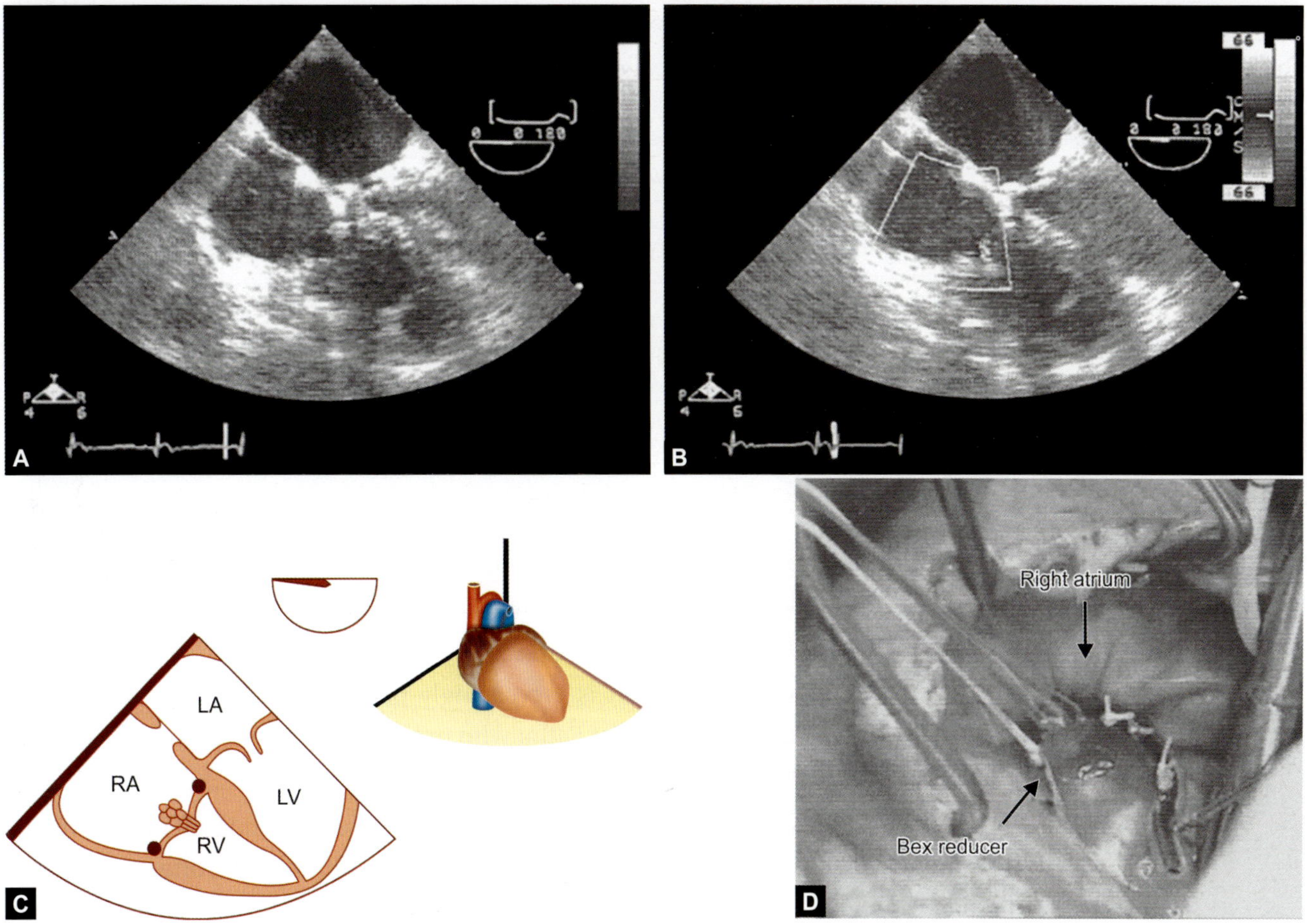

Figures 8A to D

Tricuspid annuloplasty in a 56-year-old woman (A to C) midesophageal four-chamber view at 0° demonstraining the normal appearance of the prosthetic annulus. Midresidual tricuspid regurgitation was present postoperatively; (D) Intraoperative view of the Bex reducer on the anterior and septal leaflets

TRICUSPID VALVE REPLACEMENT

The American College of Cardiology and the American Heart Association established in 1998 guidelines for the management of patients with valvular heart disease.[11] The recommendations for tricuspid surgery are summarized in **Table 3**.

The surgical decision to replace the TV is usually made preoperatively on the basis of extensive leaflet disease. Such is the case in Ebstein's anomaly, mixed or predominantly stenotic degenerated calcified leaflets, or extensive destruction by endocarditis. However, TV replacement does carry a higher operative mortality compared with repair, partly because it is often performed in light of previous cardiac surgery. In a series from our center spanning 20 years, mortality approached

Table 3: Recommendations for surgery for tricuspid regurgitation		
S. No.	*Indication*	*Class*
1.	Annuloplasty for severe TR and pulmonary hypertension in patients with mitral valve	I
2.	Valve replacement for severe TR secondary to diseased/abnormal tricuspid valve leaflet	IIa
3.	Valve replacement or annuloplasty for severe TR with mean pulmonary artery pressure <60 mm Hg when symptomatic	IIa
4.	Annuloplasty for mild TR in patients with pulmonary hypertension secondary to mitral valve disease requiring mitral valve surgery	IIb
5.	Valve replacement or annuloplasty for TR with pulmonary artery systolic pressure <60 mm Hg in the presence of a normal mitral valve, in asymptomatic patients, or in symptomatic patients who have not received a trial of diuretic therapy	III

Source: Benow et al.
Abbreviation: TR, tricuspid regurgitation.

22 percent with about the same percentage of patients also requiring permanent pacing. This underscores the close relationship of the tricuspid annulus to the conduction system.[12]

Pulmonic valve replacement is increasingly performed especially in patients with previous repair of tetralogy of Fallot who present with right ventricular volume overload from severe PV regurgitation.

It is also done with implantation of a heterologous aortic homograft in pulmonary position of as a part of the Ross procedure, a treatment for congenital aortic stenosis (AS) in childhood and adolescence. In this procedure, AoV replacement is done by transplanting the normal PV and root to the aortic position, thus avoiding the need for long-term anticoagulation while allowing stenosis of the prosthetic heterologous aortic homograft in pulmonary position is a late complication **(Figs 9A to F)**, sometimes difficult to diagnose by TTE alone.

Tricuspid Valvectomy

In the setting of significant echocarditis, total valvectomy is sometimes necessary and is surprisingly hemodynamically well tolerated initially. Once the infection is brought under control, a second stage procedure with tricuspid prosthetic valve implantation is performed to prevent wide-open TR progression to severe right heart failure. This technique has a define place in the treatment of Abcede tricuspid or PV endocarditis in intravenous drug abusers.[13]

Types of Valve Prosthesis

Bioprosthesis have been the most commonly implanted valves in the tricuspid and pulmonic position, usually in the setting of refractory right-sided endocarditis.

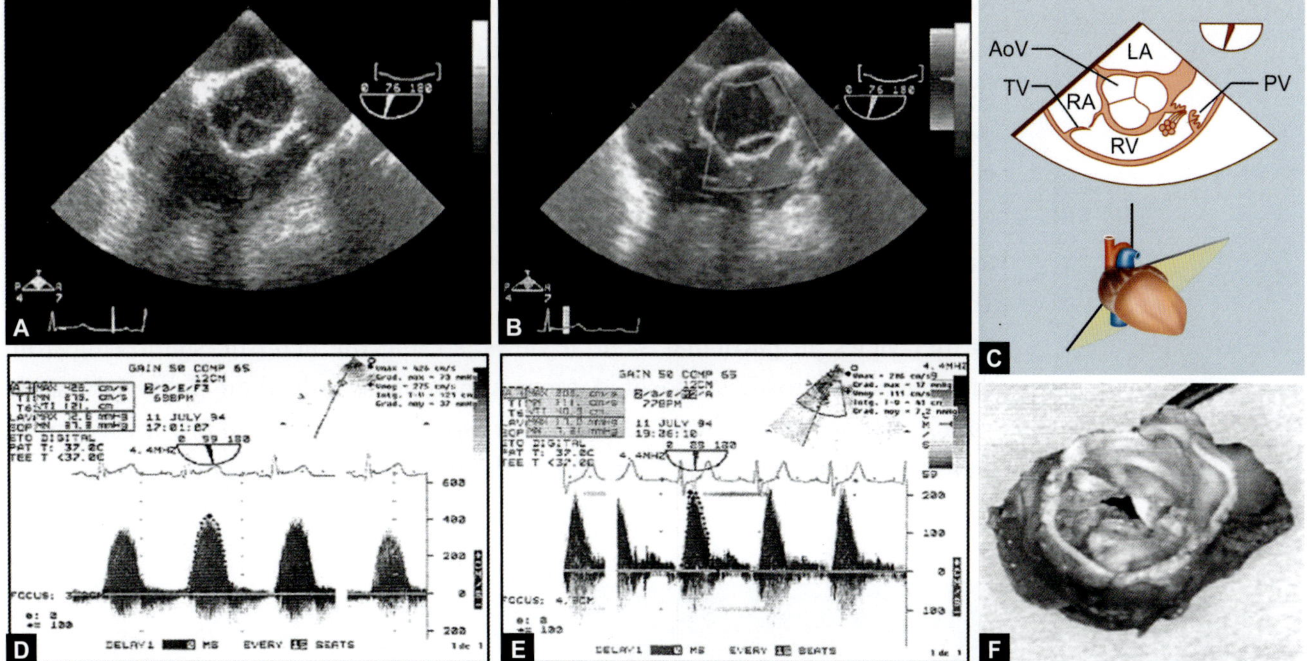

Figures 9A to F

Reoperation for stenotic pulmonary homograft (from a Ross procedure initially for congenital aortic stenosis). (A to C) Mid-esophageal right ventricular inflow-outflow view of the thickened pulmonic valve (PV) (D and E) The pressure gradient (PG) across the PV decreased from 37.3 to 7.2 mm Hg after the procedure; and (F) Intraoperative findings showing the excised stenotic pulmonary homograft

The need for chronic anticoagulation is avoided in subjects at high-risk of bleeding or deemed unreliable to benefit overall from such therapy. Unfortunately, bioprosthetic valve failure occurs in 50 percent of patients at 10 years postoperatively and may require reoperation.[14]

Mechanical valve replacement offers greater durability but requires chronic anticoagulation.[15] This may not be any more a significant issue in patients with rheumatic or degenerative disease where mitral valve involvement and atrial fibrillation are commonly associated with TV pathology and warrant anticoagulation by themselves. However, mechanical prosthesis in tricuspid position prevents the implantation of endoventricular pacemaker leads in this group of patients in which atrioventricular block is common.

In view of the specific RV geometry, it was believed that the lower profile and the lesser procoagulant tendency of bioprosthesis in the setting of a low-pressure system would reduce thrombotic complications compared with mechanical values. The poor performance of tilting-disk valves in 1980s appeared to support this point but more recent data on the good long-term performance of the low-profile bileaflet mechanical valves may outweigh the risk of long-term tissue valve failure in patients likely to be reliable in taking anticoagulation therapy.[16] A new approach has been the implantation of a mitral homograft in tricuspid position with adjustment of papillary muscle tension obtained by two ventriculotomy apertures through which each papillary muscle is inserted.[17]

Transesophageal echocardiography assessment of TV prosthesis begins as for native valves in the mid-esophageal four-chamber view **(Figs 10A to D)**. The presence of coexisting mitral and aortic prostheses requires the use of further views, in particular sagittal views, so that the acoustic shadowing from the left-sided prosthesis located more superoposteriorly than their right-sided counterparts are circumvented. The atrial aspect of the tricuspid prosthesis can be shown with relative ease at 30 to 120° in the midesophageal and in the transitional

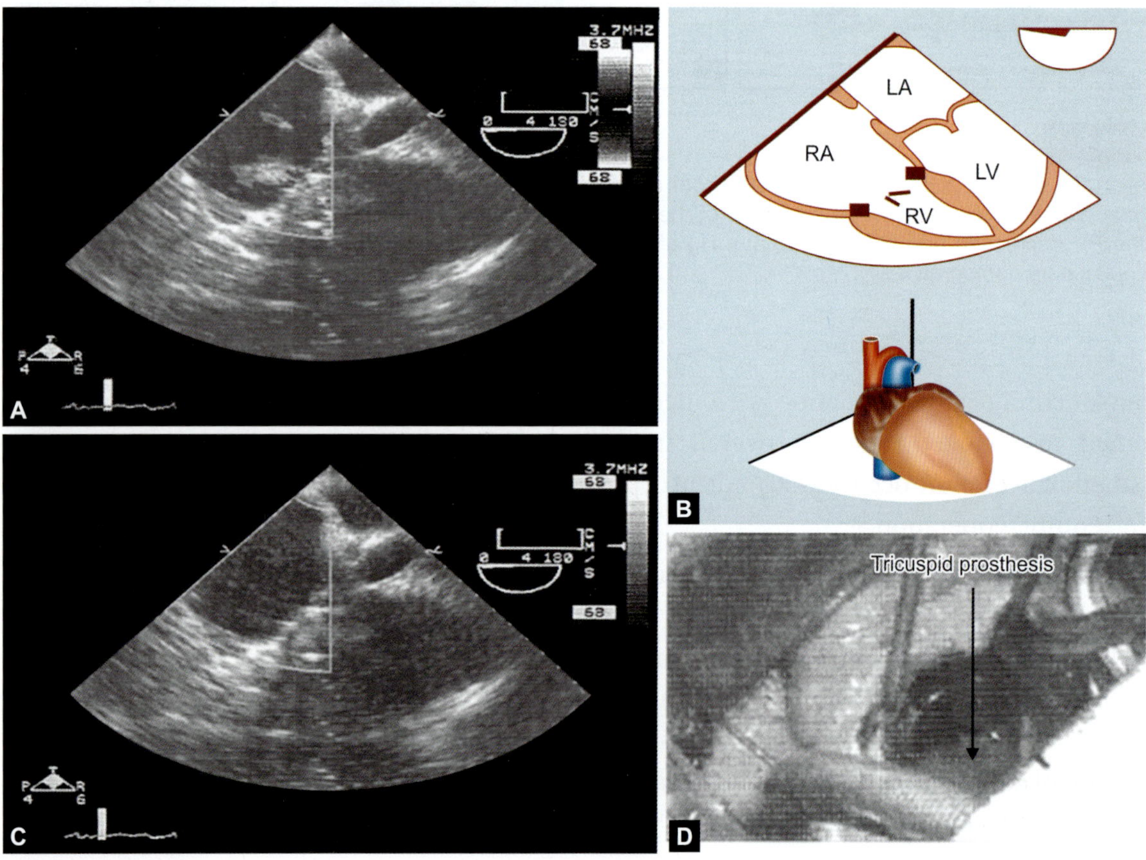

Figures 10A to D

A 41-year-old man operated on for tricuspid bileaflet prosthetic valve dysfunction. Midesophageal four-chamber view showing dilated right atrium (RA) and right ventricle (RV). Mid-tricuspid regurgitation is present. The lateral wall of the open position

gastroesophageal view. The transgastric views at 60 to 120° can also be used to inspect the diaphragmatic aspect of the TV. The normal tricuspid bioprosthesis has thin leaflets (2–4 mm) attached to three struts which protrude into the RV. Their appearance and movement resemble those of native leaflets. Mechanical bileaflet valve hemidisks have more linear aspects and produce characteristics linear acoustic reverberations pivoting within the annulus. In the open position, the two hemidisks appear as two parallel lines, while in the closed position; they assume a wide-open V-shape against the prosthetic annulus.

Mechanical TV thrombosis should be ruled out when full range excursion of both hemidisks cannot be demonstrated.[18] Even by TEE, thrombus within the prosthesis associated with decreased morbidity of the occlude is sometimes difficult to establish. A search for perivalvular regurgitation should be done by color flow imaging in multiple imaging planes to describe the sector, site and width of the leak.

As for its native counterpart, the assessment of the pulmonary valve prosthesis suffers from the distance between the TEE in the esophagus and the anterior position of the pulmonary valve. In the absence of shadowing from the aortic valve, the pulmonary valve can be seen in the midesophageal short axis view at 30 to 80° and sometimes in the sagittal transgastric view.

In conclusion, TEE is a useful modality in the evaluation and quantification of the tricuspid and pulmonic valves, and prosthetic dysfunction. Its intraoperative use compliments hemodynamic data from the pulmonary artery catheter and is likely to become an essential part of the postoperative evaluation of tricuspid and PV surgery.

Tricuspid Involvement in Other Etiologies

Fenfluramine-phentermine valvulopathy: It is also associated with elevated serotonin levels, so the echo findings resemble those in carcinoid syndrome.[19] The leaflets thicken, shorten, and fail to coapt. The septal leaflet may be fixed to the septum. Unlike carcinoid, however, Fen-Phen valvulopathy affects the left and right-sided valves.

Blunt chest trauma: It can lead to papillary muscle disruption and leaflet flail due to an acute increase in RV pressure.[20] Total papillary muscle disruption will affect two leaflets; partial rupture can lead to single leaflet flail. Patients typically present with severe TR, but may not present until weeks after the trauma. TV injury and subsequent TR can also occur during ICD lead or pacemaker lead extraction.[21]

EBSTEIN'S ANOMALY AND THE RIGHT HEART

Ebstein's anomaly and the right heart is characterized by apical displacement of all or part of the TV into the RV. It is diagnosed when the distance from the level of the mitral annulus to the septal leaflet exceeds 11 mm. The RA therefore appears larger and the RV, smaller. TR is the predominant clinical manifestation. *AV canal defects* may be associated with TR since the septal leaflet and the anterior mitral leaflet both are derived from the endocardial cushions.

Percutaneous Tricuspid Valve

To date, there have been few reports describing percutaneous approaches to tricuspid valve disease. In 2005, Boudjemline et al.[22] described a novel percutaneous tricuspid valve consisting of a bovine jugular venous valve mounted to a self-expanding nitinol frame consisting of 2 disks. The device was deployed through an 18F sheath in the right internal jugular vein, with right ventricular and right atrial disks deployed sequentially to sandwich the native tricuspid valve **(Figs 11A to C)**.

The device was successfully implanted in seven normal sheep, but no further work has been done with this device. As percutaneous approaches to valvular heart disease emerge, lessons gained from prior surgical experiences are relevant. Concomitant surgical repair of TR at the time of mitral valve surgery should be

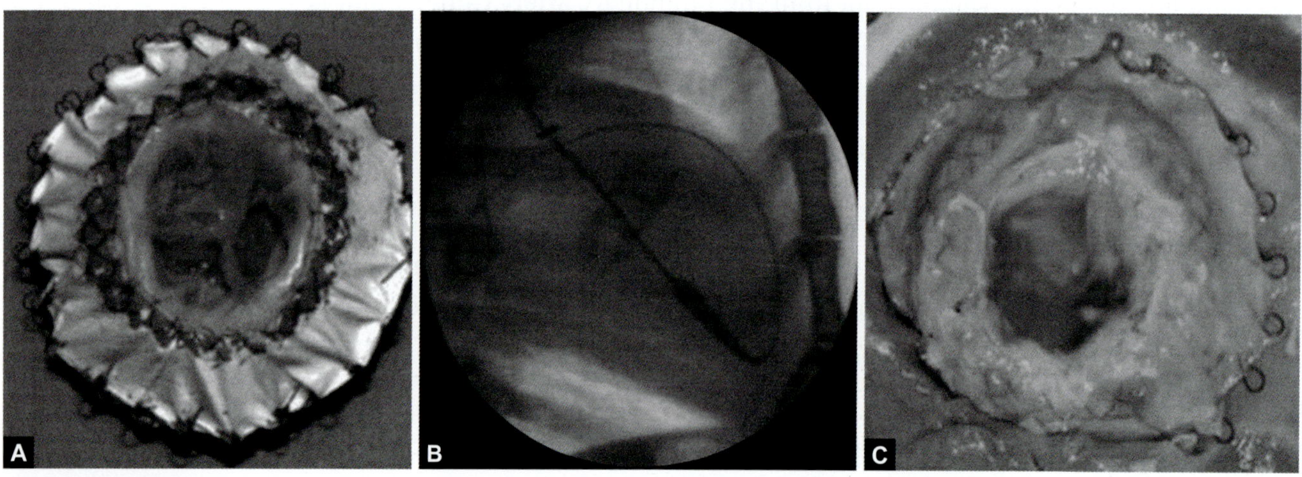

Figures 11A to C

Percutaneous tricuspid valve replacement. (A) Novel nitinol stent-based percutaneous tricuspid valve. An 18 mm bovine jugular venous valve is mounted in the central part of the stent, with a polytetrafluoroethylene membrane sutured to the ventricular disk to assist in sealing; (B) Percutaneous tricuspid valve delivered in an ovine model via an 18F sheath in the internal jugular vein under fluoroscopic and echocardiographic guidance; (C) Gross appearance of valve explanted at 1 month after implantation showing neoendocardial coverage of the stent (atrial view) (*Source:* Boudjemline et al. copyright © 2005, with permission from Elsevier)

considered standard of care, as this approach has been shown to result in improved perioperative outcomes, functional class, and survival. Surgical correction of isolated TR can significantly improve right ventricular volumes and ejection fraction.[23] It is currently estimated that as many as 500000 people in North America have clinically significant congestive heart failure-associated or functional mitral regurgitation. This constitutes the clinical need on which current percutaneous approaches to functional mitral valve repair are based. There would appear to be an associated need in many these patients for some manner of percutaneous tricuspid annuloplasty/repair or replacement.

Unique challenges for emerging percutaneous approaches to the tricuspid valve include the lack of convenient adjacent structures for device placement (such as the coronary sinus and its relationship to the mitral valve) and the relatively low-flow state in the right heart, which may promote thrombus formation. The coronary sinus ostium, atrioventricular node, and inferior vena cava are adjacent structures that must not be covered by any potential therapeutic devices. The presence of pre-existing transtricuspid pacemaker or defibrillator leads will undoubtedly require unique percutaneous solutions.

REFERENCES

1. Javier G Castillo, David H Adams, Gregory W Fischerb. Absence of the tricuspid valve due to severe carcinoid heart disease. Rev Esp Cardiol. 2010;63(1):96.
2. Connolly HM, Nishimura RA, Smith HC, Pellikka PA. Mullany CJ, Kvols LK. Outcome of cardiac surgery for carcinoid heart disease. J Am Coli Cardiol. 1995;25(2):410-6.
3. Connolly HM, Schaff HV, Mullany CJ, Abel MD, Pellikka PA. Carcinoid heart disease: impact of pulmonary valve replacement in right ventricular function and remodeling. Circulation. 2002;106(12 suppl 1):151-6.
4. Nishimura RA, Pieroni DR, Bierman FZ, Colan SD, Kaufman S, Sanders SP, et al. Second natural history study of congenital heart defects. Pulmonary stenosis: echocardiography. Circulation. 1993;87(suppl 2):173-9.
5. Gatzoulis MA, Balaji S, Webber SA, Siu SC, Hokanson JS, Poile C, et al. Risk factors for arrhythmia and sudden cardiac death late after repair of tetralogy of Fallot: a multicentre study. Lancet. 2000;356(9234):975-81.
6. Zoghbi WA, Enriquez-Sarano M, Foster E, Graybum PA, Kraft CD, Levine RA, et al. Recommendations for evaluation of the severity of native valvular regurgitation with two-dimensional and Doppler echocardiography. J Am Soc Echocardiogr. 2003;16(7): 777-802.
7. ACC/AHA guidelines for the management of patients with valvular heart disease. A Report of the American College of Cardiology/American Heart Association. Task Force on Practice Guidelines (Committee on Management of Patients with Valvular Heart Disease). J Am Coll Cardiol. 1998;32(5):1486-588.
8. Yiwu L, Yingchun C, Jianqun Z, Bin Y, Ping B. Exact quantitative selective annuloplasty of the tricuspid valve. J Thorac Cardiovasc Surg. 2001;122(3):611-4.

9. Rabago G, Fraile J, Martinell J, Artiz V. Technique and results of tricuspid annuloplasty. J Card Surg. 1986;1(3):247-53.

10. Abe T, Tukamoto M, Yanagiya M, Morikawa M, Watanabe N, Komatsu S. DeVega's annuloplasty for acquired tricuspid disease: early and late results in 110 patients. Ann Thorac Surg. 1989;48(5):670-6.

11. Bonow RO, Carabello B, de LA Jr, Edmunds LH Jr, FedderJy BJ, Freed MD, et al. Guidelines for the management of patients with valvular heart disease: executive summary. A Report of the American College of Cardiology/American Heart Association Task Force on Practice Guidelines (Committee on Management of Patients with Valvular Heart Disease). Circulation. 1998;98(18):1949-84.

12. Do QB, Pellerin M, Carrier M, Cartier R, Hebert Y, Page P, et al. Clinical outcome after isolated tricuspid valve replacement: 20-year experience. Can J Cardiol. 2000;16(4):489-93.

13. Arbulu A, Holmes RJ, Asfaw I. Tricuspid valvulectomy without replacement. Twenty years' experience. J Thorac Cardiovasc Surg. 1991;102(6):917-22.

14. Glower DD, White WD, Smith LR, Young WG, Oldham HN, Wolfe WG, et al. In-hospital and long-term outcome after porcine tricuspid valve replacement. J Thorac Cardiovasc Surg. 1995;109(5):877-83.

15. Scully HE, Armstrong CS. Tricuspid valve replacement. Fifteen years of experience with mechanical prostheses and bioprostheses. J Thorac Cardiovasc Surg. 1995;109(6):1035-41.

16. Singh AK, Feng WC, Sanofsky SJ. Long-term results of St. Jude Medical valve in the tricuspid position. Ann Thorac Surg. 1992;54(3):538-40.

17. Hvass U, Baron F, Fourchy D, Pansard Y. Mitral homografts for total tricuspid valve replacement: comparison of two techniques. J Thorac Cardiovasc Surg. 2001;121(3):592-4.

18. Shapira Y, Sagie A, Jortner R, Adler Y, Hirsch R. Thrombosis of bileaflet tricuspid valve prosthesis: clinical spectrum and the role of nonsurgical treatment. Am Heart J. 1999;137(4 Pt 1):721-5.

19. Connolly HM, Crary JL, McGoon MD, et al. Valvular heart disease associated with fenfluramine-phentermine. NEJM. 1997;337:581-8.

20. Van Son JA, Danielson GK, Schaff HV, et al. Traumatic tricuspid valve insufficiency. Experience in thirteen patients. J Thorac Cardiovasc Surg. 1994;108:893-8.

21. Assayag P, Thuaire C, Benamer H. Partial rupture of the tricuspid valve after extraction of permanent pacemaker leads: detection by transesophageal echocardiography. PACE 1999;22:971.

22. Boudjemline Y, Agnoletti G, Bonnet D, Behr L, Borenstein N, Sidi D, Bonhoeffer P. Steps toward the percutaneous replacement of atrioventricular valves an experimental study. J Am Coll Cardiol. 2005;46:360-5.

23. Mukherjee D, Nader S, Olano A, Garcia MJ, Griffin BP. Improvement in right ventricular systolic function after surgical correction of isolated tricuspid regurgitation. J Am Soc Echocardiogr. 2000;13:650-4.

III

MULTIPLE CHOICE QUESTIONS

rajiv juneja
section editor

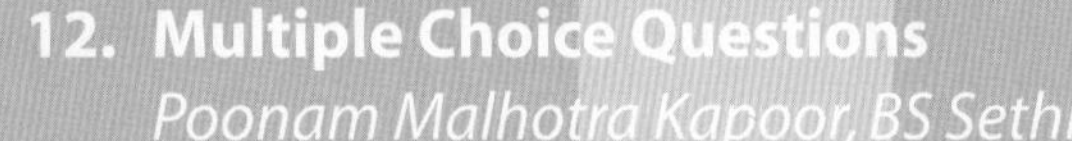

12 Multiple Choice Questions

Poonam Malhotra Kapoor, BS Sethi

1. The LA dimensions on M-mode are best measured at:

a. End-systole

b. End-diastole

c. Both

d. Neither a nor b

2. The left ventricular short-axis diameter can be obtained from a transgastric midpapillary view as shown in the figure.

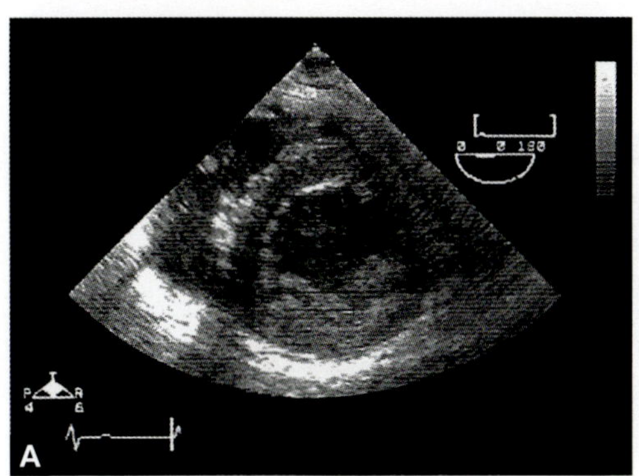

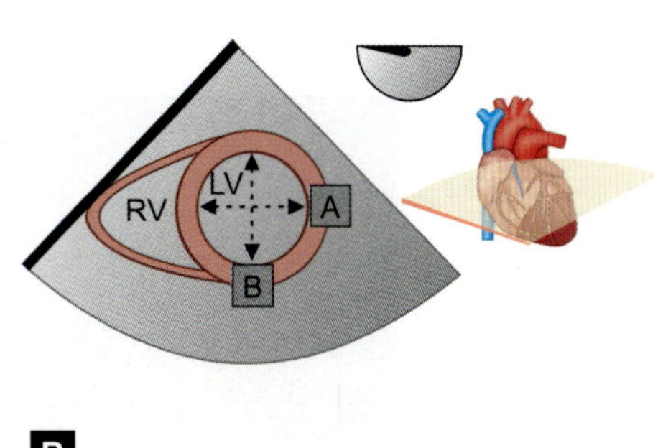

B

Measurements are made from:

a. Inner to outer edge

b. Outer to outer edge

c. Inner to inner edge

d. Outer to inner edge

1. a 2. c

3. The dimensions showed in the figure are all for a normal adult. They are:

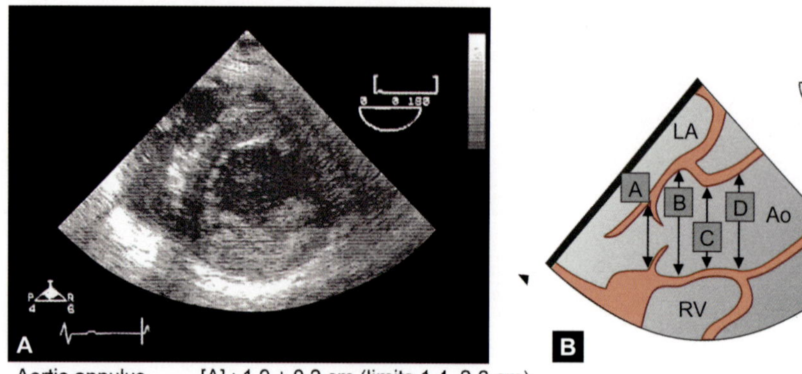

Aortic annulus [A] : 1.9 ± 0.2 cm (limits 1.4–2.6 cm)
Sinus of Valsalva [B] : 2.8 ± 0.3 cm (limits 2.1–3.5 cm)
Sinotubular junction [C] : 2.4 ± 0.4 cm (limits 1.7–3.4 cm)
Ascending aorta [D] : 2.6 ± 0.3 cm (limits 2.1–3.4 cm)

Mid-esophageal long-axis view of the left ventricular outflow tract (LVOT) and various parts of the ascending aorta (Ao). The LVOT diameter is measured at the aortic annulus (LA, left atrium; RV, right ventricle).

a. Correct
b. Incorrect
c. First and second are correct
d. Third and fourth are correct

4. The view represents RV inflow-outflow tract in which two measurements can be done—the RVOT and:

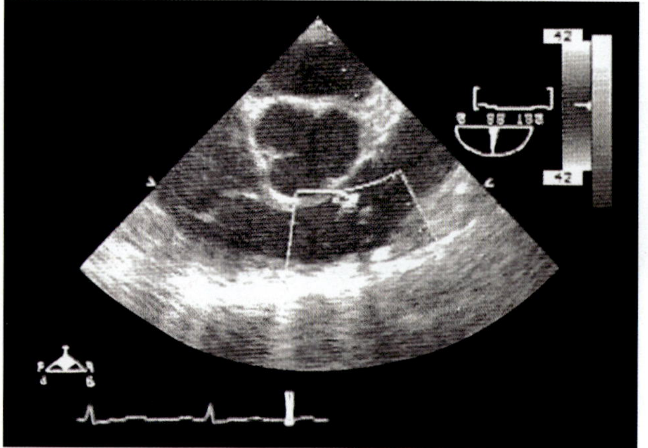

RVOT : 2.7 ± 0.4 cm (Limits 1.8–3.6 cm)
MPA : 3.6 ± 0.7 cm (Limits 2.7–4.5 cm)

a. LPA
b. RPA
c. MPA
d. None of the above

3. a 4. c

5. **The TV annulus diameter is obtained from the four-chamber view in the mid-esophageal position at:**

a. 0° b. 20°
c. 120° d. 90°

6. **LV volume = D^3 wherein the D represents:**

a. LVEDD b. LVEDS
c. Both assumed together d. Either

7. **Low-esophageal four-chamber view of the coronary sinus (CS) wherein the CS diameter is measured:**

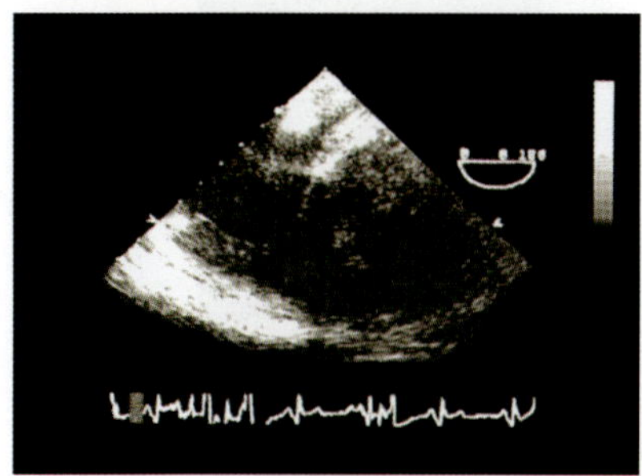

CS diameter : 0.7 ± 0.2 cm (Limits 0.4–1.1 cm)

A

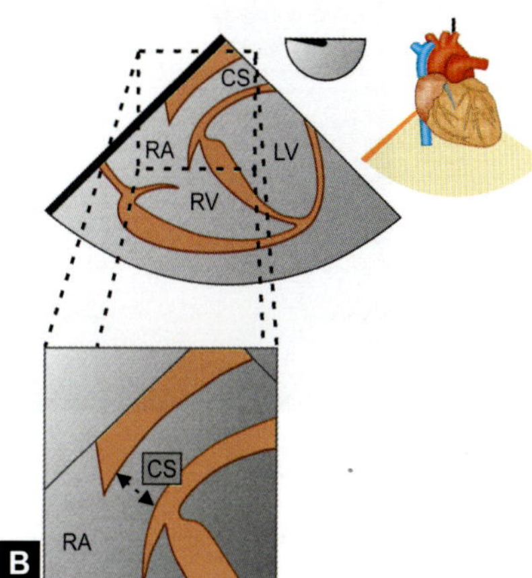

B

a. 1 cm proximal to where it enters the RA
b. 2 cm proximal to where it enters the RA
c. 3 cm proximal to where it enters the RA
d. 4 cm proximal to where it enters the RA

8. **The empty box in the table above represents which one of the following: Echocardiographic estimation of right atrial pressure (RAP). Using IVC diameter and hepatic venous Doppler profile.**

Size of IVC (cm)	*Collapse with sniffing*	*Hepatic vein Doppler profile*	*Suggested mRAP (mm Hg)*
< 1.5	≥ 50%	S + AR > 0	5
< 1.5	< 50%	S + Ar > 0	10–14
> 2.0	≥ 50%	S + AR < 0	15–20
—	< 50%	S + AR < 0	> 20

a. >2.0 b. >3.0
c. >2.5 d. >4.0

5. a 6. d 7. c 8. a

9. At a IVC diameter of < 1.5 cm with ≥ 50% collapse on sniffing, the suggested mRAP is:

   a. 0 to 5 mm Hg
   b. 10 to 15 mm Hg
   c. >20 mm Hg
   d. 15 to 20 mm Hg

10. The picture shows a:

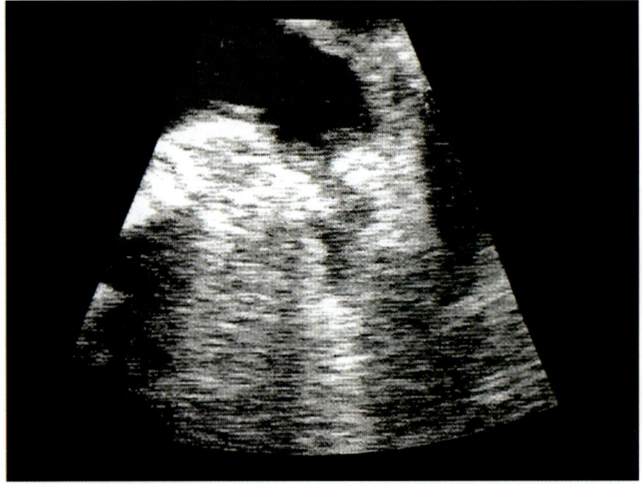

   a. LAA thrombus
   b. Pectinate muscles
   c. Coronary sinus
   d. LA clot

11. The figure shown is:

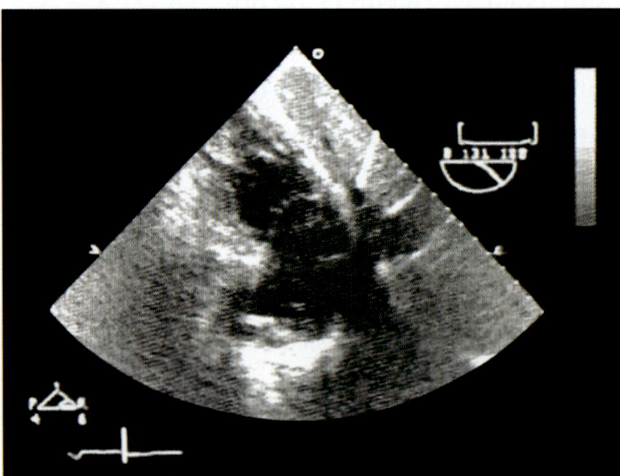

   a. Deep TG LAX
   b. TG LAX
   c. TG midpapillary view
   d. TG basal

9. a   10. a   11. a

12. In modified transgastric basal view of the RV, the leaflets of the TV seen are:

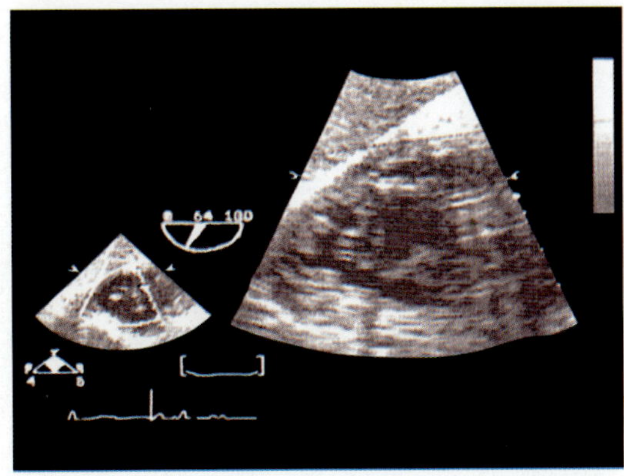

a. Anterior, posterior and septal
b. Anterior posterior
c. Septal and posterior
d. Septal and anterior

13. This view shows a mass on which leaflet of the TV.

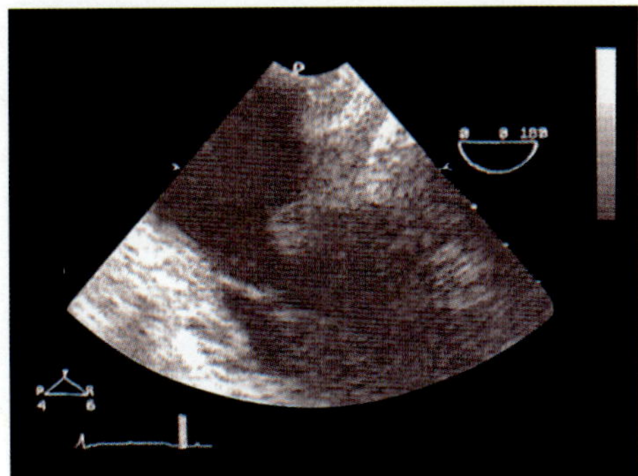

a. Anterior
b. Septal
c. Posterior
d. No mass seen

14. The diameter of the TV as shown in the figure, shows:

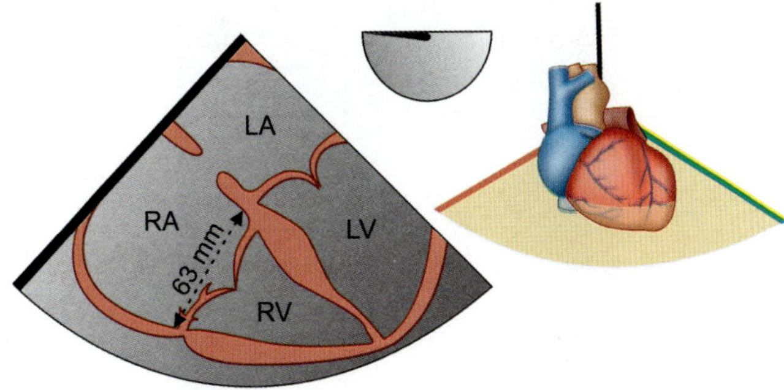

a. Functional TR
b. Organic TR
c. Normal TV dimension
d. Fit for annuloplasty

12. a 13. b 14. d

15. **This figure shows:**

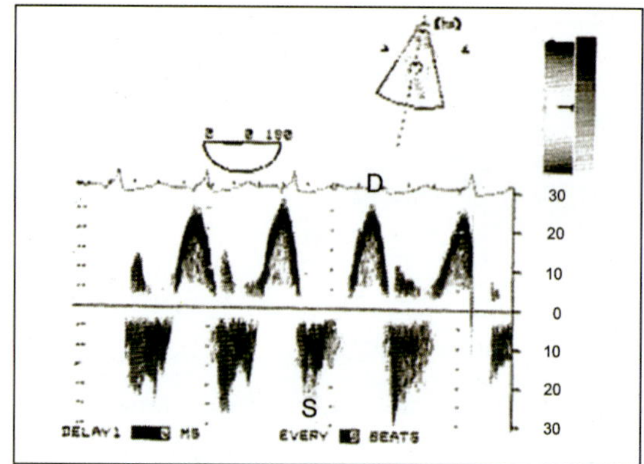

a. Normal hepatic vein pattern
b. Systolic dominance
c. Diastolic dominance
d. Systolic flow reversal

16. **This view called:**

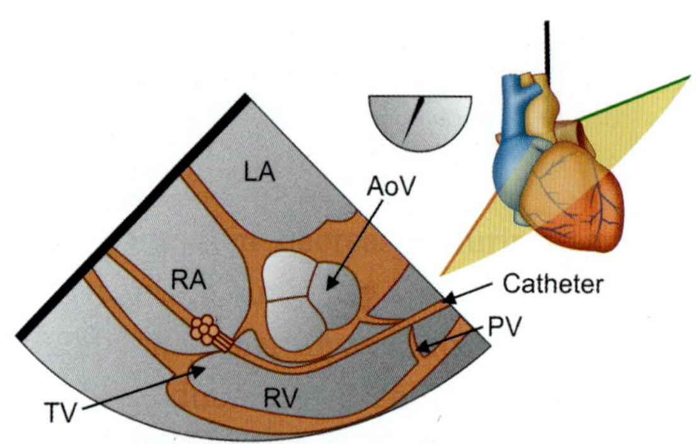

a. ME four-chamber view
b. ME five-chamber view
c. ME aortic SAX
d. ME RV inflow-outflow view

17. **Dilated ____________ heart border is seen in severe TR:**

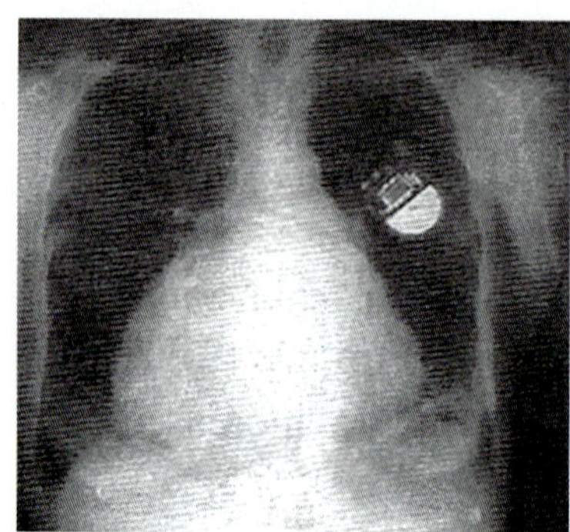

a. Right
b. Light
c. Base
d. None

15. d 16. d 17. a

18. Systolic blunting of hepatic vein flow is seen in:

a. Mild TR
b. Moderate TR
c. Severe TR
d. None of the above

19. PISA method has the advantage of being:

a. Qualitative
b. Quantitative
c. Specific for TR
d. Well validated

20. Best view to see a pacing lead vegetation of the TV is :

a. ME four-chamber view
b. ME five-chamber view
c. ME bicaval view
d. ME LAX

21. This view show transverse view of:

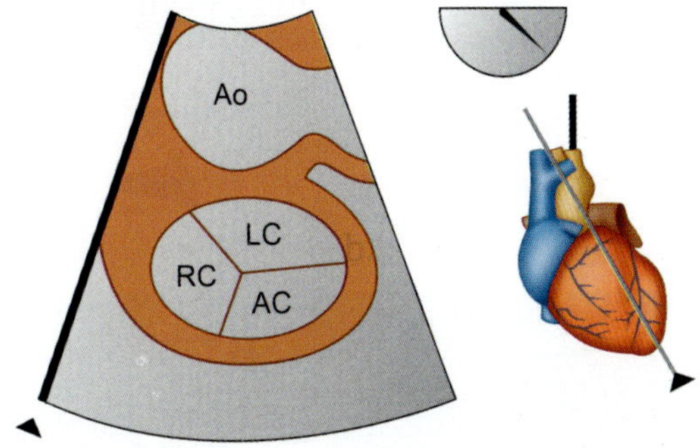

a. Aortic valve
b. Tricuspid valve
c. Mitral valve
d. Pulmonic valve

22. The above represents M-mode of a:

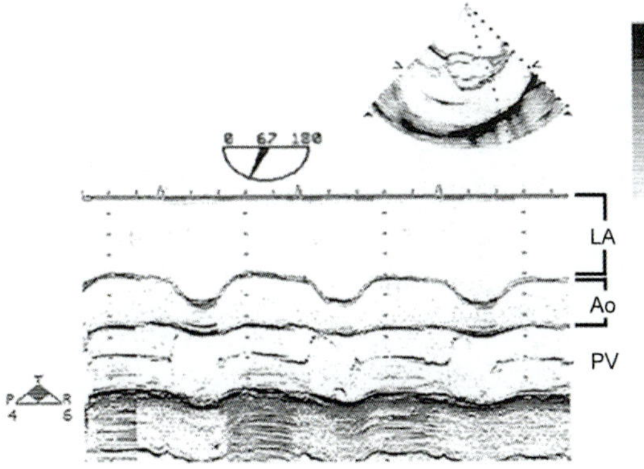

a. Normal PV
b. Pulmonary regurgitation
c. Pulmonic stenosis
d. Tricuspid stenosis

18. b 19. b 20. a 21. d 22. a

23. The figure represents a:

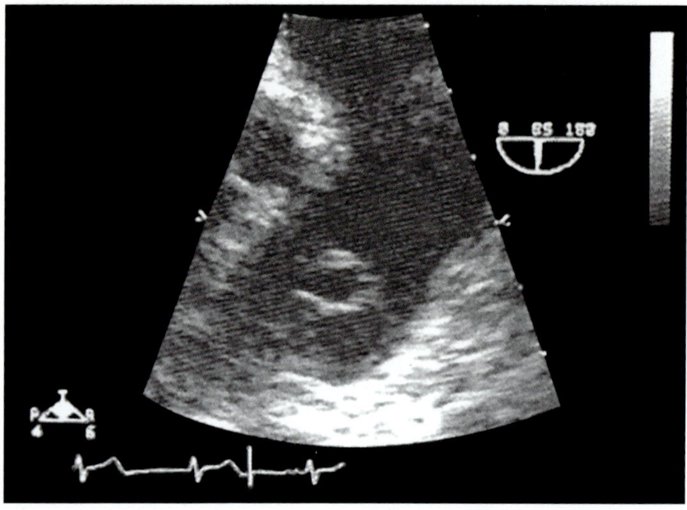

a. Bicuspid PV
b. Tricuspid PV
c. Unicuspid PV
d. Quadricuspid PV

24. The figure shows a 3D face view of:

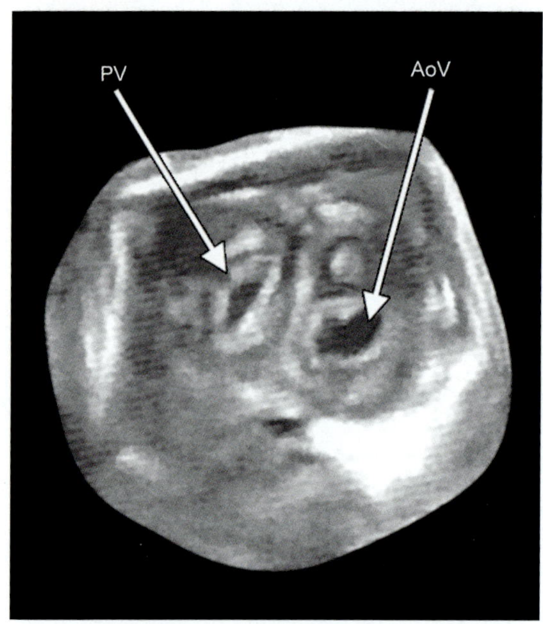

a. Atrial stenosis
b. Pulmonary stenosis
c. Mitral stenosis
d. Tricuspid stenosis

23. a 24. b

25. This figure represents a double purse string technique of Vegas annuloplasty of the:

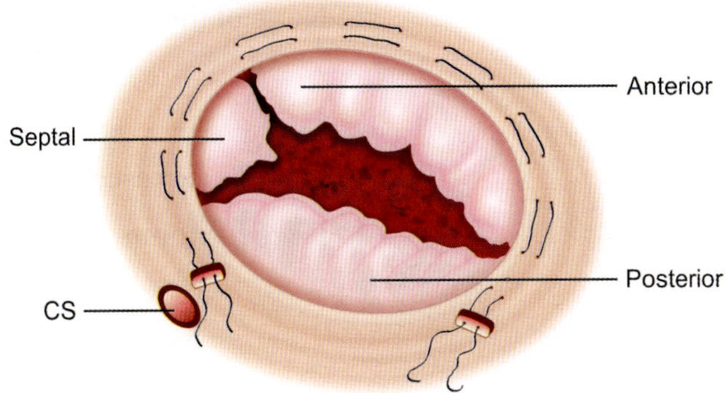

a. TV
b. AOV
c. PV
d. MV

26. A soft slow deceleration on CWD with a soft jet density is a hallmark of:

a. Mild PR
b. Moderate PR
c. Severe PR
d. None of the above

27. In surgery for TR, annuloplasty for severe TR and pulmonary hypertension in patients with mitral valve disease requiring mitral valve surgery is a class:

a. I recommendation
b. IIa recommendation
c. IIb recommendation
d. III recommendation

28. Surgically, induced PR is common after:

a. TOF
b. CCP
c. Dilated CMOP
d. MV repair

29. The cursor to obtain this view is placed at:

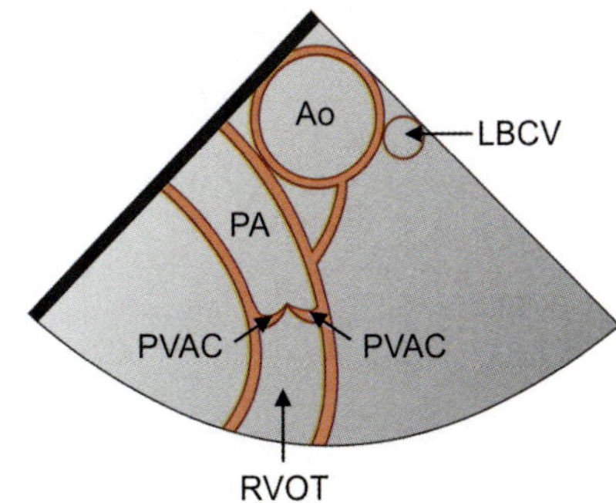

a. 60 to 70°
b. 5 to 10°
c. 90°
d. 120°

25. a 26. b 27. a 28. a 29. a

30. Straddling the TV leaflet is generally the:

a. STL
b. ATL
c. PTL
d. None of the above

31. The following tumors on semilunar valves are all benign except:-

a. Angiosarcoma
b. Lambl's excrescences
c. Lipoma
d. Fibroelastoma

32. The arrowhead in this live 3D TTE shows a left atrial myxoma. The arrowhead points to a:

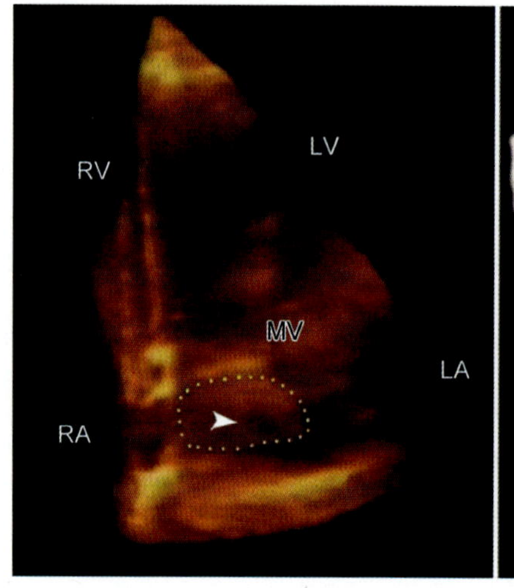

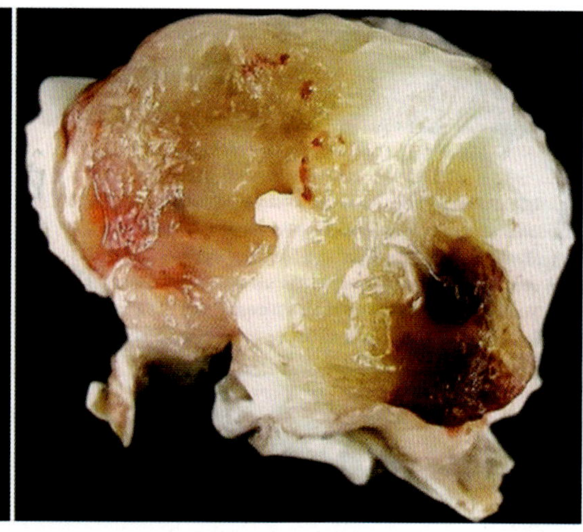

a. Infarct
b. Abscess
c. Thrombus
d. Hemorrhage

33. What view for this mass in the RV:

a. RV myxoma
b. RV thrombus
c. RV fibroelastoma
d. RV infarct

30. a 31. a 32. d 33. a

34. **What view does the figure represent:**

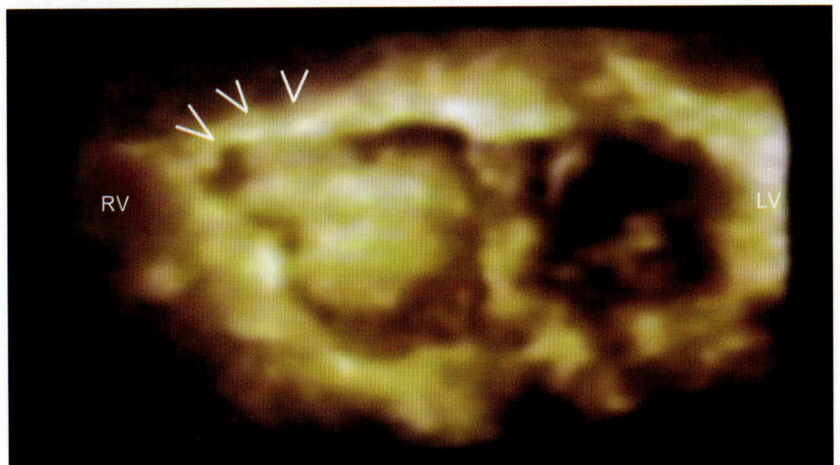

a. Deep TG view
b. Parasternal SAX view
c. TG RV outflow view
d. TG long-axis view

35. **Lipomas are markedly:**

a. Echogenic
b. Echolucent
c. Dense and multiple
d. Opaque and multiple

36. **Figure of 3D echo shows a:**

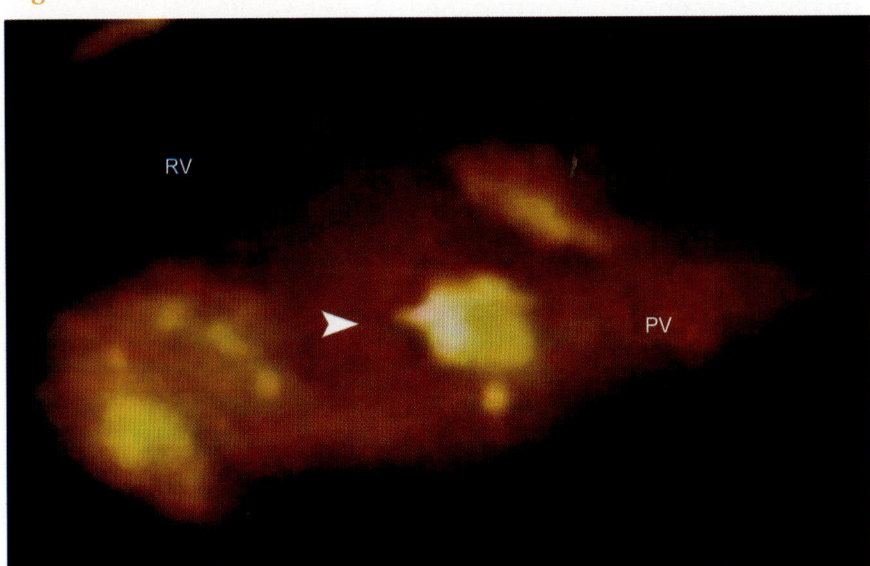

a. PV angiosarcoma
b. PV hemangioblastoma
c. PV fibroelastoma
d. PV infarct

34. a 35. b 36. c

37. **The above tumor has dense inner core and multiple finger projections. It is a hallmark of:**

a. PV angiosarcoma
b. PV hemangioblastoma
c. PV fibroelastoma
d. PV infarct

38. **The innermost portion of the hydatid cyst is called the:**

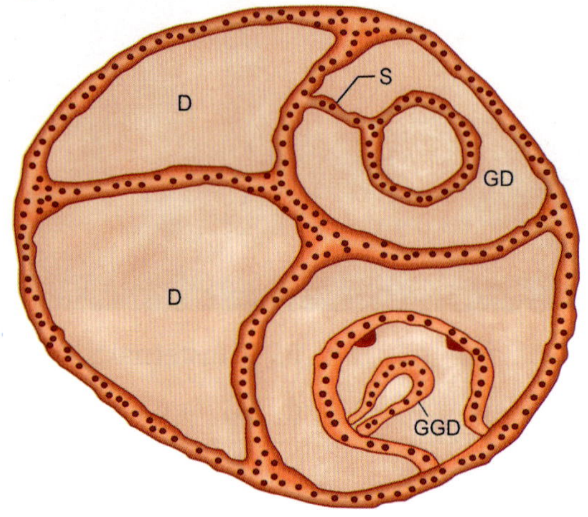

a. Daughter cyst
b. Son cyst
c. Granddaughter cyst
d. Great granddaughter cyst

39. **This sea anemone like structure showing multiple founds like structure is:**

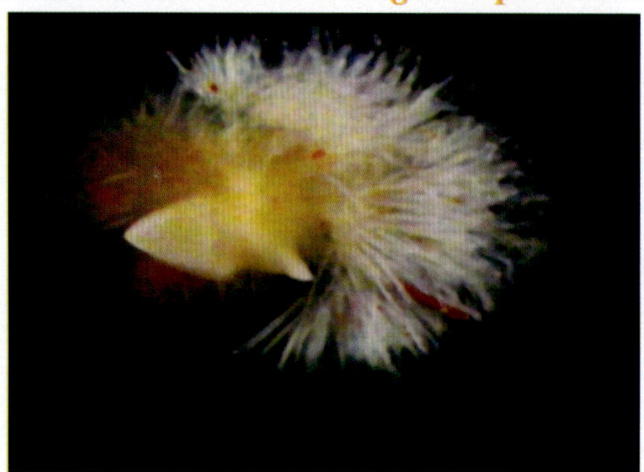

a. Rhabdomyosarcoma
b. Angiosarcoma
c. Fibroelastoma
d. Hemangioma

40. **In a RA thrombus, there is all of the following, except:**

a. Absence of lysis
b. Complete lysis
c. Intact platelets
d. Homogenous deposits

37. c 38. d 39. c 40. b

41. One of the following is correct nomenclature for TV leaflets.

a. Anterior, posterior, septal
b. Anterior, inferior, lateral
c. Posterior, inferior, lateral
d. Septal, lateral, inferior.

42. One of the following is correct statement regarding TV leaflets size:

Largest	*Smallest*
a. Anterior	Septal
b. Posterior	Anterior
c. Lateral	Anterior
d. Septal	Posterior

43. In the diagram of TV after incision through the acute margin of the right heart shows the term FC. FC stands for:

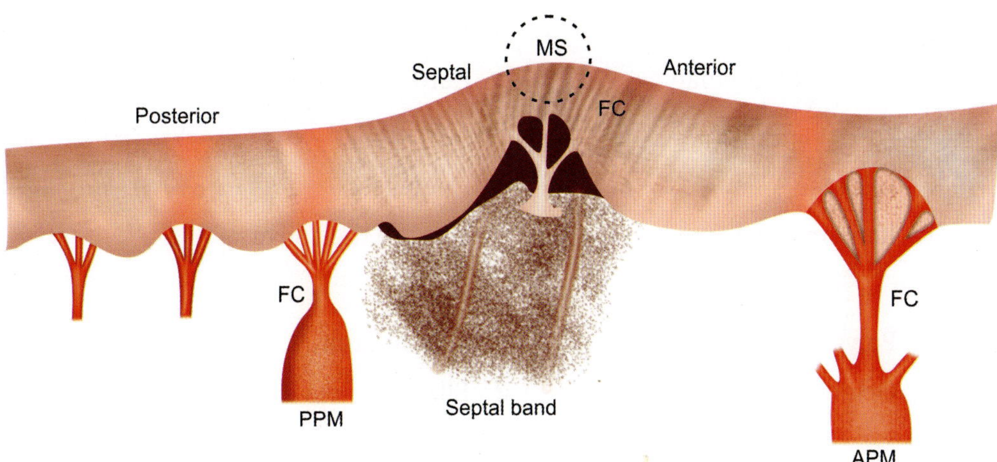

a. Deep chordae
b. Fan-shaped chordae
c. Free edge chordae
d. None of the above.

44. The normal circumference of the tricuspid valve annulus in adult is:

a. 7 to 9 cm^2
b. 11 to 12 cm^2
c. 12 to 14 cm^2
d. 5 to 7 cm^2

45. The moderator band in the RV arises from the:

a. Posterior papillary muscle
b. Anterior papillary muscle
c. Septal papillary muscle
d. RV free wall

41. a 42. a 43. b 44. b 45. b

46. **The normal pulmonic valve in relation to the aortic valve is:**
    a. Perpendicular and anterior
    b. Paralled and anterior
    c. Perpendicular and posterior
    d. Paralled and posterior.
47. **The contraction of the RV following a specific __________ pattern with the outflow tract:**
    a. Ribbed
    b. Peristaltic
    c. Tortuous
    d. Perpendicular
48. **During the process of spontaneous respiration all of the following increase, except:**
    a. PA flow
    b. RV stroke volume
    c. RVEDV RV preload
    d. Cardiac tamponade.
49. **During inspiration the RV after load:**
    a. Increase
    b. Decreases
    c. Remains the same
    d. None of the above
50. **The shape of the RV is thought to be like that of:**
    a. Polygen
    b. Tetrahedron
    c. Octahedron
    d. Ellipsoid

46. a 47. b 48. d 49. a 50. b

TRUE AND FALSE QUESTIONS

Imaging Artifacts and Pitfalls

1. Pectinate muscles are parallel muscular ridges typically observed in the inner surfaces of both atrial appendages.

   a. True b. False

2. A fenestrated membrane attached across the orifice of the coronary sinus is the Eustachian valve.

   a. True b. False

3. The validity of M-mode measurements is based upon the perpendicular alignment of the structures of interest with the line of examination represents by the M-mode cursor.

   a. True b. False

4. End-diastole is measured as the onset of the QRS complex on the ECG.

   a. True b. False

5. The normal aortic root measurement in a young adult is 1.0 – 1.8 cm/m^2

   a. True b. False

6. LVEF $= \frac{SV \times 100}{LVEDV}$ is true/false.

   a. True b. False

7. LAP = SBP-4V^2 (V = VMR) is true/false for measurement of left atrial pressure?

   a. True b. False

8. The Chiari network is an embryologic remnant found in 10 to 15 percent of normal hearts.

   a. True b. False

9. Persistent left SVC presents as an echo-free space between the LAA and left upper pulmonary vein.

   a. True b. False

10. Lipomatous hypertrophy is closely related to the position of the fossa ovalies on a bicaval view.

    a. True b. False

1. a 2. b 3. a 4. a 5. a 6. a 7. a 8. b 9. a 10. a

11. **During the clamping of the LAD the PWD transmitral pattern changes from a predominant. A wave to predominant E velocity with short decleration time suggesting a restrictive pattern.**

a. True b. False

Before LAD clamping

TMF

E A

During LAD clamping

TMF

A E

After LAD unclamping

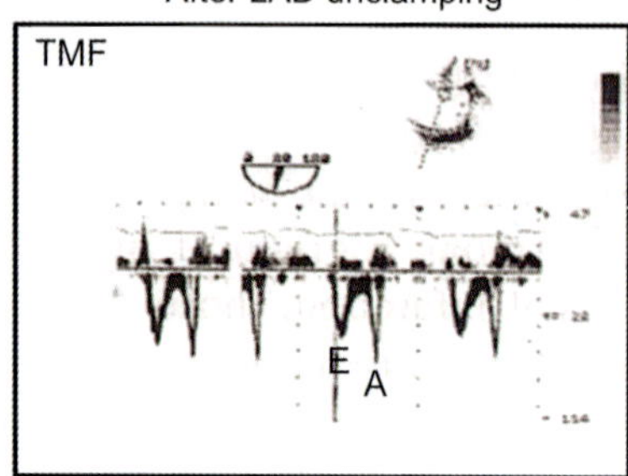

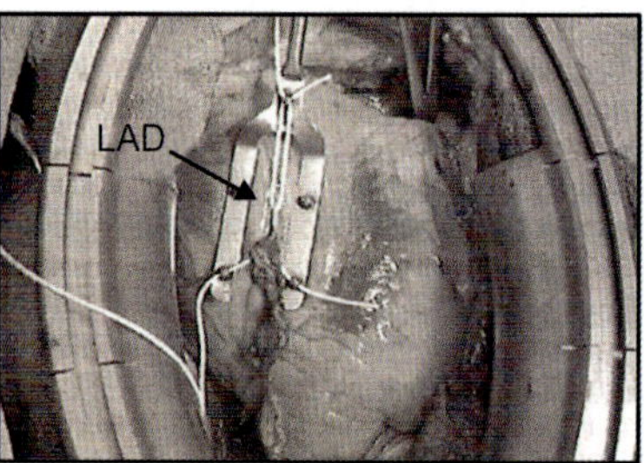

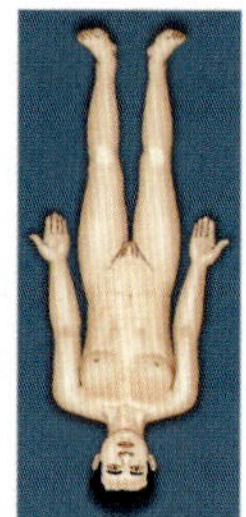

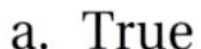

12. **At 120°, rightward rotation of the probe shaft, yields the equivalent of a transthoracic parasternal long-axis RV inflow view which shows the TV anterior and posterior view.**

a. True b. False

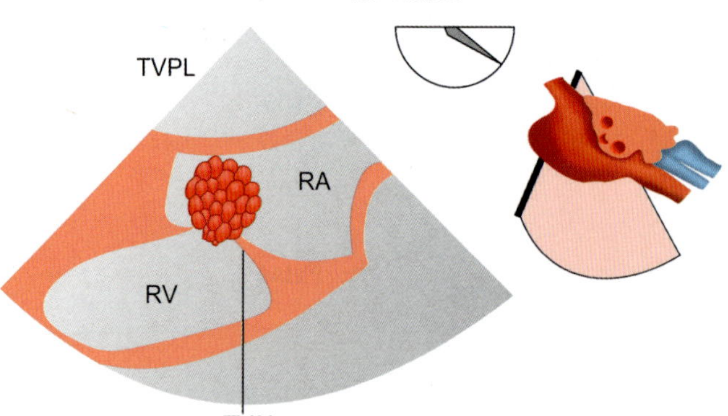

13. **For a TR jet, a color flow area more than 9 cm^2 is deemed significant, while a jet area less than 4 cm^2 is viewed as mild.**

a. True b. False

11. a 12. a 13. a

14. An eccentric jet makes grading of TR difficult.

a. True b. False

15. It was Tribowlloy et al who reported that a vena contracta >6 mm best predicted severe TR.

a. True b. False

16. Dilated right heart border on chest X-ray shows mild TR.

a. True b. False

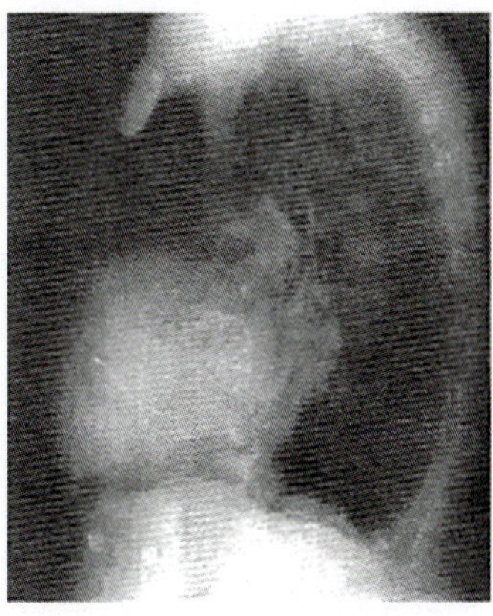

17. The hepatic vein is seen to join the IVC and RA.

a. True b. False

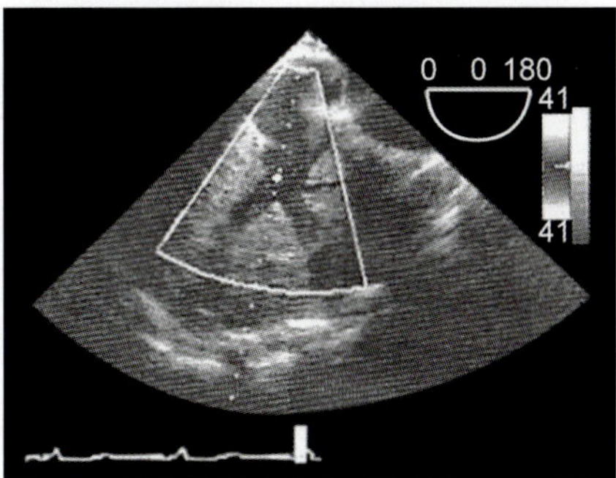

18. Paradoxical septal motion showing signs of severe TR is not specific for TR.

a. True b. False

19. Hepatic vein flow in TEE is influenced by RA pressure, but not atrial fibrillation.

a. True b. False

14. a 15. a 16. b 17. a 18. a 19. b

20. Systolic dominance in hepatic vein flow is seen in severe TR.
    a. True b. False
21. Vegetation on a pacemaker lead on the TV can be well viewed in a MV commissural view.
    a. True b. False
22. A soft slow deceleration with termination of the diastolic flow is seen in the mild PR.
    a. True b. False
23. On PWD, the pulmonary systolic flow is increased in severe PR.
    a. True b. False
24. The PA catheter could be accidentally entrapped during closure of the RA in TV surgery.
    a. True b. False
25. The normal tricuspid bioprosthesis has thin leaflets (2 – 4 mm) attached to three struts which probude into the RV.
    a. True b. False
26. Endocarditis of right-sided valves has become a common problem with the advent of intravenous access used in various forms of therapies in patients.
    a. True b. False
27. Vegetation on TV appear as a chaotically, mobile echodense mass attached on the low-pressure aspect of a valve leaflet.
    a. True b. False
28. TTE more than TEE provides a super characterization of vegetation size and extent as well as a greater specificity for endocarditis.
    a. True b. False
29. CFD has become the principal method to grade regurgitation severity on TEE.
    a. True b. False
30. Pulmonary embolism can give rise to functional TR.
    a. True b. False

20. b 21. b 22. b 23. a 24. a 25. a 26. a 27. a 28. b 29. a
30. a

31. Vena contracta width of >0.75 cm² represents a torrential TR

a. True   b. False

32. Severe TR can follow heart transplant surgery.

a. True   b. False

33. The dense and triangular TR jet intensity and contour on CWD suggests mild TR.

a. True   b. False

34. A less than 25 percent shortening of TV annulus is suggestive of severe TR.

a. True   b. False

35. A PISA estimated EROA of ≥40 mm² represents severe TR.

a. True   b. False

36. A maximum TV annulus diameter in diastole >38 mm is severe TR.

a. True   b. False

37. Carcinoid heart disease has thinned out TV leaflets.

a. True   b. False

38. Laminar TR, following CPB is not true TR.

a. True   b. False

39. DCRV and DORV can both have a functional TR developing due to TV annulus dilatation.

a. True   b. False

40. E velocity in CCP patients may show an increase, when TR develops.

a. True   b. False

41. While the other three cardiac valves are in fibrous continuity, the pulmonic valve stands alone separated by the infundibulum.

a. True   b. False

42. The pulmonic valve, being the most anterior valve, is well see by transthoracic approaches but not TEE.

a. True   b. False

31. a 32 a 33. b 34. a 35. a 36. a 37. b 38. a 39. a
40. a 41. a 42. a

43. The pulmonic leaflets are thinner than those of the aortic valve, due to it beging present on the lower pressure right side of the aortic valve.

a. True b. False

44. The nodules of arauti and the lunula are seen in both the PV and AV .

a. True b. False

45. The area of the pulmonary valve is 2 cm^2/m^2.

a. True b. False

46. A strong muscle band 3 divides the RV cavity into parts.

a. True b. False

47. The surface of the RV outflow tract is trabeculated.

a. True b. False

48. The outflow tract is a remnant of the bulbar cordis.

a. True b. False

49. The impedance of the pulmonary vascular bed represents the after load of the right ventricle.

a. True b. False

50. There is no close relation between pulmonary vascular resistance and systolic function of the right ventricle.

a. True b. False

43. a 44. a 45. a 46. b 47. b 48. a 49. a 50. b

Index

Page numbers followed by *f* refer to figure and *t* refer to table